Dedicated to
David Dunn and John Farndon
for their pioneering spirit, infectious enthusiasm and friendship

Surgery
Diagnosis and Management

Edited by

Nigel Rawlinson

FRCS (Ed), FFAEM, Dip Th
Consultant in Emergency Medicine
Bristol Royal Infirmary
Bristol

Derek Alderson

MD, FRCS
Barling Professor of Surgery
University of Birmingham
Birmingham

Fourth edition

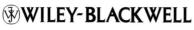
WILEY-BLACKWELL

A John Wiley & Sons, Ltd., Publication

This edition first published 2009, © 2009 by Blackwell Publishing Ltd
Previous editions: 1985, 1991, 1999

Blackwell Publishing was acquired by John Wiley & Sons in February 2007. Blackwell's
publishing program has been merged with Wiley's global Scientific, Technical and Medical
business to form Wiley-Blackwell.

Registered office: John Wiley & Sons Ltd, The Atrium, Southern Gate, Chichester, West
Sussex, PO19 8SQ, UK

Editorial offices: 9600 Garsington Road, Oxford, OX4 2DQ, UK
　　　　　　　　The Atrium, Southern Gate, Chichester, West Sussex, PO19 8SQ, UK
　　　　　　　　111 River Street, Hoboken, NJ 07030-5774, USA

For details of our global editorial offices, for customer services and for information about
how to apply for permission to reuse the copyright material in this book please see our
website at www.wiley.com/wiley-blackwell

Library of Congress Cataloging-in-Publication Data

Rawlinson, Nigel.
　　Surgery : diagnosis and management / Nigel Rawlinson, Derek Alderson. — 4th ed.
　　　　p. ; cm.
　　Rev. ed. of: Dunn's surgical diagnosis and management. 3rd ed. 1999.
　　Includes indexes.
　　ISBN 978-1-4051-2921-3 (alk. paper)
　　1. Diagnosis, Surgical—Handbooks, manuals, etc.　2. Surgery—Handbooks,
　　manuals, etc.　I. Alderson, Derek.　II. Dunn, David C. (David Christy). Dunn's
　　surgical diagnosis and management.　III. Title.
　　[DNLM: 1. Diagnostic Techniques, Surgical—Handbooks. 2. Surgical Procedures,
　　Operative—Handbooks. WO 39 R261s 2009]
　　RD35.D75 2009
　　617'.075—dc22
　　　　　　　　　　　　　　　　　　　　　　　　　　　　　　　　2008006106

ISBN: 978-1-4051-2921-3

A catalogue record for this book is available from the British Library.

Set in 8.5/10.5pt Minion by Graphicraft Limited
Printed in Singapore by Fabulous Printers Pte Ltd

1　2009

Contents

Contributors

Professor D. Alderson

Barling Professor of Surgery
Queen Elizabeth Hospital
Birmingham B15 2TH
Chapter 8

Dr R. Amirfeyz

Specialist Registrar Trauma
and Orthopaedics
Bristol Royal Infirmary
Bristol BS2 8HW
Chapter 1

Mr T. Burge

Department of Plastic Surgery
Frenchay Hospital
Bristol BS16 1LE
Chapter 13

Miss E. Cusick

Department of Plastic Surgery
Bristol Childrens Hospital
Bristol BS2 8BJ
Chapter 14

Mr R. H. Hardwick

Consultant Surgeon
Upper GI Surgery
Addenbrooke's Hospital
Cambridge CB2 0QQ
Chapter 7

Mr P. Kent

Consultant Vascular Surgeon
Leeds General Infirmary
Leeds LS1 3EX
Chapter 12

Professor T.W.J. Lennard

Professor of Breast and
Endocrine Surgery
University of Newcastle upon Tyne
Newcastle upon Tyne NE2 4HH
Chapter 4

Mr T. Leslie

Clinical Lecturer in Urology
Churchill Hospital
Oxford OX3 7LJ
Chapter 2

Mr Nigel Mercer

Department of Plastic Surgery
Frenchay Hospital
Bristol BS16 1LE
Chapter 13

Mr A. Morgan

Thoracic Surgical Unit
Bristol Royal Infirmary
Bristol BS2 8HW
Chapter 6

Professor N.J.M. Mortensen

Clinical Reader in
Colorectal Surgery
John Radcliffe Hospital
Oxford OX3 9DU
Chapter 9

Mr S. Nicholson

York Breast Unit
York Hospital
York YO31 8HE
Chapter 5, Chapter 10

Revd Mr N. Rawlinson
Consultant in Emergency Medicine
Bristol Royal Infirmary
Bristol BS2 8HW
Chapter 15

Dr S. Thomas
Consultant Maxillofacial Surgeon
Bristol Royal Infirmary
Bristol BS2 8HW
Chapter 3

Mr T. Whittlestone
Consultant Urologist
Bristol Royal Infirmary
Bristol BS2 8HW
Chapter 11

Preface to the fourth edition

The fourth edition of this general surgical textbook, now renamed *Surgery: Diagnosis and Management*, has been aimed at the same readership. We believe there is still an important role for one book describing the general surgical care that a final year student will need to learn and a doctor in the first 2 or 3 years after qualifying will need to practice. This book also has relevance for all professional groups, and so contributes to the development of interprofessional practice.

While this book is primarily aimed at helping the recently qualified doctor joining a surgical department in the foundation years, we also hope that it benefits senior medical students and those individuals who have chosen to begin a specialist training in surgery. For simplicity we have referred to all of these individuals using the term **junior surgical trainee**.

Every section has been revised by a specialist in the field. There are new sections on medical ethics, including informed consent and the procedure for intimate examination.

There is clearly a risk that between this review and publication new developments lead to further change. We ask our readers to be patient and alter the text where needed.

The text has also been revised to reflect the changing role of junior surgical trainees, especially those making the transition to the foundation years after qualification.

One major change that has happened in the last few years is the relationship between preoperative assessment clinics and admission for surgery, and the availability of cross-matched blood. In the preoperative assessment clinic there is an opportunity to take blood to 'group and save' serum. Provided that patients do not have unusual antibodies, most hospital transfusion services can provide cross-matched blood at short notice (within an hour). For this reason many elective procedures where transfusion may be required are commenced using the group and save sample taken in the clinic, and blood subsequently cross-matched as needed.

In specific circumstances it may be necessary to cross-match blood beforehand and recommended volumes are recommended in each procedure profile. Individual practice varies, so check with the surgeon doing the operation.

The layout of this book has been simplified while retaining the uniformity of structure that has been its characteristic feature.

Derek Alderson
Nigel Rawlinson
2008

Preface to the first edition

The stimulus to the production of this book has been the repeated demands of our medical students and housemen for a concise practical text which lists the methods of diagnosis and management of the main general surgical conditions they will have to deal with. It has been derived from a popular series of seminars in surgery given in Cambridge.

The combination of authors is unusual. One (DCD) has been a consultant since 1974 and the other (NR) was his houseman when the work started. We hope that this combination has helped us to concentrate on a layout which answers the needs of the houseman and medical student, needs which have often become obscure to senior doctors. Most surgical texts, for instance, fail to deal with questions which regularly confront the houseman, such as how much blood should be cross matched for an operation, and how long patients will be in hospital and off work.

The book is designed to be easy to use for rapid reference and a similar layout is used for each subject, with headings suggested by the questions our students ask, such as:

What is that condition?

What makes you think that the diagnosis is likely?

How will you prove whether you are right or not?

What is the management, before, during, and after the operation?

What do I tell the patient when I'm obtaining his consent?

We have tried hard to make sure that the facts in the book are as accurate as possible and are grateful to our many colleagues who have checked the text. Inevitably, some errors may have crept in and we hope that our readers will write to us about these so that they may be corrected later.

The housesurgeon and patient have generally been described as 'he' in this book, a choice which is merely convenient and one which we hope will not upset our many excellent female junior staff.

Both authors have found the exercise of co-operating on this book to be interesting and illuminating. We hope our readers will also benefit from what we have produced.

David C. Dunn
Nigel Rawlinson
1985

Acknowledgements

We would like to thank everyone who has contributed to the revision of the text. Surgery is continually developing and changing. Consultants are becoming more specialized. This general surgical text includes most specialties except orthopaedics, and cardiac, thoracic and neurosurgery. We hope that we have produced a general surgical text with up-to-date specialist facts.

Several of our colleagues have also helped with comments and encouragement. This includes Sarah Woolley, consultant colleague in emergency medicine who looked at Chapter 15, and the several years of undergraduate students in the Bristol and Birmingham Medical Schools who have enjoyed and critiqued the text.

Our secretaries, Christine Carter and Helen Ali have been invaluable in typing (and retyping) the text.

David Dunn, formerly consultant surgeon at Addenbrookes Hospital Cambridge, was the senior author of the first edition. He is remembered as an outstanding teacher and surgeon. He inspired many people during his 23 years as consultant both at Addenbrookes Hospital and at St John's College, University of Cambridge. He died as the third edition was being created.

John Farndon, formerly professor of surgery in Bristol, died suddenly in the medical school in 2002. He was highly respected as a surgeon and academic and mentored many (including Derek Alderson and Nigel Rawlinson) with wisdom, encouragement and humour. He is remembered with great affection and respect.

Layout of this book

The first two chapters deal with the routine of patient management before, during and after any operation. In the subsequent chapters individual surgical conditions and their management are described.

Management depends on diagnosis, and diagnosis depends on history, examination and special investigation.

Each condition is presented with the following structure.

Condition title
A brief descriptive outline of the condition is given, including any characteristic issues. Pathology is included when it has a direct influence on management, for example tumour staging.

Recognizing the pattern
When an experience clinician is faced with a patient complaining of a symptom the diagnosis is made by taking an accurate history and by a careful examination. As you do this you are constantly comparing the findings of the patient with the typical picture you associate with various diseased states. When you recognise one of several familiar patterns of symptoms and signs you will ask subsidiary questions to strengthen or weaken your developing hypothesis as to the underlying cause, and so come to a clinical diagnosis. This process depends on the background knowledge of the typical pattern of each disease. In this section such typical patterns are presented, and for each condition the presenting symptoms (from the history) and signs (from the examination) are described.

Proving the diagnosis
The usual investigations necessary to prove the diagnosis are given.

Management
The general management of each condition is discussed. Because this is a surgical text book this would usually involve an operative

procedure. A brief description of any preoperative preparation is followed by a short account of the operation itself. Detail varies. There is sufficient to enable the junior surgical trainee to understand what is going on and speak in an informed way to patients and relatives. Other procedures, where it is possible the junior surgical trainee may have a more involved role, are described in greater detail.

After each operation we have tabled a 'procedure profile'.

Procedure profile

Blood requirement
Anaesthetic
Operation time
Hospital stay
Return to normal activity

The idea of this procedure profile is to provide the junior surgical trainee with some guidelines for answering those questions that frequently arise at the time of any operation. It is recognized that this is not uniform but depends on the advances in surgery and the practice of individual consultants. We hope, however, that they will be useful guides. The tables are designed to allow room to write in the practice of your particular unit.

Blood requirement

Many elective procedures are now commenced with a sample of serum that has been 'group and saved'. Transfusion laboratories can cross-match the blood quickly (within 1 hour) and will do this if blood is required during an operative procedure. In specific circumstances it may be necessary to cross-match blood beforehand. These are usually operations where blood loss is expected. Recommended volumes are indicated in each procedure profile. However, individual practice does vary so check with the surgeon during the operation.

Anaesthetic
Procedures may be done under general, local or regional anaesthesia.

Operation time
There is variability here for many operations. However, it is still a good indicator of whether a procedure is minor or major.

Hospital stay
Although this is now shorter, with patients being discharged to recover in the familiar and safer environment of home, away from hospital infections, some procedures still require lengthy admission.

Return to normal activity
For some this may be the time required before they may return to work. Others will do different activities. The change in title from the previous editions reflects the increasing number of retired people who will be under our healthcare.

1 The daily management of patients in surgical wards

1.1 Admitting the surgical patient

The first two chapters of this book deal with the daily tasks a junior surgical trainee has to perform. They will also help medical students to understand what is going on in a surgical ward and to prepare themselves for their first few years of work after qualifying as a doctor.

Managing people who need operations

Many people tend to assume that young doctors are trained to regard the human body as a collection of mechanical tubes and pipes and that they overlook the importance of the 'individual'. In fact, most doctors find their work fascinating because they are dealing with a human body enclosing a mind and a spirit as well as complex, delicate biological systems.

The management of patients in surgery is dominated by this difference between the mechanical and the human, the difference between a technician and a surgeon. To obtain good results in surgery the mechanics must, of course, be correct. The anastomosis must not leak, the wound must heal and the electrolytes must be kept in the correct range. Over and above this, however, the patient has to believe in their management and obtain confidence from their carers. Efforts spent on developing a trusting, friendly and honest relationship can pay huge dividends during the patient's illness. Every practising doctor knows this and has experience of patients surviving by their own will or dying because they have just given up. Maintaining a patient's

---

Surgery: Diagnosis and Management, 4th edition. Edited by N. Rawlinson and D. Alderson. © 2009 Blackwell Publishing, ISBN: 978-1-4051-2921-3

morale can be just as important as maintaining their blood pressure. The ability to develop good relationships with patients will transform the knowledgeable bad doctor into the excellent and successful practitioner whom most students aspire to be.

The junior surgical trainee plays an indispensable role in the organization of a surgical firm. While the more senior members of the firm have to split their time between the ward, the outpatient department and theatre, the junior surgical trainee's main priority is the ward. He or she is the link between the patient, relatives, surgical staff, nurses and paramedical staff, and will coordinate all aspects of patient care.

The daily ward work

Routine ward work can be split into five parts:
- admitting the patient
- preparing the patient for operation (see p. 18)
- organizing the operating list (see p. 10)
- the junior surgical trainee in theatre (see p. 28)
- conducting regular postoperative ward rounds (see p. 30).

Admitting the patient

Remember the underlying principle of clinical practice. Management depends on diagnosis, and diagnosis depends on history, examination and investigation.

Make sure that you have seen the outpatient notes and the consultant's letter before you start the routine clerking. A working or definitive diagnosis may have been made, but always make your own assessment critically and independently. Avoid blindly following a predetermined diagnostic pathway. Check that any X-rays, scans and other specific investigations taken previously are available on the ward. By keeping an open mind you will be able to spot problems that may have been missed in a hurried outpatient assessment.

A full clerking is then carried out on all patients. Some points require special attention when an operation is being planned. The junior surgical trainee plays an important role in the medical assessment of the surgical patient. You are looking for any indication that the patient may not be fit for surgery or may be liable to develop problems postoperatively. Particular points are listed below.

History
CHEST
Look for the following.
- Pre-existing chest disease.
- Shortness of breath on minor exertion or at rest.
- Cough, and is it productive?
- History of asthma. Beware prescribing non-steroidal anti-inflammatory drugs (NSAIDs).
- Smoking habit.

CARDIOVASCULAR SYSTEM
Is there a history of the following.
- Chest pain or angina?
- Symptoms of cardiac failure (such as oedema, nocturnal dyspnoea, orthopnoea or palpitations)?

ALIMENTARY AND GENITOURINARY SYSTEMS
Ask about the following.
- Anorexia and weight loss. Malnutrition increases risks of complications after many types of surgery. Does this require correction to get the patient safely through a particular treatment schedule?
- Bowel habit. Might a planned treatment lead to constipation? Consider the need for laxatives to keep the bowels moving.
- Heartburn and reflux. A patient with reflux may have an increased risk of aspiration during induction of anaesthesia. Consider the need for a proton pump inhibitor (PPI) and warn the anaesthetist.
- Peptic ulcer disease. Beware of prescribing NSAIDs.
- Micturition. Poor stream, nocturia or hesitancy may be a clue to postoperative retention or infection. Bladder distension may be difficult to detect in the presence of a recent lower abdominal incision.
- Periods. Heavy periods are a common cause of anaemia in women.

LOCOMOTOR SYSTEM
- Does the patient suffer from arthritis?
- Are there any particularly stiff joints?
- Intubation may be difficult in the presence of cervical joint disease.
- It may be difficult or impossible to put patients in the lithotomy position on the table when they have fixed deformities or stiff hips, knees or back.
- In the case of rheumatoid arthritis anteroposterior (AP) and lateral C-spine views (in flexion and extension) might be necessary to rule out an atlantoaxial instability.

PAST MEDICAL HISTORY
Find out about the following.
- Previous operations, and whether they were followed by any complications such as deep venous thrombosis or infection.
- Previous anaesthetics. Were there any problems such as drug reaction, excessive vomiting, or malignant hyperpyrexia?
- Previous history of rheumatic fever that may have damaged the heart valves. With such a history you must examine the heart carefully. Prophylactic antibiotics may be needed for a significant valvular lesion.
- Previous history of jaundice.
- Medical conditions. Does the patient suffer from any other diseases that will influence your management? These are dealt with in section 1.3 and include diabetes, heart disease and chest disease.
- Methicillin-resistant *Staphylococcus aureus* (MRSA) status. This may be important for patients who have been in hospital or institutional care for some time before surgery, for those who are immunosuppressed and for patients with existing wounds. Specific measures are discussed below.

DRUG HISTORY
Many drugs interfere with anaesthetic agents. Some may lead to electrolyte abnormalities (e.g. diuretics). Care must be taken with those on anticoagulants. The antiplatelet effect of aspirin lasts up to 7 days and combination of aspirin with other antiplatelet agents can cause excessive bleeding after surgery. Many

hospitals have specific written policies for elective procedures, but patients requiring urgent or emergency surgery are particularly at risk.

There is controversy regarding the oral contraceptive in the perioperative period. We advise offering deep venous thrombosis prophylaxis to all young women on the pill.

ALLERGIES

Ask about allergies to:

- anaesthetics
- antibiotics
- applications (e.g. iodine, elastoplast, latex rubber).

Check whether the allergy is genuine by determining what sort of reaction the patient had when they were exposed to the agent. Many patients say they are allergic to antibiotics because they felt ill or nauseated at the time they took them. Where there is any possibility of allergy the patient's record should be marked and that drug avoided. Latex sensitivity is common and this requires special packaging of equipment and the use of non-latex gloves and tubes in the operating theatre.

Whenever any allergy is noted, this should be clearly marked on the operating list.

FAMILY HISTORY

Is there a family history of reaction to an anaesthetic? If positive, inform the anaesthetist.

SOCIAL HISTORY

Important points are as follows.

- The patient's job. This will determine when the patient can go back to work.
- Support. What sort of support is available from the family or friends postoperatively? This can be important in cases for day surgery.
- Habits. Check how much the patient drinks and smokes. A heavy drinker may be resistant to the normal doses of anaesthetic agents. A heavy smoker will be very liable to develop a chest infection postoperatively and preoperative physiotherapy may be indicated to minimize this risk.

Examination

Always try to improve on the findings made during the out-patient assessment. Finding a supraclavicular lymph node, for instance, may save a patient with gastric cancer from an unnecessary abdominal operation (see pp. 146, 296).

Details in the general examination that may be important are as follows.

GENERAL CONDITION

Look for signs of dehydration, anaemia, jaundice, lymphadenopathy or cachexia. These may require correction before operation is undertaken.

MENTAL STATE

Any patient will be anxious about the operation and in some this anxiety is extreme. Careful explanation and reassurance is required. A mild hypnotic or tranquillizer given on the night before operation is sometimes helpful.

CARDIOVASCULAR SYSTEM

Perform a full examination and inform the anaesthetist of any significant abnormalities. Pay particular attention to the blood pressure. If it is elevated come back and check it later. Often it normalizes once the patient settles into their new environment.

CHEST

Assess the shape of the chest looking for signs of emphysema. Check for scars and that there are no signs of pleural fluid, lung consolidation or bronchospasm.

ABDOMEN

The presence of abdominal scars provides a useful check on the patient's history. They may also indicate that a routine operation will be more difficult than usual and require more operative time because of adhesions.

All patients should have a rectal examination before abdominal surgery. In males note the size of the lobes of the prostate. This information will be of value if the patient develops urinary problems postoperatively. Once in retention, the size of the prostate is much more difficult to assess.

JOINTS AND TEETH

The presence of false teeth or crowns, limitation of movement of the neck and micrognathia will make intubation more hazardous. These features should be brought to the attention of the anaesthetist.

Investigations

The following five investigations should be considered pre-operatively.

- Urea and electrolytes. These should be performed if:
  - the patient is on intravenous fluid therapy
  - the patient is on diuretics or steroids
  - the patient has acute or chronic renal disease
  - the patient is diabetic
  - there is a history of heart disease or hypertension
  - there has been recent significant fluid loss
  - you anticipate postoperative fluid therapy to continue for more than 24 h.
- Full blood count. This should be performed if:
  - anaemia is suspected
  - there is a history of malignancy
  - there is a history of cardiac or vascular disease
  - there is haematological disorder like sickle cell trait/disease or a coagulopathy
  - there is a potential for major blood loss.
- Chest X-ray. This is indicated in:
  - suspected malignancy or possible TB
  - likely admission to ITU (major upper abdominal or thoracic surgery)
  - cardiothoracic surgery
  - those with signs or symptoms of significant cardiac or pulmonary disease (excluding asthma) and the very elderly.
- Electrocardiogram (ECG). This should be performed:
  - in known cardiovascular disease (including hypertension)
  - in males over 50 and females over 60 years
  - in those with diabetes or hyperlipidaemia.
- Liver function tests. The serum albumin gives some indication of the state of nutrition of the patient. Other liver function tests may form part of the work-up for general liver disease such as hepatic metastases or cirrhosis.

Other investigations can be considered depending on the operation intended, or findings from the history and examination.

Some common pitfalls in surgical diagnosis and management

Avoid accepting the diagnosis with which the patient has been labelled, until you have confirmed or altered this as a result of your own history and examination.

When taking the history do not blindly accept non-specific terms used by the patient. Define the symptoms they are trying to describe. While a patient might tell you they have had pleurisy, simple questioning may reveal that this included haemoptysis, shortness of breath and pleuritic chest pain (more indicative of a pulmonary embolus) and this will affect your management. Be careful with words like 'diarrhoea' or 'indigestion'. Get the patient to explain carefully what they mean.

Be aware of the patient's previous medications. Find out which can be stopped, which must continue (using alternative forms if appropriate) and which may have affected the patient's electrolyte balance (such as diuretics).

1.2 Preparing the patient for operation

Preoperative management

The following is a useful checklist to run through for each patient on the next day's operating schedule.

Identification

Check that the *correct* patient is having the *correct* operation on the *correct* side.

The As, Bs and Cs

ANAESTHETIST

The anaesthetist needs to be told a number of facts on the afternoon of the day before surgery.

- A brief summary of the patient's general health, outlining any relevant problems, past medical history, drugs and examination findings.
- The proposed surgery.
- The position of the patient on the list.
- When the patient last ate or drank (in emergency cases). The anaesthetist also needs to be asked.
- If he or she will be writing up the premedication.
- If he or she requires any further preparation.

ANTIBIOTICS
Is cover required? See p. 103.

ANTICOAGULATION
Does the surgeon require the patient to have prophylactic anticoagulation? See p. 105.

ALLERGY
Latex sensitivity and known drug allergies should be clearly indicated on the operating list.

BLOOD
Is the haemoglobin available?

BIOCHEMISTRY
Are the electrolytes available and within the normal range? Regular blood sugar results should be available in diabetics.

BACTERIOLOGY
Make sure the results of culture swabs are available on any patients who have preoperative sepsis. Check MRSA if relevant.

CROSS-MATCH
Many patients scheduled for elective surgery attend preoperative assessment clinics. This provides an opportunity to take blood for group and save. Provided that patients do not have unusual antibodies most hospital transfusion services can provide cross-matched blood at short notice (within an hour). For this reason many elective procedures where transfusion may be required are

commenced using the group and save sample and blood subsequently cross-matched as needed.

In specific circumstances it may be necessary to cross-match blood beforehand and recommended volumes are indicated in each procedure profile. Individual practice varies so check with the surgeon doing the operation.

CHEST X-RAY
If required.

CARDIOGRAM
If required.

CONSENT AND MARKING
Make sure an appropriate member of the team obtains the patient's consent to the procedure (see p. 124). Check that the patient and their main carers (usually relatives) understand what is going to happen over the next few days. Each operative procedure is described and profiled in this book to help you do this. Mark such things as hernias, lumps in the breast, varicose veins and small 'lumps and bumps' using a permanent skin marker.

Investigations

Make sure that the results of all the diagnostic investigations that have been asked for preoperatively are available before the operation starts. These often contain some surprises that affect what should be done.

Organizing the operating list

Having admitted each individual patient, you should check that the operating list has been organized and submitted. Other departments may need to be contacted (e.g. radiology and pathology).

The following headings summarize the main steps and may be used as a checklist. This should be done on the day before the operations are scheduled.

SURGEON
Be sure you know the following from the surgeon.
- All the patients on the list.
- What operation is intended for each patient. Check you know the precise description and the most complicated alternative procedure likely to be performed. Find out whether any special instruments or preoperative investigations will be needed.
- The order of the list.
- What time the surgeon wants to start.
- In cases where you are uncertain, check whether blood is required.

ANAESTHETIST
Is he or she fully informed as on p. 8?

ASSISTANT
One assistant of adequate experience should be available (some procedures will require more).

THEATRE
All the information collected needs to be passed on to the theatre staff. This is done by providing an operating list (Fig. 1.2.1). They need to know the following.
- The surgeon's name.
- The anaesthetist's name.
- The name and age of the patients (children require special instruments).
- The order of the list. Write clearly with no abbreviations. Always indicate the side of the operation in capital letters. Indicate any allergies or conditions that pose extra risks to healthcare personnel or where special decontamination of equipment might be needed.
- The operation intended, and any alternatives thought likely.
- Any special equipment needed, e.g. nerve stimulator.

WARDS
A copy of this list is sent to all the wards involved.

LIST OF OPERATIONS

DATE 24. 12. 91   SURGEON: Mr Cutfaster   ANAESTHETIST: Dr Snooze

TIME 8.30 a.m.   THEATRE 8

Number	Patient's name	Number	Age	Ward	Operation
1	Andrew SMITH	54321	6 months	D2	LEFT inguinal hernia (baby)
2	Jane BLOGGS	68624	55	D8	Cholecystectomy and exploration of common bile duct. Operative cholangiogram.
3	Susan McARTHUR	72643	60	D8	Laparotomy for abdominal mass. ?RIGHT hemicolectomy ? oophorectomy.
4	Henry SMITH	629953	39	D8	RIGHT nephrectomy for hypernephroma ? Exploration of inferior vena cava.

Fig. 1.2.1 Specimen operating list.

PEROPERATIVE INVESTIGATION

The relevant departments need to be informed of any special investigations that will be undertaken during an operation, such as histopathology for frozen section, radiology for operative cholangiogram.

BLOOD

Blood should be considered a potentially hazardous item, and should be transfused only if absolutely necessary.

1.3 The management of patients with pre-existing medical diseases

It is important to identify any patients with an illness that could influence the postoperative course, and to do so in time to allow adequate treatment before the operation. The procedure may have to be delayed until the patient is made as fit as possible.

The following medical conditions and patients will be considered in this chapter:

- respiratory disease: acute and chronic
- cardiovascular disease
- diabetes
- patients on steroids

- patients on anticoagulants
- haemophilia and other coagulation disorders
- blood-borne diseases
- acquired immune deficiency syndrome (AIDS).

Respiratory disease

ACUTE

Coughs, colds, sore throats and acute infections are all contraindications to elective surgery. Recovery usually takes place very quickly, especially in children, and unless the operation is urgent it should be delayed until the patient is fit. This usually means a delay of 2–4 weeks. The final decision as to whether a patient is fit for anaesthetic is left to the anaesthetist.

CHRONIC

Any patient with chronic obstructive pulmonary disease (COPD) has an increased risk of developing problems after an operation. Factors adversely affecting the chest include immobility, abdominal distension, inability to cough due to pain and suppression of the cough reflex by analgesics.

The risks are increased by certain factors.

- The nature and extent of the disease. Chronic airways obstruction is more of a problem than restrictive chest disease.
- The severity of the operation. A prolonged anaesthetic or postoperative recovery enhances the risk of chest infection.
- The site of the operation. Chest problems are more common after thoracic or abdominal operations, where coughing is very painful in the absence of suitable analgesia.
- Type of anaesthetic. General anaesthetics potentially cause more problems than local anaesthetics.
- Continued smoking. Increased secretions occur if smoking continues up to the time of surgery. Postoperative atelectasis is therefore more likely to occur.

Assessment

Patients at risk should be recognized and the severity of their condition assessed by history (How far can you walk on the level?

Can you climb a flight of stairs? Is it usually shortness of breath that stops you?), examination and special investigation.

- Full blood count. The haemoglobin may be elevated reflecting secondary polycythaemia due to chronic hypoxia. This indicates severe respiratory impairment.
- Blood gases. Both hypoxia and hypercapnia in a blood gas sample reflect severe respiratory impairment.
- Chest X-ray. This is an important preoperative baseline investigation for comparison with later postoperative X-rays, especially for patients with pre-existing lung disease.
- Respiratory function tests.
  - Spirometry measures the rate at which a patient can exhale. The patient is instructed to take a full inspiration and then blow as hard and for as long as possible into the mouthpiece. The instrument plots the volume exhaled against time. From the best plot obtained one can determine the volume of air exhaled in the first second (FEV1 = forced expiratory volume in the first second) and the total volume exhaled (FVC = forced vital capacity).
  - The peak expiratory flow rate (PEFR) is another simple measurement and is related to the FEV1. Normal values depend on age, weight and sex, and nomograms are available.
  - A useful measure from the graph is the ratio of FEV1 to FVC. (Normal value is above 75%.)
  - Airways obstruction or volume restriction affects the shape of the graph in a characteristic way (Fig. 1.3.1). Airways obstruction reduces the rate at which air can be expelled more than the total volume. Thus the ratio of FEV1 to FVC is less than 75%. If it is less than 50% significant obstruction is present and an attempt should be made to improve the situation before anaesthesia. Previous vitalographs may also be useful for comparison.
  - Restrictive airways disease (e.g. fibrosing alveolitis). The vital capacity is decreased more than the FEV1 and the ratio may therefore be above 75%.

Management
PREOPERATIVE
- The patient should stop smoking at least 1 month before surgery. The attempt to stop must therefore be made from the

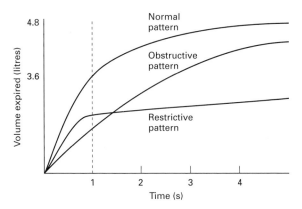

Fig. 1.3.1 The vitalograph plots the volume exhaled against time.

outpatient appointment. Explain that they are likely to develop pneumonia after their anaesthetic if they continue smoking. Most patients understand this and try to do something about it.

- Preoperative treatment may be possible and may be available from the physiotherapy department. This consists of the following:
  - physiotherapy – this may be both active (breathing exercises and loosening of secretions) and passive (postural drainage)
  - bronchodilators – there is usually an element of reversible airways obstruction and bronchodilators are therefore used. Nebulized salbutamol (2.5 mL 0.1% solution 4-hourly by inspiration) is effective. Aminophylline suppositories at night help nocturnal dyspnoea and bronchospasm
  - perioperative steroid use could be considered
  - antibiotics – these may be given if surgery is necessary in a patient with chronic pulmonary sepsis, but in general should be avoided as they encourage emergence of resistant strains.
- If possible, perform procedure under local or regional rather than general anaesthesia.
- Consider the risks and benefits carefully when a prolonged operation might be needed or one that exposes the lungs to additional risk (e.g. reperfusion of the lower limbs in arterial reconstructive surgery).

POSTOPERATIVE
- Encourage early mobilization as this will improve chest expansion and decrease ileus.
- Continue active physiotherapy.
- Good analgesia enables an effective cough to clear secretions. Various excellent postoperative systems are available, including epidurals and patient-controlled analgesia. A pain team may be available to help monitor postoperative pain.
- Examine the chest regularly to identify atelectasis and sputum retention.
- Bronchodilators.
- Prompt treatment of infection. Watch for signs of infection such as increased respiratory rate, pyrexia, purulent sputum and shortness of breath. Give broad-spectrum antibiotics after taking appropriate cultures. Change if necessary once sensitivities are known.

Asthma

Asthma is characterized by reversible airways obstruction. It may be precipitated by an allergen, exercise or cold. There may be no obvious precipitating factors.

Assessment
Find out about the following.
- Any known precipitating factors.
- The frequency and severity of attacks and the treatment needed to reverse them.
- What normal maintenance treatment is required to prevent attacks.

Management
- A mild well-controlled asthmatic is rarely a problem.
- Severe asthmatics may need to be admitted early to allow time for assessment and for the patient to settle on the ward.
- Reassurance and good premedication are important as anxiety may precipitate an attack.
- Discuss the case with the anaesthetist and ask if he or she wants any particular preoperative medication, such as nebulized salbutamol or steroid cover.

• Listen for bronchospasm postoperatively and treat it early. Similarly, treat any developing chest infection quickly.

Cardiovascular disease

The following problems will be considered.
• Myocardial ischaemia:
  ◦ infarction
  ◦ angina.
• Hypertension.
• Left ventricular failure.
• Cardiac dysrhythmias, e.g. atrial fibrillation.
• Heart murmurs.
  These pre-existing conditions should be identified during the history and examination. If present, a full cardiovascular assessment is required.

Assessment
All patients with a cardiovascular abnormality should have the following investigations.
• Haemoglobin to exclude anaemia.
• Biochemistry (urea and electrolytes) to exclude electrolyte imbalance.
• Chest X-ray:
  ◦ assess heart size and shape
  ◦ look for pulmonary congestion
  ◦ look for unfolding of the thoracic aorta (seen in longstanding hypertension)
  ◦ look for calcification in the cardiac valves or aorta.
• ECG:
  ◦ look for evidence of dysrhythmia
  ◦ look for changes of ischaemia
  ◦ look for conduction defects.

Management
MYOCARDIAL INFARCTION
An elective operation should not be undertaken in the first 6 months after a myocardial infarct, as there is a substantial risk

of perioperative re-infarction and death during this time. The risk is increased if the patient is hypertensive, if the operation is likely to be prolonged or if the operation involves thoracic or abdominal surgery. Patients who have had a myocardial infarction more than 6 months previously have a small risk of re-infarction.

ANGINA
- Assess its severity using the following parameters:
  - the frequency of attacks
  - the duration of attacks
  - the state of improvement with rest or glyceryl trinitrate
  - how severe the circumstances were that brought on the attack.
- Inform anaesthetist and surgeon. If appropriate, refer to a cardiologist for consideration of investigation, and delay operation.
- Intraoperatively severe swings of blood pressure should be avoided.
- Postoperatively give adequate analgesia and avoid fluid overload.

HYPERTENSION
Patients receiving treatment for hypertension usually stay on this treatment while in hospital. It is important that the anaesthetist knows which drug is being used as it will influence the management (e.g. β-blockers may mask any sympathetic response to hypotension). He or she will also have to decide whether any alternative therapy should be given when the patient is taken off oral drugs just before operation. Sudden cessation of certain drugs can lead to rebound hypertension.

Check the blood pressure is well controlled. It may need to be taken on at least two occasions preoperatively.

If the patient is on long-term diuretics check the electrolytes. Such patients are often sodium- or potassium-depleted.

Look for secondary effects such as left ventricular hypertrophy, myocardial ischaemia, ECG changes and impaired renal function.

LEFT VENTRICULAR FAILURE
If this is acute it should be brought under control prior to surgery. The help of medical colleagues should be sought. If it is chronic, the following must be done.

- Assess the present degree of failure. An ECG is helpful to determine left ventricular function and to exclude ischaemia as the cause of failure. A transoesophageal echocardiogram provides additional quantitative information about ventricular function and gradients across valves.
- Note the treatment the patient is receiving.
- Check the urea and electrolytes and relay this information to the anaesthetist.
- Postoperative fluid management is difficult. It may be an advantage to run the patient rather more dehydrated than usual.

DYSRHYTHMIA (e.g. ATRIAL FIBRILLATION)
Acute dysrhythmias are often precipitated by surgical emergencies and the treatment of these is best discussed with the anaesthetist. Chronic dysrhythmias are usually stable but the anaesthetist should be informed of current treatment.

HEART MURMURS
Define the murmur by clinical assessment and evaluation of the ECG, chest X-ray and echocardiogram. If you are in any doubt about the interpretation of the murmur seek expert advice. Check the patient's notes for evidence of previous problems.

VALVULAR DISEASE AND SEPTAL DEFECTS
- Treat any cardiac failure or dysrhythmia.
- Antibiotics. Any diseased valve may act as a site for subacute bacterial endocarditis. Its surface may be colonized by organisms during a transient bacteraemia. Therefore prophylactic antibiotics are given to those patients with a murmur who are having the following procedures:
  ○ upper respiratory tract, oral or dental surgery (*Streptococcus viridans*)
  ○ interventional GI endoscopy
  ○ biliary surgery
  ○ large bowel surgery
  ○ cystoscopy, prostatectomy, genitourinary surgery (*S. faecalis*)
  ○ abortion (*S. faecalis*).

Follow local protocols for prophylactic antibiotics.
- As in all cardiac disease, avoid any hypovolaemia or fluid overload.

Diabetes

Diabetic treatment is normally planned and adjusted for the individual patient to follow their usual lifestyle, while maintaining a normal blood sugar. Admission for a surgical operation disturbs this balance of 'treatment versus lifestyle', due to the catabolic response to surgery. Diabetics also have an increased risk of developing problems at the time of surgery due to the following factors.

- Infection.
- Cardiovascular disease.
- Renal disease: diabetic nephropathy may affect the elimination of drugs by the kidney.
- Autonomic neuropathy: this causes postural hypotension, affects the bladder causing retention, and has been implicated in sudden cardiorespiratory arrest in diabetics undergoing surgery.

Assessment
Determine the severity and stability. In addition look for evidence of diabetic complications. Assess the following.

- Cardiac function (by history, examination, chest X-ray and ECG).
- Renal function (by measurement of the blood pressure, looking for the presence of oedema, testing the urine for protein and checking the serum urea and electrolytes).
- The neurological system (look for autonomic neuropathy by taking the blood pressure lying and standing).

   Ideally, diabetic patients needing major surgery should be admitted 24 h before the operation for assessment and stabilization. More time will be needed if their method of diabetic treatment is to be changed (see below).

Management
The aim of management is to maintain good control and prevent ketoacidosis and hypoglycaemia. Ketoacidosis is prevented by supplying adequate calories and insulin, and hypoglycaemia is prevented by ensuring that the insulin given is covered by sufficient glucose input. Hypoglycaemia is to be strenuously

avoided. If it occurs under anaesthetic and is not picked up, brain damage may occur.

Patients can be divided into three main groups:

- diabetics controlled by diet
- diabetics controlled by oral hypoglycaemics
- insulin-dependent diabetics.

Procedures can be divided into:

- minor operations, where the patient may eat as soon as they wake up
- major operations, where the patient may have no oral intake for a variable length of time postoperatively.

The precise management will depend on which combination of these factors is present.

DIABETICS CONTROLLED BY DIET

- Minor operations: no specific measures.
- Major operations.
  - Measure the blood sugar just before anaesthetic.
  - Regular 3–4-hourly blood sugar measurements postoperatively for 24 h.
  - Usually there is no problem, but the combination of stress and bed rest may cause a rise in blood sugar and make the patient temporarily insulin-dependent (p. 22).
  - For patients withdrawn from oral feeding, a standard intravenous regime (e.g. 1 L of normal saline, 2 L of 5% dextrose, each with 20 mmol potassium) will give the patient 100 g of carbohydrate. Insulin may or may not be added to this.

DIABETICS CONTROLLED ON ORAL HYPOGLYCAEMICS

- Minor operations.
  - No hypoglycaemics on the day of operation.
  - Measure blood sugar just before anaesthetic, postoperatively and 4 h later.
  - Restart oral hypoglycaemics as soon as oral intake is established.
- Major operations.
  - Patients must be stabilized and managed on short-acting insulin. Ideally they should be admitted 24–48 h before the operation for conversion to a short-acting soluble insulin.

◦ Further management is then as for patients on insulin.
◦ The effects of oral hypoglycaemics may last many hours and insulin requirements will vary. Therefore use a sliding scale of insulin.

INSULIN-DEPENDENT DIABETICS

Discuss the preoperative management with the anaesthetist. There are different ways of managing such diabetics and the anaesthetist may well have a preference.

- Minor operations.
  ◦ If possible plan the operation early in the list.
  ◦ Omit any long-acting insulin the night before the operation.
  ◦ Omit the morning dose of insulin. Set up an intravenous infusion for the pre- and perioperative period of 1 L of 5% dextrose with 16 units Actrapid and 20 mmol KCl, infused at 100 mL/h. Patients having small operations later in the day can have a light breakfast covered by half the normal dose of insulin in the morning. They are then starved and an infusion is set up as above.
  ◦ Check the blood sugar before operation, immediately after operation and 4-hourly until the patient is eating normally.
  ◦ As soon as oral intake is re-established after the operation, restart the insulin.
- Major operations. There are many possible regimes for intravenous insulin administration. One regime is shown in Table 1.3.1, but your anaesthetist may prefer to use a different one.
  ◦ Plan the operation early in the list.
  ◦ The day before the operation give the patient their normal dose of insulin in short-acting form.
  ◦ On the morning of the operation start an intravenous infusion of 5% dextrose (1 L) with 16 units Actrapid and 20 mmol KCl, infused at 100 mL/h.
  ◦ Postoperatively, the insulin is given by continuous infusion from an insulin pump 'piggy-backed' into the side of the drip. 50 units Actrapid in 50 mL 0.9% saline (strength 1 unit/mL) are administered according to the scale shown in Table 1.3.1. One litre 5% dextrose is infused intravenously concurrently over 8–10 h. The saline requirement is given through a second line. Potassium requirements can be added as usual.

Table 1.3.1 Sliding scale for insulin infusion rate according to hourly blood sugar measurement.

Ward glucometer test (mmol/L)	Insulin i.v. (units/h)
< 2	Give 50 mL 50% glucose i.v
2–5.9	None
6–8.9	0.5
9–10.9	1.0
11–16.9	2.0
17–28	4.0

- This system needs good nursing care as the glucose and insulin are given independently and there is a risk that they may get out of phase (in particular, there is a danger of hypoglycaemia).
- An insulin infusion is ideal, especially for a long period of care when the patient is going to have no fluid or restricted fluid by mouth.
- Once the patient begins to drink and becomes re-established on a diet, a twice- or thrice-daily soluble insulin regime can be restarted and adjusted according to blood sugar levels.
- The initial total daily insulin should roughly equal the patient's preoperative dose. It should be increased by about 20% in the presence of infection or when the patient is taking high-dose steroids. The dose may need doubling or quadrupling if the patient is severely ill.
- Measure the blood sugar hourly postoperatively until stable, adjusting the infusion rate according to the above chart. Once stable, measure it 2–4-hourly. Monitor the potassium levels.

EMERGENCY SURGERY IN DIABETICS
- Diet-controlled diabetics and those on oral hypoglycaemics can usually be managed by putting up a 5% dextrose infusion and administering subcutaneous Actrapid, according to a sliding scale.

- Insulin-dependent diabetics and those who are extremely ill should have an insulin dextrose infusion as outlined. It is usually better to run the blood sugar a little too high, rather than a little too low.
- Ketoacidosis can mimic the acute abdomen. Therefore patients should be stabilized and reassessed prior to operation.

Patients on steroids

If the patient has been on regular steroids in the 6 weeks preceding the operation they may have adrenal suppression and be unable to respond to stress and trauma in the usual way. Additional steroid cover is then required.

The dose given is influenced by the severity of the operation and the length of the previous steroid treatment. A commonly used regime for a major operation is listed below.

- Hydrocortisone 100 mg i.m. with premedication.
- Hydrocortisone 100 mg 8-hourly over the day of the operation.
- Hydrocortisone 50 mg 8-hourly on the second postoperative day.
- Hydrocortisone 50 mg 12-hourly on the third postoperative day.
- Then 25 mg 12-hourly gradually decreasing to the patient's normal dose over a further week. It is useful to remember that 5 mg of prednisolone is equivalent to 20 mg of hydrocortisone.
- If the patient's blood pressure falls postoperatively and other causes have been excluded, suspect adrenal insufficiency and give extra hydrocortisone (100 mg hydrocortisone i.v.) until the blood pressure is restored.

Patients on anticoagulants

The precise management depends on the policy of the local surgical unit, anaesthetists and haematologists. Patients are usually on anticoagulants as prophylaxis against venous thrombosis or arterial emboli. In each case a fine balance needs to be kept between effective anticoagulation and minimal risk of haemorrhage during surgery.

The anticoagulant effect of both heparin and warfarin can be reversed. The action of heparin is reversed with protamine sulphate. The action of warfarin is reversed with fresh frozen plasma (FFP) and vitamin K.

The management of a patient on warfarin will depend on the reason for warfarinization. Those with prosthetic heart valves should be managed more precisely than those on warfarin for atrial fibrillation.

In some patients it may be suitable to omit warfarin for 2–3 days and operate when the international normalized ratio (INR) falls to approximately 1.6. Others may need to be fully stabilized on heparin prior to elective surgery. In the emergency setting use FFP and small doses of intravenous vitamin K (in consultation with the haematologist) to achieve an INR of less than 2.

Antiplatelet agents like aspirin or clopidogrel may need to be stopped a week before the operation in discussion with the surgeon and the anaesthetist.

Haemophilia and other coagulation disorders

Classical haemophilia is due to a deficiency of factor VIII. Christmas disease is due to a deficiency of factor IX. The severity of the condition varies between different patients, but all need special management when surgery has to be undertaken. Capillary bleeding initially ceases due to platelet aggregation (primary haemostasis). Because of the factor deficiency, the clotting cascade is inadequately activated and insufficient fibrin is produced to stabilize the clot. Continued bleeding therefore occurs in the postoperative period unless replacement therapy is given.

Management
This should be discussed with the haematologist pre- and perioperatively.

It is increasingly recognized that congenital and acquired disorders of coagulation are common causes of postoperative thrombosis. Such conditions, frequently due to a reduction of the level of naturally occurring anticoagulants (such as protein C, protein S and antithrombin III) will require careful pre- and postoperative management. Once again a personal or family history of deep venous thrombosis or pulmonary embolism, especially before the age of 40 years, will give a clue as to whether further detailed investigations are required.

Blood-borne diseases

Healthcare professionals have quite rightly become concerned about the transmission of certain diseases from patients to those dealing with them or with their specimens. Contamination with human immunodeficiency virus (HIV) and hepatitis B and C most commonly require consideration. As doctors we are at particular risk of transmission from patients' blood, either from needle-stick injuries during cannulation or from major contamination in theatre. Blood-borne disease does not gain entry through intact skin.

For some diseases all those at risk can be immunized (e.g. hepatitis B), and occupational health departments are active in ensuring this. Other diseases, while detectable, have no known vaccine, and new diseases may have emerged by the time you read this book.

The only practical solution therefore, is to minimize the risk of exposure by adopting certain 'universal' precautions.
- Cover all open wounds with appropriate dressings.
- Wear gloves when coming into contact with patient body fluids.
- Avoid contact with sharps. Avoid resheathing needles, use sharps bins for needles, syringes and scalpel blades, and use other instruments when manipulating sharps (no-touch technique).
- In theatre use a sharps receiver to pass scalpels and needles to one another.
- In theatre wear eye protection to avoid contamination via the conjunctiva.

OCCUPATIONAL EXPOSURE TO HIV
Report needle-stick injuries immediately to the relevant authority. Recent evidence suggests that the risk of acquiring HIV after a contamination incident is reduced by postexposure prophylaxis with indinavir, lamivudine and zidovudine. You and the

patient may then be tested after relevant counselling. If you do have the misfortune to acquire a disease, testing will enable you to prove your seroconversion was occupationally related. This could be important in future compensation or insurance claims.

Acquired immune deficiency syndrome (AIDS)

AIDS, caused by HIV, is a major disease which has profound implications for both patients and staff. Infection can be acquired by drug abuse, sexual intercourse or treatment with blood products contaminated with HIV.

Transmission of the disease occurs with difficulty and requires intimate contact with infected human blood, serum or semen. Once infection has occurred, the virus may remain dormant for many years. Eventually, most, if not all, carriers develop immune deficiency syndrome in which there is an absence of T-cell helper activity. This syndrome can present in a wide variety of ways due to lowered resistance to other infections. These may involve any of the surgical specialties. Among the common presentations are atypical pneumonia (pneumocystis), orogenital candidiasis, progressive lymphadenopathy and Kaposi's sarcoma. Although at the time of writing there is no cure for this infection, active treatment can improve the patient's length and quality of life. Patients have a right to confidentiality, particularly as there is still intolerance by society to this diagnosis.

Recognizing the pattern
The diagnosis should be considered in any patient presenting with an unusual condition who might be in a high-risk group for infection. The main high-risk groups are:

- homosexual males
- bisexual males
- intravenous drug users
- haemophiliacs
- recipients of blood products before 1985 (when HIV testing of donated blood started)
- residents of African countries south of the Sahara
- sexual partners of any of the above

- children of infected mothers
- prison inmates, past or present.

Heterosexual transmission is now increasingly recognized.

Proving the diagnosis

Check for antibodies (the patient's informed consent must be obtained before HIV testing). HIV antibodies appear in serum up to 3 months after infection. The patient can transmit infection during the seronegative phase. HIV antigen can also be detected in serum, but this test is less widely available than that based on the antibody.

Management

It is unethical for a doctor to refuse treatment to a patient infected with HIV on the grounds that there is a risk of the doctor becoming infected (General Medical Council 1988). Therefore adequate precautions must be taken to prevent cross-infection from any patient by the means listed under 'Blood-borne diseases' (p. 26).

1.4 The operation and afterwards

The junior surgical trainee in theatre

As junior surgical trainee you should ensure that the operating list runs as smoothly as possible. Hospitals and surgical units vary in their requirement for you to be present in theatre for the list. Although the surgical ward is often busy, we believe that there is also an important role to play in theatre, as well as vital training for anyone hoping to specialise in surgery.

When possible, visiting the operating theatre to observe part of a procedure will provide you with a far better impression of what was done than you will get from reading an operation note.

Before scrubbing up do the following.
- Check whether the patient requires a bladder catheter.
- Check that any necessary preoperative antibiotics have been given.
- Fill in a histology form for frozen section if this is required.

- If the operating list is running late, inform any other department that might be affected, e.g. those providing peroperative radiology or frozen section histology.

Pagers and mobile telephones can be distracting to the surgeon and should not be worn in theatre.

ASSISTING AT OPERATION

The principle of assisting is to make the operation as easy as possible for the surgeon. If you are the first assistant try and follow the operation, imagining you were having to do it yourself, and thus anticipating what is required.

When sutures are being tied have a pair of scissors ready to cut the ends when asked to do so. Always use the tips of the scissors. If you use the blade higher up there is a danger of inadvertently cutting neighbouring structures as the tips close. Skin sutures should be cut so that the ends are as long as the distance between each suture. In this way they can be seen easily for removal, but are not in the way of the next knot. For internal sutures ask how long the surgeon would like the ends cut, as this will vary with the type of material used.

Ensure that the area the surgeon is operating on is as well exposed as possible, using suitable retractors or forceps to display the structures. Keep the field clear of blood using swabs or suction.

Never try and 'dictate' what the surgeon should do next; simply make it as easy as possible for them to achieve what they have decided to do.

There is usually less to do as a second assistant. With most modern retractor systems there is little need for someone to stand holding a retractor for hours on end. In some complex procedures, though, a second assistant can be a great help. Good demonstration of the operative field may make all the difference between a successful or unsuccessful operation for your patient. Do it willingly and cheerfully.

THE IMMEDIATE POSTOPERATIVE PERIOD

The junior surgical trainee should check the following things after each operation.

- Laboratory specimens. Have they been labelled and the forms signed? Make sure any microbiology specimens have gone to the laboratory.

- Operation note. Has it been written? Are instructions to recovery and ward staff clear?
- Prescription chart. Check this in order to be certain that:
  ○ adequate analgesia and night sedation are written up
  ○ an intravenous fluid regime is written up if the patient requires it.
- Intravenous lines, arterial lines, drains and catheters. After a large operation make a mental note of the position of these. Are they all necessary in the postoperative period and how long will the surgeon require them to be left in?
- Nursing observations. Note which observations are required postoperatively and inform the nurses of any particular problems such as the presence of a chest drain or drains requiring measurement of output.

Conducting regular postoperative ward rounds

The junior surgical trainee should see every patient under his or her care at least once a day. This enables you to keep in touch with the patient's progress, and to pick up any postoperative problems as they arise.

The following is a basic plan for such a round, designed to check quickly on every aspect of patient care. If you find something positive the methods of management can be followed up in sections 1.5–1.9.

HISTORY
Ask about pain and vital functions.
- Pain: if the patient has any new or unexpected pain, identify the cause. Ask particularly about pain in the legs or chest (thromboembolism), or increasing pain in the wound (wound infection). Has adequate analgesia been prescribed?
- Breathing: shortness of breath, cough, haemoptysis.
- Eating: appetite, nausea, vomiting.
- Bowels: passage of flatus, motions.
- Urine: has the patient passed urine? Has the patient had any dysuria or difficulty?

EXAMINATION
Check the following.
- Temperature charts for pyrexia, change in pulse rate, blood pressure and respiratory rate.
- Chest: examine for signs of infection, collapse or oedema.
- Wound: check for developing localized tenderness.
- Bowel sounds (after abdominal surgery).
- Legs: check for localized tenderness over the soleal muscles.
- Mental state.

FLUID BALANCE
Examine the fluid chart and check the input (oral, i.v.) against the output (urine, nasogastric tube, drains and insensible loss). Is the patient in positive or negative fluid balance?

DRAINS AND TUBES
Check the position of intravenous lines, drains and any urinary catheter. Are they all draining? Can any be removed? Have any become infected?

DRUGS
Check the prescription sheet for any unnecessary drugs which can be deleted.

INVESTIGATIONS
Order any tests which may be necessary (e.g. haemoglobin, urea and electrolytes, serum proteins). These should all be clearly documented in the notes.

1.5 Postoperative complications: presenting symptoms

Some of the common problems you will be called upon to deal with in the postoperative period are dealt with in this section. They are listed in Table 1.5.1. Further notes on subsequent management are given in sections 1.6–1.9.

Table 1.5.1 Common postoperative problems.

Common presentations	Causes	Page
Pyrexia	Pulmonary collapse or bronchopneumonia	43
	Wound infection	65
	Intra-abdominal abscess	
	(pelvic or subphrenic)	70
	Urinary tract infection	58
	Inflamed drip site	70
	Thromboembolism	52
	Blood transfusion reaction	47
	Septicaemia	77
Postoperative pain	Wound haematoma or infection	65
	Chest	35
	Abdomen	35
	Legs	35
Discharging wound	Abscess	65
	Fistula	64, 74
	Dehiscence	68
Nausea and vomiting	Drugs	35
	Intestinal obstruction	308, 370
	Acute dilatation of the stomach	42
Constipation	Paralytic ileus	41
	Drugs	36
Breathlessness	Pulmonary collapse	43
	Bronchopneumonia	43
	Pulmonary embolism	54
	Left ventricular failure	50
	Pneumothorax	45
Confusion		37
Collapse	Inhalation of vomit	45
	Haemorrhage	46
	Septicaemia	77
	Pulmonary embolus	54
	Myocardial infarction	49
	Stroke	50
Oliguria/anuria	Postrenal, renal and prerenal failure	61
	Retention of urine	59

Postoperative pyrexia

The temperature chart is a very good indicator of developing postoperative problems and should be inspected every day. The time of onset of the fever will help you decide the cause.

Early postoperative fever, days 0–2

A mild pyrexia in the first 24 h after operation is commonly due to tissue damage and necrosis, or haematoma formation at the operative site. A higher and more persistent pyrexia may be due to pulmonary collapse, or specific infections related to the surgery, e.g. urinary infection after bladder surgery or biliary infection after a cholecystectomy. A fever due to blood transfusion may also appear in this early period.

Fever, days 3–5

A pyrexia developing in this period is likely to be due to either developing sepsis (e.g. wound infection or pelvic or subphrenic abscess formation) or bronchopneumonia.

Fever, days 5–7

Problems presenting at this time include those associated with failure of a bowel anastomosis, e.g. leakage and fistula formation, and a fever due to venous thrombosis either in the limbs or in the pelvic veins.

Fever after the first week

This is less likely to be due to a problem directly related to the operation, although the development of wound or deep sepsis can be delayed if the patient has received prophylactic antibiotics. Other causes include the development of distant sepsis such as a hepatic abscess or cerebral abscess. Thrombotic disease may also be delayed in onset and appear at this time.

If you cannot find an adequate explanation for a fever at any time, assume that something has gone wrong with the operation (e.g. a leak) until you can prove conclusively otherwise.

Recognizing the pattern
Carry out the following routine.

- Ask about symptoms of cough, sputum, dysuria, urinary frequency or calf pain.
- Examine:
  - the respiratory and pulse rates
  - the chest
  - the wound
  - the drip site and drain sites
  - the calves for tenderness localized over the soleus muscle
  - the abdomen if an abdominal operation has been performed.
- Investigations: culture specimens of sputum, urine, blood (if temperature above 38°C), take a wound swab and perform a chest X-ray.

Management
Some common causes of postoperative pyrexia are shown in Table 1.5.1. Further details of these conditions are given in subsequent chapters.

Postoperative pain

Pain relief is almost always required in the postoperative period and analgesic therapy is discussed on p. 98. The cause of any pain must be determined in the same way as in other circumstances but there are certain characteristics in a postoperative patient.

Wound pain
Pain in the wound is worse on movement and is usually maximal in the first 72 h. Thereafter it usually settles. If the pain is getting worse after this, check for signs of a wound infection, either superficial or deep. Occasionally, patients suffer quite severe 'spasms' of pain in an abdominal wound. This is more common in those who are excessively tense.

Management
Appropriate analgesia for wound pain. Diazepam 2 mg 8-hourly is helpful for muscle spasms.

Chest pain

Excluding any pain due to a thoracic wound, two other significant types of chest pain occur postoperatively.

- Pleuritic. Sharp, localized and severe pain increased by inspiration. This may be due to infection involving the pleura or pulmonary infarction after an embolus (see pp. 43 and 54).
- Cardiac pain due to myocardial ischaemia. The patient may complain of crushing central chest pain with or without radiation into the neck and arms (see p. 49).

Abdominal pain

Possible causes of increasing abdominal pain include:

- intra-abdominal sepsis (see pp. 70–74)
- anastomotic leakage (p. 74)
- retention of urine (p. 59)
- constipation (p. 36)
- new intra-abdominal pathology, e.g. ischaemic bowel, intussusception, intestinal obstruction (pp. 308, 370).

Legs

- Deep or superficial venous thrombosis (p. 52).
- Sciatica.
- Postoperative arterial thrombosis or embolism.

Discharging wound

A copious discharge from the wound may be due to the release of a wound abscess. You should also consider the possibility of the development of an intestinal fistula (p. 74), a urinary fistula (p. 64) or a deep wound dehiscence (p. 68).

Nausea and vomiting

The common causes of postoperative vomiting are as follows.

- Drugs:
  - analgesics (opiates)

- ∘ anaesthetic agents
- ∘ other drug therapy, e.g. digoxin toxicity.
- Intestinal obstruction:
  - ∘ paralytic ileus
  - ∘ mechanical.

Recognizing the pattern
- Note which drugs the patient has received.
- Check possible drug interactions.
- Assess the oral input and listen for bowel sounds. Nausea and vomiting when the patient has just started drinking after abdominal surgery may be due to a persistent paralytic ileus. In this case the abdomen will be distended and bowel sounds absent.
- If nausea and vomiting occur after the patient has been tolerating oral fluids, consider the possibility of a mechanical obstruction. Here there is usually colicky pain with active bowel sounds. An abdominal X-ray will show distended loops and fluid levels with paucity of distal gas on the erect film.

Management
- Pass a nasogastric tube to drain the stomach.
- Paralytic ileus (p. 41).
- Mechanical obstruction (pp. 308, 370).
- Drug-induced vomiting. Treat with an antiemetic (e.g. prochlorperazine 12.5 mg i.m. 4–6 hourly, or metoclopramide 10 mg i.m./i.v. 8 hourly). Cyclizine and ondansetron could be considered in resistant cases. Stop the responsible drug if possible.

Constipation

Constipation occurs frequently after an operation and can cause great discomfort to the patient. A rectal examination is essential. Faecal impaction causes considerable distress and the cause is not always apparent to the patient. The early use of laxatives while the patient is still immobile often avoids the need for enemas or manual evacuation later on.

Opiate analgesics are a major cause of such constipation.

Breathlessness

Breathlessness in a postoperative patient is usually due to one of the following factors.

- Pulmonary collapse (p. 43).
- Bronchopneumonia (p. 43).
- Pulmonary embolism (p. 54).
- Left ventricular failure either due to fluid overload or myocardial infarction (p. 50).
- Pneumothorax (p. 54). This occasionally complicates the insertion of a central venous pressure (CVP) line or intercostal anaesthetic blocks, or may occur spontaneously.

Confusion

It is quite common for a surgical patient, often elderly, to become confused after an operation. This is distressing both for the patient and the relatives. There is usually a cause that may well be amenable to treatment. Causes include:

- hypoxia (bronchopneumonia, pulmonary embolus) – easily the most common
- infection (sepsis, urinary tract infection, chest infection)
- drugs (analgesics, sedatives, steroids)
- withdrawal (alcohol or drug)
- electrolyte imbalance
- uraemia
- pain (wound, retention of urine).

Recognizing the pattern

The symptoms of confusion are disorientation and agitation. Review with the above causes in mind. Always examine the chest. Bronchopneumonia is a frequent cause of confusion in the elderly. Check for a past history of alcohol abuse and see what drugs have been given. Remember that more than one of the causative factors may be operating.

Proving the diagnosis

The investigations may include:

- haemoglobin and haematocrit
- urea and electrolytes
- blood sugar
- blood gases
- microbiology where appropriate, e.g. blood cultures, samples of sputum and urine
- appropriate X-rays.

Management
- Talk to the patient. Gentle reassurance is required. A confused, elderly patient is usually aware of their own strange behaviour and terrified they are going to be permanently insane. Reassure the patient, and also the relatives, as they are usually more upset than the patient (who will not remember the events when they recover).
- Check the drug chart for anything that may be causing the confusion and, if possible, stop the drug concerned.
- Treat any organic cause found.
- If the patient is still agitated or potentially hostile despite the above measures, then sedation may be required, but before you do this, be certain that the problem is not hypoxia. There is no ideal drug to recommend; however, small incremental doses of haloperidol may be used.

Collapse

When a patient suddenly collapses after an operation there is often a degree of panic and it is important to take charge and make a careful assessment.

The collapse is usually associated with cerebral impairment, either due to cerebral depression by anoxia, toxaemia or drugs, or due to a fall in the cerebral blood supply. Whatever the initial cause, the final picture tends to be similar as one system failure results in failure of another (Fig. 1.5.1).

Common primary causes to think of include the following conditions.
- Hypoxia:
  - inhalation of vomit (p. 45)

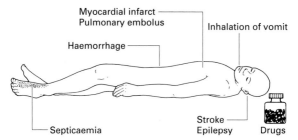

Fig. 1.5.1 Postoperative collapse.

- bronchopneumonia (p. 43)
- pulmonary oedema due to fluid overload in patients with left-sided heart failure
- respiratory depression secondary to opiates or anaesthetic drugs.
- Central circulatory failure:
  - myocardial infarction (p. 49)
  - pulmonary embolism (p. 54).
- Peripheral circulatory failure:
  - haemorrhage (reactionary or secondary) (p. 46)
  - third-space fluid loss (e.g. pancreatitis, mesenteric infarction).
- Toxaemia:
  - septicaemia (p. 77)
  - drug overdose (e.g. opiates, digoxin).
- Cerebral causes:
  - stroke (p. 50)
  - epilepsy.

Recognizing the pattern
Make a quick appraisal of the following.
- Check the airway
- Breathing and oxygenation. Respiration. Rate and character. Quiet or dyspnoeic? Laboured? Tracheal tug? Are there any physical signs in the chest? Pink or cyanosed?
- Circulation. Blood pressure, pulse rate and character. Jugular venous pulse (JVP). Listen to the heart.

- Are the extremities warm (vasodilated) or cold (vasoconstricted)?
- Cerebral function. Level of consciousness.

If the blood pressure and pulse are adequate then the cause is anoxia, toxaemia or a cerebral problem such as a stroke. If there is circulatory collapse (low blood pressure and tachycardia), then you have to decide whether this is due to central (cardiac) failure or peripheral failure (third-space loss or vasodilatation). In central failure there is venous hypertension (raised JVP, peripheral oedema, pulmonary oedema). Peripheral failure may be due to inadequate blood volume (in which case the patient is cold and sweating and the peripheries are vasoconstricted), or due to toxic vasodilatation (in which case the blood pressure is low but the peripheries are warm and well perfused).

Proving the diagnosis
The following investigations may help in making further progress:

- haemoglobin and white cell count
- electrolytes and blood glucose
- ECG
- chest X-ray.

While arranging these remember to cross-match blood if this is likely to be needed.

Management
Initial management involves attention to the airway, high flow oxygen, and setting up an intravenous infusion as necessary. The further management depends on the cause of the collapse.

Oliguria/anuria

It is not uncommon for a patient to have a diminished urine output after a major operation, due to the effects of fluid and blood loss and the physiological response of the adrenal cortex to stress (see intravenous fluid therapy, p. 90). This temporary oliguria should recover after 12–24 h. An output of less than 0.5 mL/kg/h is not satisfactory and should be investigated. It may reflect a deliberate act to prevent fluid overload and this can be accepted if pulse and blood pressure are both normal.

There are three possible causes to consider for poor postoperative urine output:

- retention of urine
- prerenal failure
- acute renal failure.

These are dealt with in section 1.8. Retention of urine is diagnosed by finding a full bladder on examination and confirming this by catheterization. If no evidence of retention is found then renal failure must be suspected and appropriate steps taken.

1.6 Gastrointestinal and respiratory complications

Paralytic ileus

Paralytic ileus is atony of the intestine causing intestinal obstruction. It has a complex aetiology and is common after any operation when the stomach or bowel have been handled, or where there has been peritonitis. The condition is exacerbated by chemical derangement (hypokalaemia, uraemia, diabetes), by reflex sympathetic inhibition (e.g. after retroperitoneal haematoma or injury) or by anticholinergic drugs. It is much less problematic after a laparoscopic procedure.

There may be an ileus for a variable period after open abdominal surgery. Oral feeding can only be restarted once bowel function has returned and you will be called upon to make a decision about this.

Management

Surgeons differ widely in their attitudes towards reintroducing fluids an diet after abdominal operations. Immediately after the operation, unless a nasogastric tube is present, the patient is either kept 'nil by mouth', or only allowed small volumes of water to drink (e.g. 15 mL/h) or ice to suck occasionally. The fluid requirements are given intravenously. The nasogastric tube should be aspirated regularly. You should check that it is draining freely and not blocked. If in doubt, test by giving fluid to drink and then reaspirating it up the tube.

Recovery from ileus is demonstrated by:
- the return of bowel sounds, often accompanied by colic
- passage of flatus
- the patient beginning to feel hungry
- a decrease in the nasogastric aspirate
- an increase in the urinary output as fluid is absorbed from the bowel.

Listen to the abdomen daily. When bowel sounds return, oral intake may be increased. The nasogastric tube can be removed. As the ileus recovers the patient frequently has some abdominal distension and 'wind' pains, and will require reassurance about these. They are relieved when flatus is passed.

If the ileus persists for more than 4 days, there may be some other cause operating such as continuing peritonitis, intra-abdominal abscess formation, anastomotic leakage or mechanical intestinal obstruction. Providing none of the above causes are apparent, encourage the patient to mobilize, pushing their drip stand before them. Rectal suppositories may help. Metoclopramide (10 mg i.m./i.v.) is a good antiemetic, as it not only has central action but also helps gastric emptying. A prolonged ileus may eventually necessitate the introduction of intravenous feeding.

Simple constipation

This is dealt with on p. 36.

Acute dilatation of the stomach

This is a rare complication of any laparotomy. It is occasionally seen in the diabetic patient. There is massive distension of the stomach, which contains several litres of fluid, mucus and air. As distension progresses the duodenum becomes kinked, causing mechanical obstruction to outflow.

Recognizing the pattern
The most important factor is to think of the possibility. Do not be misled by the presence of a nasogastric tube as this may not have been aspirated efficiently. The patient complains of

progressive distension, hiccups and vomiting. The vomiting becomes effortless, and is of dark brown fluid. On examination the upper abdomen is distended. The patient may be dehydrated with a tachycardia and hypotension.

Proving the diagnosis

The diagnosis is proved by successful aspiration of large volumes of dark-coloured fluid.

An abdominal X-ray shows a very large gastric air bubble. A chest X-ray may show a raised left hemidiaphragm and some basal collapse.

The following investigations are important:
- urea and electrolytes to check the potassium
- haematocrit to assess the degree of hypovolaemia.

Management

- The nasogastric tube is left in place and aspirated regularly to keep the stomach empty. The patient immediately feels better. The gastric ileus recovers rapidly once the stomach is decompressed.
- Intravenous fluid is given to provide both the body requirement and to replace that lost by vomiting and aspiration. This should correct the hypovolaemia. Watch the potassium level.

Pulmonary collapse and bronchopneumonia

Pulmonary collapse, or atelectasis (Fig. 1.6.1) is due to the blockage of bronchi with retained secretions and absorption of air from the distal segment. It usually happens within 48 h of operation. If the sputum plug persists then secondary bronchopneumonia ensues.

Recognizing the pattern

The patient may complain of shortness of breath and a dry cough. They may feel there is something they want to cough up but are unable to. On examination the most constant feature is an early postoperative pyrexia which may be quite high (e.g. 39°C). If initial treatment fails to dislodge this blockage, the pyrexia remains high and eventually purulent sputum is produced. The

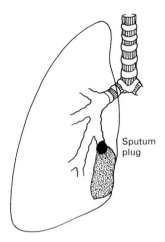

Sputm
plug

Fig. 1.6.1 Pulmonary collapse.

patient has a raised respiratory rate and a tachycardia. Examination of the chest usually fails to show anything very significant in the early stages.

Proving the diagnosis

The collapsed segment may be visible on chest X-ray after a few days. As soon as a sample of sputum is produced it should be sent off to the microbiologists for culture in case antibiotics are required later.

Management

The condition may be prevented by adequate analgesia and encouraging coughing in the first few hours after operation. If it occurs, however, physiotherapy is used to help the patient cough. This is both active (chest percussion and breathing exercises) and passive (postural drainage). Adequate analgesia is essential if this is to be successful. Nebulized saline can make the mucus less tenacious.

In severe cases bronchoscopy and suction may be indicated. If the pyrexia persists for more than 48 h then antibiotic therapy should be instituted to treat secondary infection.

Inhalation of vomit

This usually occurs in the early postoperative period and may be associated with acute gastric dilatation or a pre-existing hiatus hernia with reflux. Inhalation of vomit causes an aspiration pneumonitis (Mendelson's syndrome). The chemical inflammation causes bronchospasm, pulmonary oedema, and respiratory and circulatory collapse, the extent of which depends on the volume and the acidity of the aspirate.

Recognizing the pattern

There is often a history of unconsciousness, vomiting or difficult intubation. There is progressive deterioration in respiratory function with cyanosis, tachycardia and dyspnoea. There is generalized bronchospasm, poor air entry and diffuse crepitations in the chest. The blood pressure is low and the peripheral vessels are vasoconstricted.

Proving the diagnosis

A chest X-ray shows widespread pulmonary infiltrates.

Management

- Clear the airway.
- Give oxygen.
- Notify the anaesthetist or intensive care team.
- Commence broad-spectrum antibiotics.
- Consider using hydrocortisone and bronchodilators.
- Monitor oxygenation with a pulse oximeter or serial blood gases. If the oxygen saturation deteriorates, consider mechanical ventilation.

Pneumothorax

Pneumothorax can occur during or after an operation. It can arise:

- spontaneously
- due to rupture of the lung occurring during positive pressure ventilation

- following insertion of a CVP line
- if the pleura has been opened accidentally (e.g. in nephrectomy or cervical sympathectomy).

  Tension pneumothorax is described on p. 626.

Recognizing the pattern
The chest on the affected side is immobile and hyperresonant with decreased breath sounds.

Proving the diagnosis
The air in the pleural space is visible on a chest X-ray.

Management
A pneumothorax large enough to impair breathing is treated by aspiration or chest drainage. The emergency insertion and management of a chest drain is discussed in section 6.1.

1.7 Cardiovascular complications

Haemorrhage

The condition of postoperative haemorrhage may be one of the following.
- Primary: bleeding at the time of operation from uncontrolled vessels.
- Reactionary: occurs within 24 h of operation. This is from uncontrolled vessels after vasospasm relaxes. Such haemorrhage also occurs as the blood pressure rises after recovery from anaesthesia, and with increases in venous pressure on moving and coughing.
- Secondary: occurs 7–14 days after operation and is due to reopening of a vessel by separation of the thrombus or to erosion due to infection. Such haemorrhage is often preceded by a 'warning' minor bleed.

Recognizing the pattern
The pattern of presentation depends on the rate of bleeding.

MINOR BLEED

With a slow haemorrhage there will be a tachycardia with mild hypotension made worse by an upright posture. The patient often notices blood in the bed or a blood-soaked dressing.

MAJOR BLEED

Acute severe haemorrhage presents as collapse. The patient becomes semiconscious, appearing restless, pale, cold and sweaty. The pulse is weak and there is tachycardia with a low blood pressure and low JVP/CVP.

Look for external bleeding (e.g. from the wound) or increasing abdominal distension suggesting intra-abdominal haemorrhage. Check whether there is blood issuing from any drains.

Early detection of haemorrhage is important as it significantly reduces morbidity and mortality. Regular reliable observations should be carried out on any patient at risk, half- to one-hourly, for at least 12 h after an operation.

Management

- Stop the bleeding. Pressure dressings may help. If the loss is rapid the patient may need to go back to theatre for laparotomy or exploration of the wound. Wound dressings must be changed regularly as blood-soaked dressings are a good medium for infection.
- Replace the lost blood volume. Insert two large-bore cannulae (14 or 16 gauge). Cross-match some blood urgently. Initial fluid replacement can be with crystalloid, plasma expanders or blood as discussed on p. 85. Give oxygen and catheterize the patient to monitor the urine output.
- A chronic slower bleed may require blood transfusion over the next 24 h.

Blood transfusion reactions

A reaction to blood transfusion is quite common and occurs for a number of reasons. The most serious, though least common reaction, is that following transfusion of incompatible blood due to an error of identification. This causes intravascular haemolysis with haemoglobinaemia and haemoglobinuria and later circulatory collapse, acute renal failure and jaundice. Disseminated intravascular coagulation and a bleeding tendency can develop.

More commonly, milder reactions occur due to the presence of pyrogens in the donor blood, or recipient antibodies to donor white cells. This results in a mild febrile reaction. Atopic individuals may have antibodies to exogenous antigen, e.g. milk or egg protein present in the donor plasma, which may cause an urticarial reaction. This very occasionally causes acute anaphylactic shock.

Recognizing the pattern

A mild pyrexia (37.5–38.0°C) commonly occurs during or within 2 h of blood transfusion. It is usually harmless, lasting a few hours, and the patient is otherwise well. Sometimes, an itchy urticarial rash may develop. There may be a past history of allergy.

The symptoms and signs of a haemolytic reaction include pain in the transfused limb, constricting pain in the chest and pain in the loins. On examination there is flushing, pyrexia, rigors, hypotension and bronchospasm. There may be persistent bleeding, and this can be the first indication of incompatible blood transfusion during operation.

Management

The following guidelines may be helpful.
- Mild pyrexia with no other symptoms or signs:
  - leave the blood transfusion running
  - watch for any deterioration in the routine observations
  - reassure the patient.
- Pyrexia with an itchy urticarial rash, no other abnormalities:
  - slow the transfusion down
  - the itching and rash may be relieved by antihistamine drugs. Chlorpheniramine (10 mg i.m.) can be used. If patients have a past history of repeated urticarial reactions to blood they may be started on chlorpheniramine (4 mg orally 8-hourly) before transfusion
  - if the rash persists, remove the unit of blood.
- Patients with more serious symptoms that suggest either a haemolytic reaction or anaphylactic shock:

∘ take the blood and the giving set down. Send it with a fresh sample of the patient's blood and urine to the laboratory for analysis
∘ hydrocortisone (200 mg i.v.)
∘ adrenaline (1 : 1000: 0.5–1.0 mL i.m.)
∘ oxygen (mask with reservoir bag)
∘ watch the pulse, blood pressure, clotting time and urine output very carefully and treat accordingly with i.v. fluid.

Overall, if you are in doubt, change the blood being transfused.

Myocardial infarction

Myocardial infarction may occur after operation. People who have a past history of infarction or angina are particularly at risk, as are those undergoing vascular surgery.

Recognizing the pattern
The history is of central crushing chest pain which may radiate down the arms or into the neck. Note that in diabetics it can be pain free (silent MI).

Usually the patient is pale, cold, clammy and tachycardic. Postoperative infarction may be silent, or simply present as an unexplained hypotensive episode.

Proving the diagnosis
The ECG shows:
• ST elevation
• T-wave inversion
• Q waves.

Cardiac enzymes are elevated over the next few hours. Troponin I needs to be checked immediately and repeated 12 h later.

Management
Initial management is analgesia with diamorphine, aspirin, nitrates, oxygen and bed rest. An urgent cardiology/medical review is required. Although thrombolysis is contraindicated after major surgery, reperfusion by emergency angioplasty is increasingly available.

Left ventricular failure

Left ventricular failure occurs in surgical patients who have been overloaded with fluid, particularly where there is a past history of heart failure or myocardial ischaemia. When the left ventricle fails the lungs become oedematous and the patient dyspnoeic.

Recognizing the pattern

The patient, who is often elderly, complains of shortness of breath. This may come on acutely or slowly, and is worse on lying flat. Urine output may be poor.

On examination the patient is dyspnoeic, often very distressed and cyanosed. There is a tachycardia with a triple rhythm, and bilateral fine basal crepitations with or without bronchospasm in the lungs. In the absence of chronic obstructive airways disease, acute bronchospasm in the elderly is often due to pulmonary oedema.

There may also be associated signs of right heart failure, such as a raised JVP, hepatomegaly and peripheral oedema.

Proving the diagnosis

A chest X-ray shows hilar congestion. An ECG must be performed. In severe cases blood gas measurements are helpful.

Management

Sit the patient up and give oxygen. Intravenous diuretics (e.g. frusemide 80–120 mg) and diamorphine (5–10 mg i.v.) are effective in the acute attack. Ask for a cardiology/medical opinion.

Preventative measures are important. The elderly need less fluid (sometimes with the aid of CVP monitoring) and this must be remembered during the administration of intravenous fluid therapy (see section 2.1). Blood transfusion should be undertaken with caution. At night the patient should be propped up in bed.

Stroke

A stroke is due to intracerebral haemorrhage, thrombosis or embolism with subsequent ischaemia or infarction of cerebral tissue. Preoperative predisposing factors include hypertension and vascular disease. During or after operation severe hypovolaemia may result in intracerebral thrombosis. Emboli may arise from the myocardium, heart valves, great vessels, or carotid and basilar arteries.

Recognizing the pattern

The patient usually suffers a sudden collapse and becomes unconscious.

On examination there may be neurological signs of hemiplegia (e.g. paralysis on one side, upgoing plantar responses, difficulties with speech). There may also be evidence of raised intracranial pressure such as a progressively slowing pulse, rising blood pressure and the appearance of papilloedema and pupil dilatation.

Proving the diagnosis

This is usually made obvious by the neurological deficit. CT scan will show intracerebral haemorrhage, and after 12 h any cerebral infarct.

Management

- If a CT scan shows a large haemorrhage with brain shift and compression, a neurosurgical opinion is sought. Acute craniotomy and decompression is only done as a last resort.
- Normally the initial management is conservative, comprising nursing care, catheterization, attention to fluid balance and regular observations.
- Treat any excessive hypertension with care, as a sudden massive fall in blood pressure to normal levels can sometimes result in a cerebrovascular event.
- The patient may be referred acutely to the neurologists for further management. They may decide to treat raised intracranial pressure.
- Most patients who have had a stroke have long-term problems and are going to be dependent on others for some time. A team consisting of occupational therapist, physiotherapist, social worker and physician for the elderly will be available to help with ongoing issues of mobilization, rehabilitation and placement.

Deep venous thrombosis

Virchow's triad describes three predisposing factors for thrombosis:
- increased coagulability of the blood
- decreased flow in the vessel
- local injury to the intima.

Once a localized thrombus has formed in a vein it may extend proximally and there is a danger that fragments of the clot will break off as emboli.

Thromboembolism is common after any surgical procedure since the criteria of the triad are all likely to be fulfilled. There is an increase in blood viscosity after an operation, associated with dehydration and alteration in the serum proteins. The patient is immobile and there may be local injury to vessels while lying on the operating table or during abdominal and pelvic surgery. In addition, there is an increase in blood coagulability following the physiological response to trauma.

The risks are particularly increased by long operations in the pelvic or hip regions. Other risk factors include a past history of deep venous thrombosis or pulmonary embolus, obesity, smoking, carcinomatosis, congenital predispositions and taking the contraceptive pill.

Common sites of postoperative phlebothrombosis are in the pelvis and in the venous plexus in the soleal muscles of the calf.

Recognizing the pattern

A characteristic sign of venous thrombosis is a persistent tachycardia and a mild 'rumbling' fever. Other signs depend on the site of the thrombus formation.
- Pelvic phlebothrombosis is difficult to diagnose. Apart from the systemic signs, there is little to find.
- Acute thrombosis of the iliac veins or femoral veins leads to a grossly swollen painful leg. There is localized tenderness over the involved vein.
- Axillary vein thrombosis similarly presents with a marked swelling of the arm.

- When thrombosis occurs in the soleal plexus there is tenderness in the soleal muscle, which is swollen and turgid compared with the other side. The enlargement can be measured accurately with a tape measure.

Proving the diagnosis
D-dimers are degradation products from fibrin mesh and are produced during the organization of a thrombus. They will therefore be elevated. However, this is non-specific after surgery.

The best non-invasive investigation is a duplex scan of the femoral veins. Although iliac and calf veins are difficult to see, isolated calf venous thrombosis is unlikely to lead to massive embolization and a normal femoral vein usually excludes iliac vein disease.

A venogram is performed:
- where duplex is not available
- to detect clot in the iliac venous segments or inferior vena cava
- for placement of a caval filter.

Management
PREVENTION
Identify any patient who is at risk (see above). During the operation avoid prolonged calf compression (rest the heels on a pad to elevate the calves; do not lean on the calves). It is also possible to aid venous return by compression stockings or intermittent calf compression with inflatable stockings. Subcutaneous low molecular weight heparin should be given to 'at-risk' patients (5000 units subcutaneously 8-hourly). The timing of the first dose may be influenced by the type of anaesthetic, particularly if an epidural catheter is to be inserted. Be sure you are familiar with local policy. Prophylaxis should be continued until the patient is fully mobile. Passive leg exercises should be encouraged whilst the patient is in bed, and the foot of the bed should be elevated to increase the venous return. Early mobilization should be the rule for all surgical patients.

In certain procedures the surgeon may not wish to give subcutaneous heparin because of the risk of bleeding and you should always check with him or her before starting therapy.

TREATMENT
If deep venous thrombosis is proven, full anticoagulation with intravenous heparin is the treatment of choice, followed by oral warfarinization.

Compression stockings, analgesia and mobilization when comfortable, are important factors in treatment.

Pulmonary embolus

Pulmonary embolism occurs when a thrombus from the peripheral venous system becomes detached, passes through the right side of the heart, and impacts in the pulmonary arterial circulation. The consequences depend on the size of the embolus and the site at which it lodges.

A small embolus causes a localized pulmonary infarction and pleurisy if the periphery of the lung is involved (Fig. 1.7.1a). Small emboli may herald larger ones; repeated small emboli can cause pulmonary hypertension.

A large embolus blocks the main pulmonary arteries and thus causes a major block to the whole circulation. The effects are shown in Fig. 1.7.1(b). There is decreased output from the left ventricle and a rise in venous pressure.

Emboli imply the presence of deep venous thrombosis. In 50% of cases the site of the primary problem is not obvious.

Recognizing the pattern
A small embolus may cause pleuritic chest pain, haemoptysis and difficulty in breathing due to pain. However, it is often silent. A large embolus may cause collapse with cardiac ischaemic pain due to poor cardiac output. It is one of the common causes of sudden death postoperatively.

Usually there are no chest signs. The patient is almost always tachycardic. A life-threatening pulmonary embolism will give signs of a gallop rhythm, hypotension and right ventricular strain (e.g. raised JVP).

Proving the diagnosis
This is difficult and one must have a high index of suspicion.

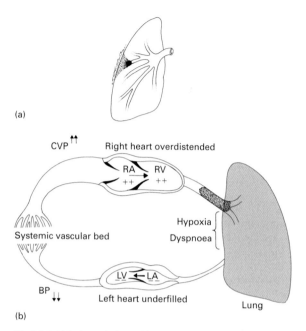

Fig. 1.7.1 (a) A minor embolus produces a pulmonary infarct. (b) A major pulmonary embolus affects the whole circulation. CVP, central venous pressure; BP, blood pressure; LA, left atrium; LV, left ventricle; RA, right atrium; RV, right ventricle.

- Arterial blood gases.
  - There will be a lowered PO_2 due to the physiological shunt present.
  - The PCO_2 will be low due to tachypnoea.
- D-dimers are degradation products from fibrin mesh and are produced during the organization of a thrombus. They will therefore be elevated. However this is non-specific after surgery.
- The ECG usually shows tachycardia, and may show an S wave in lead 1, a Q wave in lead 3 and an inverted T wave in lead 3 in the presence of right heart strain (S1, Q3, T3).

- A chest X-ray is usually normal. Subtle signs may be present such as paucity of lung markings on the affected side, or a wedge-shaped opacity in the presence of pulmonary infarction.
- Ventilation perfusion scans show areas of defects in perfusion which are not associated with defects of ventilation (V/Q mismatch). The scans report a probability that there has been an embolus. This ranges from low, to moderate, to high probability.
- Emergency CT angiography is the gold standard examination. This will show the presence of the clots in the major pulmonary arteries, confirming the diagnosis.

Management
RESUSCITATION

A large embolus can cause acute circulatory collapse and cardiac arrest. The patient may require intubating and ventilating with oxygen. An intravenous cannula should be inserted to provide a route for drugs. If the patient has a cardiac arrest, efficient heart massage may break up the clot and push it further into the pulmonary tree, thus allowing some circulation to be restored. Immediate embolectomy may be appropriate. This is discussed further below.

ANALGESIA

Non-steroidal analgesia is effective in pulmonary embolism. It may be dangerous to give any other analgesia because of the risk of exacerbating the hypotension.

ANTICOAGULATION

The patient is heparinized and anticoagulated as on p. 105. If the patient does not improve and cardiac failure persists, further measures to remove the clot are indicated. This may be attempted using thrombolytic agents or by open pulmonary artery embolectomy.

- Thrombolytic agents.
  - Many emboli can be dissolved by agents such as streptokinase, urokinase or tissue plasminogen activator. Thrombolytics may be given by direct infusion into the pulmonary artery or into the systemic circulation through a peripheral vein. They break up the embolus by activating plasminogen.

- ○ Thrombolytic therapy is dangerous in patients who are:
  - within 5 days of a major operation
  - within 10 days of a hip replacement
  - within 4 weeks of a diagnostic cannulation of a major artery
  - hypertensive
  - pregnant, within 10 days of delivery or lactating
  - in hepatic or renal failure
  - actively bleeding from the bowel or urinary tract.

  These patients may be treated by pulmonary embolectomy, but the relative risks will have to be weighed up on an individual basis.
- Pulmonary artery embolectomy. Massive pulmonary emboli can be removed surgically as an emergency. This is only indicated when the patient fails to respond to anticoagulation or thrombolytic therapy, when there is insufficient time to allow thrombolysis to work because of the patient's desperate condition, or when thrombolytic therapy is considered to be too dangerous.

  The operation may be done in one of two ways.

OPERATION: INFLOW STASIS PULMONARY EMBOLECTOMY

This operation is performed if there are no facilities for cardiopulmonary bypass. The superior and inferior vena cava are exposed through a midline sternotomy and controlled with tapes. The pulmonary artery is opened and the clot sucked out. The venous inflow can be restored and interrupted several times in order to remove all the emboli.

Procedure profile

Blood requirement	10
Anaesthetic	GA
Operation time	1–2 hours
Hospital stay	Variable
Return to normal activity	2–3 months

OPERATION: CARDIOPULMONARY BYPASS
This is the safest way to remove major emboli surgically. The sternum is split and the right atrium and aorta cannulated. After cardiopulmonary bypass has been established the pulmonary artery is opened and all clot removed.

Procedure profile

Blood requirement	10
Anaesthetic	GA
Operation time	1–2 hours
Hospital stay	Variable
Return to normal activity	2–3 months

1.8 Urinary complications

Urinary tract infection

Urinary tract infection is a common complication in the post-operative period. Urinary catheterization is an important predisposing factor, although it can occur following any episode of hypovolaemia, with decreased renal perfusion, low urinary output and urinary stasis. The organism is commonly a Gram-negative bacillus such as *Escherichia coli*. Risk factors for the development of urinary tract infections in the non-hospitalized population include:
• anatomical abnormalities leading to urinary stasis or urinary reflux into the upper tracts (ureter and kidney)
• bladder outflow obstruction with consequent residual urine
• stones
• bladder diverticulum
• bladder carcinoma
• pregnancy
• diabetes mellitus.

Recognizing the pattern

Women are more frequently affected than men. The patient complains of frequency and urgency of micturition, and burning dysuria. She is usually pyrexial and this may be the first sign if a catheter is in place. Other symptoms include suprapubic pain and pain in the renal angle due to ascending infection. Advanced infection can result in septicaemia and rigors. The urine looks cloudy and may smell offensive. There may be haematuria.

Proving the diagnosis

The white cell count is elevated with a neutrophil leucocytosis. Urinalysis shows the presence of blood, leukocytes and nitrites. Microscopic examination of a specimen of urine shows white cells and protein casts. The causative organism may be cultured.

Management

The patient is encouraged to drink up to 4 L/day. Antibiotics are commenced once the bacteriological specimen has been taken. The choice of drug is discussed on p. 104. Any indwelling catheter should be removed if this is feasible.

Further investigations, such as an ultrasound scan (USS), CT scan with contrast (CT KUB) and cystoscopy, are indicated if the infection does not settle or recurs.

Postoperative retention of urine

This is a common postoperative problem and the most frequent cause of oliguria following surgery. The patient finds it difficult to initiate micturition while under the influence of drugs, in strange surroundings, when movements are painful and when they are immobilized in bed. Benign prostatic hypertrophy is an important predisposing cause, although postoperative urinary retention also occurs in women. Patients at risk should be recognized during the initial clerking. Other causes of acute retention are mentioned on p. 452.

Recognizing the pattern

The patient in classical acute retention is anuric and in great discomfort with an intense desire to micturate. The bladder is palpable as a tender mass arising out of the pelvis.

This classic picture is not, however, always present and the condition can be difficult to diagnose.

- Elderly patients, in particular, may develop acute confusion, without other symptoms indicative of acute urinary retention.
- The patient may not be anuric. In acute retention with over-flow the patient produces urine but the amounts are small (50–100 mL) and passed very frequently. This pattern, recorded on the fluid chart, should alert you to the possible diagnosis.
- An abdominal incision covered with dressings may make it impossible to palpate the enlarged bladder and thus obscure the cause of pain. Suprapubic dullness to percussion can be a useful sign in these circumstances.
- Patients with chronic retention have a distended bladder and frequency, but may have no discomfort.

Proving the diagnosis

The diagnosis is proved by passing a urethral catheter and releasing a large volume of urine (more than 500 mL in an adult). Very occasionally an ultrasound examination can be helpful to define the enlarged bladder.

Management

Patients at risk should not be subjected to continual questions about whether they have passed urine or not. Privacy, reassurance and adequate analgesia are helpful. If retention is developing, a tranquillizer (such as diazepam 5–10 mg i.m.) can be useful and conservative measures, such as sitting in a hot bath, and allowing the patient to sit out on the toilet, should be tried.

There are two indications for catheterization:

- the patient is in pain from the distended bladder and demands relief
- there is doubt about the diagnosis and renal failure must be excluded.

In other circumstances it is always worth waiting for the patient to pass urine naturally.

The method of passing a urethral or suprapubic catheter is described on p. 453. If there is very little urine in the bladder and adequate amounts are not produced after catheterization, the patient may be in renal failure and should be managed accordingly (see below).

Patients who have been in retention should have the catheter removed after 24–48 h. In elderly males, if two trials of catheter removal are unsuccessful, the patient should be considered for a prostatectomy (p. 455).

Postoperative renal failure

Failure to produce urine after an operation, once obstruction has been excluded, may be due to prerenal failure or acute renal failure (Fig. 1.8.1).

Prerenal failure

The blood supply to the kidneys may become inadequate postoperatively due to dehydration, blood loss or systemic hypotension. These causes are reversible, but if they are not dealt with early the condition may progress to acute renal failure.

Recognizing the pattern

The minimum adequate urine output in the postoperative period is generally accepted to be 0.5 mL/kg/h (about 30 mL/h for a 70-kg man). Having established that the urine output is inadequate, if necessary by insertion of a catheter, the diagnosis of prerenal failure is made by finding concentrated urine and signs of a cause, and excluding acute renal failure.

- Examine the patient, looking for hypotension, dehydration (dry tongue, poor skin turgor) or cardiac failure (JVP, CVP). Assess the peripheral perfusion (warm or cold hands?).
- Inspect the charts, looking for a negative fluid balance, and check whether there has been any excess blood loss or a period of hypotension.
- Check the renal function and measure the urine specific gravity. In prerenal failure, the plasma creatinine should be normal, but the serum urea may be high, indicating

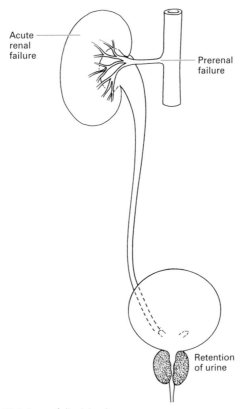

Fig. 1.8.1 Causes of oliguria/anuria.

dehydration. The urine will be very concentrated (specific gravity over 1020).

Management

Administer crystalloid or colloid fluids, or blood, intravenously, in order to restore urine output. In the elderly or those with haemodynamic instability it is wise to monitor the CVP via a central line (p. 93), aiming to get it to the upper limit of normal.

If the urine output remains poor, urine production can be stimulated by the use of an intravenous low-dose dopamine infusion (2–5 µg/kg/min) or an intravenous bolus of frusemide (20–40 mg).

Acute renal failure

In a surgical patient this usually follows a period of renal hypoperfusion (prerenal failure) as above. It can also be a complication of incompatible blood transfusion, extensive trauma or drug therapy. The condition is associated with acute necrosis of the renal tubules (acute tubular necrosis).

Proving the diagnosis

The diagnosis is made after catheterization has excluded retention, and careful fluid status assessment and correction have excluded renal hypoperfusion. If the urine output remains less than 0.5 mL/kg/h, acute tubular necrosis has occurred. This should be confirmed by finding a rising plasma urea and creatinine concentration. A urine specimen should be sent for biochemical analysis. Typical findings are low urine sodium, potassium and urea concentrations and a low osmolarity.

Management

- Insert a central line to assist with the careful management of the patient's fluid status. Aim to keep the CVP at the upper limit of normal, avoiding fluid overload.
- Administer an intravenous infusion of low-dose dopamine or an intravenous bolus of frusemide as this may restart urine production.
- Treat hyperkalaemia. If the plasma potassium concentration is dangerously high ($K^+ > 7.0$ mmol/L) administer calcium gluconate (10 mL of 10%) intravenously while monitoring the ECG. Administer an intravenous bolus of 50 mL 50% dextrose with 16 units of insulin and commence an intravenous dextrose/insulin infusion. Plasma potassium concentrations may also be reduced by administration of an enteral potassium chelating agent (e.g. calcium resonium 15 mg q.d.s. orally or rectally).
- The further management of established renal failure is complex and best described in medical textbooks. It includes:

- ∘ restricted fluid intake: 500 mL/day plus any fluid losses
- ∘ restricted protein intake (less than 20 g/day)
- ∘ adequate carbohydrate intake (3000 kcal/day)
- ∘ daily assessment of blood and urinary electrolytes and adjustment of electrolyte intake accordingly. Sodium losses are replaced but potassium is not given
- ∘ peritoneal dialysis or haemodialysis if necessary. Peritoneal dialysis can be used in a patient who has had laparotomy from about 4 or 5 days after the wound has been closed. Continuous haemofiltration is preferred in the intensively ill patient.

Urinary fistula

This follows either breakdown of a urinary tract anastomosis or accidental damage to the ureters during operation.

Recognizing the pattern
The condition presents with an increased discharge through the wound or drain site. This has a characteristic appearance and smell of urine. There is less constitutional upset than with an intestinal fistula.

Proving the diagnosis
The urea content of the fluid is high (like urine) and above the level of the patient's serum urea. If further proof is necessary it can be obtained by giving an intravenous injection of indigo carmine, which is excreted by the kidney and will appear through the fistula.

Management
A urinary fistula will close spontaneously (like bowel fistula, p. 74) providing there is no distal obstruction. Such closure may take several weeks. The presence or absence of distal obstruction can be ascertained by performing a 'fistulogram'.

If the fistula fails to heal, operation is needed and the precise nature of this depends on the site of the fistula. Free distal urine drainage must always, however, be established.

Urinoma

This occurs for the same reasons as a urinary fistula, but does not drain spontaneously. An intra-abdominal collection of urine develops. This may become infected.

Recognizing the pattern
The condition presents with abdominal discomfort due to pressure and local inflammation. The patient may have a fever and a mass may be palpable.

Proving the diagnosis
The presence of a fluid collection is best demonstrated using ultrasound or a CT scan, which will have a characteristic appearance. The diagnosis is confirmed by demonstrating urine on aspiration (see below).

Management
A suspected urinoma should be drained percutaneously, under ultrasound or CT guidance. Distal obstruction should be excluded by performing an IVU.

1.9 Infections, abscesses and fistulae

Wound infection

Infection complicates between 1 and 40% of surgical incisions, depending on the type of procedure being performed (Fig. 1.9.1). A wide variety of organisms may be involved.

Predisposing factors
- Preoperative:
  - malnutrition
  - diabetes
  - carcinomatosis
  - infection near the site of incision
  - immunosuppressive therapy.

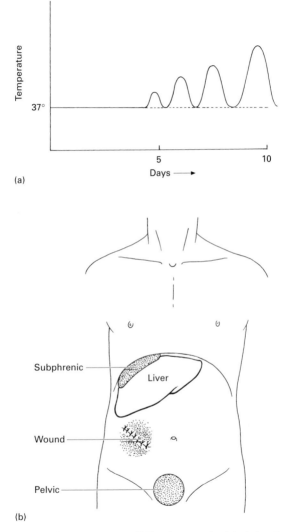

Fig. 1.9.1 (a) Postoperative sepsis. (b) Sites of postoperative abdominal sepsis.

- Operative:
  - the incidence of wound infection depends on the amount of operative contamination:
    - clean wounds: 1%
    - slight contamination: 1–5%
    - clear contamination: 5–30%
    - dirty wounds (e.g. faecal peritonitis): > 30%
  - infection from staff, instruments or air-borne agents
  - poor surgical technique, e.g. haematoma formation, devitalized tissue in wound or closure under tension
  - poor blood supply.
- Postoperative: infection on the ward (from either the patient themself, other patients or staff).

Recognizing the pattern

There is a history of increasing pain and tenderness in the wound.

On examination the patient has a climbing, swinging pyrexia with localized tenderness in the wound, which is also swollen, hot and red. There may be fluctuation on palpation or pus may discharge.

Proving the diagnosis

- White cell count. This will be elevated in active infection.
- A specimen of pus must be sent to microbiology for culture.

Management

- The collection should be drained. Remove some of the stitches and probe the wound to let out all the pus. Sometimes an anaesthetic is required to achieve adequate drainage.
- The wound is dressed daily, or more frequently if dressings become saturated. The wound is not resutured but left to heal by secondary intention.
- Analgesia.
- Antibiotics should be started on clinical grounds if the patient has systemic upset or cellulitis and changed later according to microbiology advice.

Wound dehiscence

Breakdown of the wound may be either partial or complete (Fig. 1.9.2). In partial breakdown the skin closure holds, but breakdown of the muscle layers gives rise to an incisional hernia later. In complete dehiscence the abdominal incision bursts open to reveal bowel. The aetiology is similar to that for wound infection. Exacerbating factors include:

- obesity
- raised intra-abdominal pressure (from coughing, difficulty in passing urine or constipation)
- ascites draining through the wound

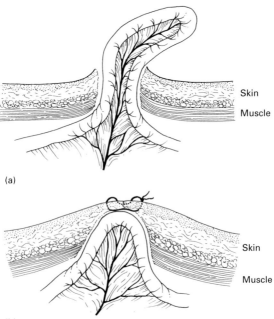

(a)

(b)

Fig. 1.9.2 (a) Complete wound dehiscence. (b) Incomplete (partial) wound dehiscence.

- wound infection
- haematoma.

However, wound dehiscence is largely due to faulty technique. Factors include pulling the sutures too tight, inserting sutures too close to the edge of the muscle, and insecure knots. Wound dehiscence is much less common since one-layer, mass closure, monofilament suture techniques have been used.

Recognizing the pattern

This occurs typically 4–10 days after operation. The patient may feel something 'give' in the wound. There is a sudden increase in pain and a pink fluid discharge from the wound. In complete dehiscence there is protrusion of loops of bowel. The patient becomes shocked and distressed.

Management

- Lie the patient down and give reassurance.
- Strong opiate analgesia is required.
- Cover the wound with a sterile pack soaked in warm saline.
- The wound requires urgent resuture in theatre with deep-tension sutures.

OPERATION: RESUTURE OF ABDOMINAL WOUND

The dressings and sutures are removed and the whole wound is reopened. All the muscle layer sutures are taken out. A laparotomy is performed and any intraperitoneal pus is removed. Bacteriological specimens are collected for aerobic and anaerobic culture. The decision whether to reclose the fascia of the abdominal wall depends upon the cause of breakdown. Resuture of the skin is generally inadvisable unless dehiscence was related solely to a technical error in fascial closure at the first operation.

Procedure profile

Blood requirement	0
Anaesthetic	GA
Operation time	1 hour
Hospital stay	2 weeks or more
Return to normal activity	6 weeks

The wound tends to discharge and may require regular dressing. Antibiotics should be started at the operation and continued as long as necessary. They can be modified according to the results of the culture.

Infected intravenous drip site

A drip site may become infected and is one of the causes of postoperative pyrexia. The organism is often staphylococcus. Spreading cellulitis suggests streptococcus.

Recognizing the pattern
The patient complains of pain in the limb that is being infused. The intravenous infusion usually slows or stops completely. The patient is pyrexial and the involved skin is red, swollen and tender. There may be spreading cellulitis over the vein proximally, and even pus around the entry of the cannula. Regional lymph nodes may become enlarged, tender and inflamed.

Management
The cannula must be removed and the tip cultured. If the infusion is still required, resite the drip in the other arm. Antibiotics are given following hospital protocol. Systemic analgesia is often needed and a poultice applied to the inflamed vein is comforting.

Subphrenic abscess

A subphrenic abscess may follow generalized peritonitis, particularly after acute appendicitis or a perforated peptic ulcer. It may also occur through infection of a haematoma after an operation such as splenectomy. Such abscesses are commonly just underneath the hemidiaphragm but may also occur beneath the liver in the lesser sac or in the hepatorenal pouch.

Recognizing the pattern
The patient initially recovers from the operation and then 7–21 days later develops a swinging fever and general malaise, nausea

and loss of weight. They may complain of pain in the upper abdomen which can radiate to the shoulder tip. They may also become breathless due to a pleural effusion above the abscess or collapse of the lower lobe of one lung.

On examination there is a swinging pyrexia for which no obvious cause is found. Occasionally, there may be tenderness or even oedema in the abdominal wall in the subcostal region. The liver may be displaced downwards and there may be physical signs of a pleural effusion or collapse of the lung.

Proving the diagnosis

The old aphorism 'pus somewhere, pus nowhere else, pus under the diaphragm' is a useful reminder of the possibility of a subphrenic abscess. The presenting symptoms and signs do not always suggest this possibility. A CT scan will reveal it.

Management

A small abscess containing thin pus may be amenable to guided aspiration and broad-spectrum antibiotics based on likely aetiology. For most patients though, the best management is CT- or ultrasound-guided percutaneous drainage. If the patient remains toxic and ill for more than 3 days, repeat scanning may reveal an undrained loculus and this may necessitate a second drain or the use of a surgical approach to achieve proper drainage.

Operation is rarely required nowadays.

OPERATION: DRAINAGE OF SUBPHRENIC ABSCESS

The abscess may be approached by a posterior or anterior route.
- Posterior approach: the patient is positioned lying on their side with the abscess uppermost. The 12th rib is removed and the subhepatic space or subphrenic space approached retroperitoneally. When the abscess is encountered it is opened and drained in the most dependent direction.
- Anterior approach: the abdomen is opened through a subcostal incision and the abscess approached extraperitoneally and drained.

Once the abscess has been opened, covering antibiotics can be given, although they are not essential. Large abscess cavities are usually drained using a large silicone tube to encourage track formation.

Procedure profile

Blood requirement	0
Anaesthetic	GA
Operation time	1 hour
Hospital stay	1–2 weeks
Return to normal activity	4 weeks

Postoperatively, if the abscess is large, a sinogram may be performed down the drain after 10 days and the progress of the cavity followed. The drain can then be gradually withdrawn as the abscess heals up behind it.

Hepatic abscess

This often occurs as metastatic infection from intraperitoneal sepsis, usually in a debilitated patient. The abscess may be single or multiple. The incidence is low since antibiotic treatment was introduced. The more common causes of hepatic abscesses include appendicitis, diverticular disease, ulcerative colitis and ascending cholangitis.

Recognizing the pattern
The patient is usually very ill with a high swinging fever and rigors. They may complain of right upper quadrant pain and develop mild jaundice. The liver may be enlarged and tender.

Proving the diagnosis
- The white cell count is raised.
- Liver function tests are abnormal. In particular the alanine transaminase (ALT) is raised.
- The abscess cavity may be demonstrated on ultrasound or CT scan.
- An erect chest X-ray shows a high right diaphragm and fluid in the pleura above it.
- Blood cultures may occasionally be positive.

Management

The patient should be given broad-spectrum antibiotics and the abscess aspirated or drained as soon as it is localized. Ideally this is done percutaneously under ultrasound or CT guidance. The same principles that apply to subphrenic colllections also apply here, although open operation is even more of a rarity.

OPERATION: DRAINAGE OF HEPATIC ABSCESS
The abscess is usually approached through an extrahepatic route over the right lobe of the liver. As the abscess is approached, oedema and fibrosis are encountered and this may be broken into, opening up the cavity in the liver. A drain is inserted.

Procedure profile

Blood requirement	2–4
Anaesthetic	GA
Operation time	1 hour
Hospital stay	14–21 days
Return to normal activity	6–12 weeks

The postoperative care is similar to that described above for a subphrenic abscess.

Pelvic abscess

This is an abscess in the rectovesical pouch commonly following peritonitis, e.g. after a pelvic appendicitis or colonic perforation. Infection of a pelvic haematoma following poor haemostasis is another common cause.

Recognizing the pattern

A patient who has had generalized peritonitis becomes unwell with pyrexia and malaise 4–10 days postoperatively. There may be a history of mucus discharged per rectum. The abscess may rupture through the rectum or vagina.

On examination the patient has a swinging pyrexia, and rectal or vaginal examination may reveal a palpable mass which may be pointing and may indeed burst on examination.

Management
Daily rectal examinations should be performed to monitor the progress of the developing abscess. The abscess may point up into the wound or down into the rectum. When a fluctuant area is felt in the rectum it can be broken into with a finger under a short general anaesthetic. If the patient has systemic symptoms antibiotics may be given but these delay the ripening and discharge of the abscess. Premature attempts to drain the abscess through the rectum may damage adjacent loops of bowel, leading to fistula formation. An alternative route for drainage in women is through the posterior fornix of the vagina.

External intestinal fistula

This is a communication between the bowel lumen and the body surface. It develops postoperatively due to the following factors.
- Disruption of a bowel anastomosis (due to tension, ischaemia, infection or distal obstruction).
- Inclusion of the bowel when suturing the abdominal wall.
- Erosion of the bowel by an abdominal drain.
- Perforation of ischaemic bowel (e.g. due to damage to the mesentery at operation or after strangulation in a hernia).

Recognizing the pattern
Five to 10 days after operation there is an increased discharge through the wound or down a drain which becomes faecal and offensive. Persistent discharge causes general malaise, dehydration, hypoproteinaemia and weight loss. If the track is not completely walled off generalized peritonitis may occur.

Proving the diagnosis
The presence of a fistula can be demonstrated by radiological studies involving the use of water-soluble contrast.

Management

Fistulae tend to heal spontaneously providing there is no distal obstruction and the patient receives adequate nutrition. Healing usually takes 3–6 weeks. A fistula will not heal where:

- the tract becomes epithelialized
- there is obstruction beyond the fistula site
- there is persistent infection (e.g. tuberculosis, a foreign body, Crohn's disease, actinomycosis or an abscess in the fistula tract)
- there is malignant disease along the tract.

In the absence of these problems, conservative management should be followed.

- Protect the skin from autodigestion (especially with a high intestinal or pancreatic fistula). This can be achieved by covering the surrounding skin with stomahesive and attaching an ileostomy bag to the fistulous opening.
- Parenteral nutrition. This has transformed the management of intestinal fistulae. When a fistula is diagnosed a central venous access line should be set up in almost all instances. It is preferable to dedicate this line to nutrition only. Oral feeding can then be restricted and the patient's nutritional state maintained until the fistula heals (see p. 91). When a fistula occurs that involves stomach or proximal small bowel, distal jejunostomy feeding may be possible , but care should be taken as fluid and electrolyte losses can be prodigious.
- Adequate fluid and electrolyte replacement of the volume lost down the fistulous track must be given. Daily electrolyte estimations should be performed.
- Octratide, a synthetic somatostatin analogue, may be used to convert a high-output fistula (> 400 mL/day) to a low-output fistula (< 400 mL/day). This makes fluid management much easier and may reduce the time to spontaneous closure.

Surgical closure may be required if the fistula fails to close off with the above conservative treatment. In that case it will be necessary to excise the fistulous track and deal with any cause of failure to heal.

OPERATION: EXCISION OF FISTULA

The skin is incised around the external opening and the track dissected out and removed. Any obstructive lesion must be dealt with. The defect in the bowel is oversewn and the abdominal wall closed. In the presence of persistent sepsis, it may be safer to bring out the bowel opening as an ileostomy (to be closed later). A repair of a large bowel fistula may need covering with a proximal colostomy.

Procedure profile

Blood requirement	2
Anaesthetic	GA
Operation time	1–2 hours
Hospital stay	10–14 days
Return to normal activity	4–6 weeks

Bed sores

Bed sores occur over pressure areas in patients who are immobilized in bed for a long period. Five factors play a part:
- pressure
- moisture
- anaemia
- malnutrition
- injury.

Making the diagnosis
The area initially becomes erythematous and does not blanch on pressure. The skin then ulcerates and may become secondarily infected.

Management
Bed sores are avoided by good nursing care with regular attention to pressure areas and regular turning in bed. The patient should not be allowed to lie on damp sheets. Sheepskin pads under the heels and sacrum help. Patients who are going to be immobilized for a long period of time should be nursed on a water bed or ripple mattress.

For established bed sores, avoid pressure on the area. Regular gentle massage to the surrounding skin is necessary. Infrared therapy may help. Keep the area dry either with dressings or by leaving the wound open to the air. Antibiotics are required if there is spreading cellulitis or systemic illness and the patient must be mobilized as soon as possible.

Extensive chronic bed sores may require excision and rotational skin grafting.

Septicaemia

This is an overwhelming infection spreading from the primary source into the bloodstream. Gram-negative organisms, staphylococci or streptococci are common culprits relating to infections in the biliary and urinary systems. Fungal septicaemia should not be overlooked in the patient who has already received antibiotics or is immunocompromised.

Recognizing the pattern
The patient is collapsed with a pyrexia (39–40°C), a tachycardia and a normal or low blood pressure. The extremities are initially warm due to vasodilatation, but may later become cold due to hypoperfusion. The patient may have rigors.

Look for a cause. Inspect the urine: is it cloudy and thick? Examine the chest and abdomen: is there a CVP line that may be infected?

Proving the diagnosis
- Blood cultures.
- Other microbiology samples should be sent depending on the suspected site of infection.
- If there is a CVP line in use and it is suspected that this is the source of the infection, it should be removed and the tip cultured. Resite it if required.
- White cell count.

Management
- Intravenous antibiotics must be started immediately after the blood cultures have been taken. The choice depends on the

sort of surgery that has been undertaken and should be chosen according to the hospital protocol or in discussion with the microbiology team.
- Intravenous support of the circulation. In severe cases a CVP line is used to monitor this.
- Watch the urine output. The patient should be catheterized.
- It is well worth while discussing the case with the microbiologists, particularly if the origin of the organism found is not known.
- Treat the cause of the septicaemia as required.

1.10 Laparoscopic and endoscopic surgery

The modern junior surgical trainee requires a working knowledge of minimal access (laparoscopic, thoracoscopic) techniques in order to explain them to patients, relatives and other health workers, and to assist in the care of patients undergoing the procedures.

GENERAL POINTS ABOUT LAPAROSCOPIC SURGERY
Because the operation is carried out through small incisions (usually less than 1 cm in diameter) there is much less trauma to the body wall. This is associated with less pain, less analgesic requirements and a more rapid recovery. There is also less scarring so the cosmetic result is superior. Patients usually enjoy a more rapid discharge from hospital. This may mean that complications then develop at home and may therefore be more difficult to diagnose, especially as such complications are rare. Before the operation the patient will need a clear explanation of what is intended. It can be very difficult for a patient to understand the gravity of their operation when they see very small scars on the skin afterwards.

TECHNIQUES
Endoscopic surgery relies on viewing the inside of the body using an image on a video screen. This image is used by the surgeon to perform the operation rather than looking at the body tissues directly, as in conventional surgery. A rod lens telescope is

connected to an external light source and to a camera that relays the image to a screen. Operating using an image has advantages. It can be obtained using a telescope through a very small incision, and is easy to magnify, facilitating very detailed surgery. The image can also be enhanced in various ways and other information can be fed to the video screen including images from X-ray machines and other equipment.

A disadvantage is that modern video screens only produce a two-dimensional image so the surgeon's ability to distinguish depth is diminished. Normal tactile feedback is lost, though it is still possible to 'feel' a certain amount through the shaft of the instruments.

ASSISTING AT LAPAROSCOPIC SURGERY

As a junior surgical trainee you may be required to hold and manipulate the camera. This is an important task as the surgeon can only carry out an accurate operation if he or she is given a good view. You should hold the camera steadily and avoid excessive movements. Only alter the position when an adjustment is required. Learn where the focusing mechanism is and keep the image in focus. Learn how to move the camera and telescope into the abdomen (zoom) and how to move it out again. With a zero degree lens, the position of the light lead does not matter, but with an angled lens, rotating the light lead will rotate the telescope, altering the field of view. The surgeon will use this facility in some operations.

POSTOPERATIVE CARE OF THE PATIENT

Generally speaking this is straightforward. Particular points are dealt with under the specific operations. Patients usually recover very quickly and have minimal pain. They may require analgesics which can usually be of the mild variety (paracetamol, codeine). Non-steroidal analgesics are useful for moderate pain but opiates are rarely needed. If the patient is discharged rapidly, tell them to get in touch with you if they develop increasing pain once they are home. This is unusual and should be taken seriously. It is often best to readmit them to check whether there is a serious problem.

1.11 The junior surgical trainee's role in the intensive care unit

Intensive care units are designed to look after the very ill. The unit is run by specialists in intensive care medicine and senior specialized nursing staff. So although the care of the patient is undertaken jointly with the intensivists, the ultimate responsibility for a surgical patient normally resides with the consultant surgeon. In the intensive care unit, the junior surgical trainee's role is to act as a coordinator and to monitor all aspects of patient care, making sure that nothing is left out. Although most of the management decisions are made by others, it is important to keep everybody in touch with events and to keep up to date with the patient's progress yourself.

The intensive care unit often seems very impersonal, with a large part of the management based on observation charts, results and machinery. In the midst of all this do not forget to examine the patient. Also remember that even if patients cannot speak (because they are intubated) they may well be able to see and hear all that is going on. Make sure you keep them fully informed about how they are progressing and avoid discussion or teaching within earshot.

A patient's family also need special care. They are understandably anxious and may find this environment intimidating. They must be reassured and care must be taken to explain all that is going on.

2 Prescriptions and other tasks

2.1 Management of intravenous fluids

The indications for setting up an intravenous infusion in a surgical patient are as follows.
- To give the normal fluid and electrolyte requirement to a postoperative patient who is unable to drink.
- To replace abnormal losses, e.g. through haemorrhage or vomiting.
- As a route for intravenous drugs.
- To give parenteral feeding.
- Access for pressure measurement and instrumentation, e.g. balloon catheters.

A useful approximation for checking the fluid and electrolyte intake against body weight is:
- 40 mL fluid/kg adult body weight (babies need more, old people less)
- 2 mmol sodium/kg
- 1 mmol potassium/kg (see Fig. 2.1.1).

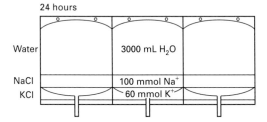

Fig. 2.1.1 Daily requirements for water, sodium and potassium ions.

Surgery: Diagnosis and Management, 4th edition. Edited by N. Rawlinson and D. Alderson. © 2009 Blackwell Publishing, ISBN: 978-1-4051-2921-3

The normal volume requirement for an adult includes:
- the 'insensible' loss of water in faeces and from the lungs – about 500 mL
- urinary output – about 1000 mL
- insensible loss from the skin plus perspiration – 500–3000 mL depending on the patient's temperature and environmental conditions.

Abnormal losses have to be added to these. They can be external or sequestrated internally within the body. External losses are usually more or less isotonic (vomiting, diarrhoea, fistulae) but may contain proteins (e.g. from nephrotic kidneys) or even blood cells. Internal losses are not immediately obvious and are often underestimated. They occur in diseases that induce a severe inflammatory reaction like pancreatitis, peritonitis and burns, but also after operative trauma. Isotonic fluid then leaks into the interstitial tissue (in wounds or generalized oedema), mesothelium-lined cavities (peritoneum, pleura) and gut (e.g. in paralytic ileus). These losses are temporary and with patient recovery the volume will be reabsorbed and excreted as urine, producing a negative daily fluid balance.

Intravenous feeding is needed in:
- patients who have no oral intake for more than 4–5 days (after major surgery)
- patients whose digestive system is not functioning because of multiple injuries or severe burns.

Commonly used intravenous fluids

Figures 2.1.2–2.1.6 in this section illustrate the contents of 1-L 'units' of fluid.

Crystalloid preparations
These are solutions of electrolytes in water. They disperse throughout the extracellular fluid space and are not confined to the circulation. They are dispensed in 500-mL or 1-L bags.
- Normal saline (0.9%) is traditionally the most commonly used. It has, however, the disadvantage of inducing hyperchloraemic metabolic acidosis if given in large volumes.

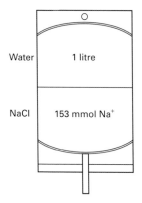

Fig. 2.1.2 One litre of normal saline.

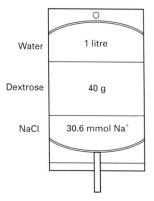

Fig. 2.1.3 One litre of 4% dextrose, 0.18% saline.

- Hartmann's solution is more 'physiological' than the others and contains potassium, calcium and lactate as well as sodium chloride. It mimics the electrolyte content of extracellular fluid, the lactate being metabolized to bicarbonate.
- Dextrose is readily taken up by cells. Pure dextrose solution is therefore effectively water, i.e. volume replacement only.

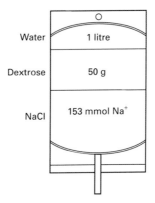

Fig. 2.1.4 One litre of 5% dextrose, 9% saline.

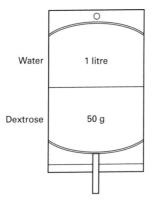

Fig. 2.1.5 One litre of 5% dextrose.

- Dextrose saline (4% dextrose + 0.18% saline) is a solution designed to simplify the continuous replacement of volume and electrolytes, and balance normal losses. There are formulations of 'dextrose saline' which are in fact 0.9% saline with 5% dextrose. They are hyperosmolar. Be aware of this and prescribe the percentage clearly on the fluid chart.

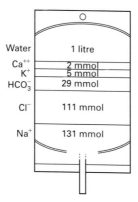

Fig. 2.1.6 One litre of Hartmann's solution.

- Any of these fluids may have additional potassium added, usually in 10-mmol aliquots of KCl.

Other types of intravenous fluid

Whereas crystalloid solutions distribute in the entire extracellular volume, colloid solutions stay in the blood circulation (unless the capillary membrane is damaged). They are therefore useful to replace losses of blood volume, though apart from blood, they have no oxygen-carrying capacity. They are electrolyte solutions that also contain albumin or other macromolecules in place of albumin (Table 2.1.1). Because of the increase in colloid osmotic pressure they draw fluid from the tissues into the circulation in addition to the actually added volume.

Table 2.1.1 Content of colloid solutions (mmol).

	Na^+	K^+	Ca^{++}	Cl^-	Protein or polyglycan
Plasma protein fraction	145	0.25	–	145	50 g (95% albumin)
Haemaccel	145	5.1	6.25	145	35 g (polygeline)
HAES 6%	153	–	–	153	60 g (pentastarch)
Dextran (in normal saline)	153	–	–	153	100 g (dextran)

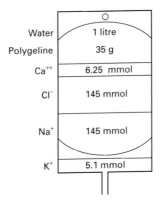

Fig. 2.1.7 One litre Haemaccel.

Plasma substitutes include the following.

- Albumin solution. Plasma protein fraction should be given through a filter . Because of the rapid turnover of albumin the effect lasts for 24–36 h only. It is therefore of little use in treating a low serum albumin.
- Gelatin solutions (Haemaccel (Fig. 2.1.7) and Gelofusine) are solutions of partially degraded gelatin. They have a half-life in the circulation of 3–4 h. There is a possibility of anaphylactic reactions because of their protein nature, but this is not as common as was previously thought.
- Etherified starch (subdivided to tetra, penta and hexa starch). HAES (hydroxyethyl starch) is made from amylopectin and because of its similarity to glycogen anaphylactic reactions are rare. HAES expands to a volume of 145–200% of the infused volume and has an effect on volume and microcirculation for 3–4 h. It is degraded by serum amylase and can lead to elevation of amylase estimation in blood.
- Dextran (40 and 70). Dextrans are polymers of glucose with an average molecular weight of either 40 or 70 kDa dissolved in either isotonic saline or 5% glucose. They have been largely superseded by the above two groups. Dextran interferes with cross-matching of blood once in the circulation and therefore

any serum for cross-matching should be taken before the infusion is started.

Blood

Blood is used to replace loss of red blood cells. Whole blood may be used, or the volume may be reduced by infusing packed red cells. The latter are useful for treating chronically anaemic patients and have the advantage that the valuable plasma protein fraction can be used for other patients.

Blood contains sodium and potassium as well as citrate, phosphate, dextrose and sometimes adenine. After several weeks storage it also holds significant amounts of cellular debris, free haemoglobin, phosphate and ammonia. It has then lost most of its clotting factors and platelets. Blood should always be given through a filter.

If large amounts of blood are transfused very quickly it is important to monitor the serum potassium. The serum calcium can also become depressed due to the infusion of excess citrate in the stored blood. More common problems are hypothermia from rapidly transfused cold blood, and alkalosis because citrate is metabolized to bicarbonate. Clotting factors are diluted by large transfusions of stored blood and should be assessed after such therapy. Additional fresh frozen plasma (FFP) with active clotting factors needs to be given during massive transfusions. Even small transfusions carry the risk of infection, transfusion reactions and immunosuppression.

Prescribing the daily requirement

When prescribing i.v. fluids think of both volume and electrolyte requirements.

Replacement of normal losses

A suitable basic intravenous requirement including electrolytes for a fit 70-kg adult is:

- water 3 L
- sodium 100 mmol
- potassium 60 mmol.

This is usually given in one of two regimes, A or B.

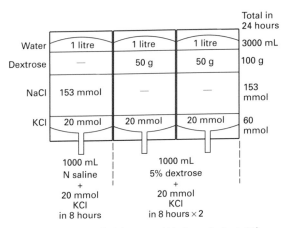

Fig. 2.1.8 Regime A: 2 L of 5% dextrose and 1 L of normal saline in 24 h – each litre bag containing 20 mmol of potassium.

REGIME A (Fig. 2.1.8)
This gives the patient some energy in the form of dextrose: 2 L of 5% dextrose solution = 100 g of dextrose, which yields 410 kcal. Although this is insufficient for energy requirements postoperatively, it is all right in the short term as the body utilizes endogenous stores. However, should the patient be off oral fluids for more than 4–5 days, intravenous nutrition must be considered.

REGIME B (Fig. 2.1.9)
An alternative regime gives the patient 3 L a day, 90 mmol of sodium, 60 mmol of potassium and 120 g of dextrose. As can be seen, this contains slightly less sodium and supplies glucose in a more continuous fashion.

Replacement of abnormal losses

In certain circumstances the above basic regimes have to be modified to take account of abnormal losses. These are replaced according to their composition. This usually means using an isotonic balanced electrolyte solution (Hartmann's). In vomiting from pyloric stenosis chloride and hydrogen ions are the main

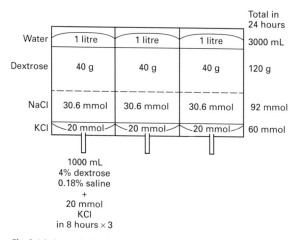

Fig. 2.1.9 Regime B: 3 L of 4% dextrose/0.18% saline in 24 h – each litre bag containing 20 mmol of potassium.

losses and are replaced with isotonic saline. Pyrexia (250 mL/ degree of fever) and artificial ventilation increase insensible losses which contain minimal electrolytes. In extensive burns the capillaries also leak proteins, and resuscitation has to include albumin.

EXTRA VOLUME AND ELECTROLYTES (CRYSTALLOIDS)
Extra electrolytes are required when the patient is suffering from losses of fluid rich in salt. This occurs in vomiting, diarrhoea and intestinal fistulae. Extracellular fluid containing electrolytes is also slowly sequestered into the peritoneum and gut after abdominal operations and into the interstitium in severe inflammatory conditions such as pancreatitis. These losses should usually be replaced with Hartmann's solution.

EXTRA VOLUME (WATER)
When the patient is pyrexial or the weather is hot, insensible salt-free losses increase. Extra water without electrolytes is required. An intake of 3000 mL/day does cover some increased losses as commonly required by postoperative patients. If more

is required the rate of infusion is simply increased and additional 5% dextrose prescribed.

LESS FLUID

In the first 24 h postoperatively the metabolic response to the trauma of surgery causes increased aldosterone and increased antidiuretic hormone release. This causes both salt and water retention and because of this some surgeons or anaesthetists prefer to give less fluid and no salt in the first 24 h, e.g. 5% dextrose 1 L 12-hourly. This is then followed by regime A or B (see above) on day 2.

EXTRA POTASSIUM

Most of the body potassium is in the cells and the serum potassium is not a good guide to overall depletion. The serum potassium may only fall when a large deficit has occurred. Those patients who may require extra potassium include the following.

- Patients receiving certain diuretics (frusemide, bendrofluazide).
- Patients with large volumes of gastric aspirate or prolonged vomiting.
- Patients with a fistula from the biliary tract or small bowel.
- Patients with diarrhoea (e.g. ulcerative colitis or villous adenoma).

The amount of potassium required depends on the volume lost. For every 500 mL of gastrointestinal loss, consider an extra 5–10 mmol of potassium.

ACUTE REHYDRATION

More intensive intravenous fluid therapy is required in the dehydrated patient, especially if an operation is imminent. Any regime for such a patient is 'tailor-made' to suit their calculated deficit as judged by the history, clinical state and biochemical results. It may be necessary to infuse, for instance, Hartmann's solution at a rate of 1 L/h for a limited period. Clearly the state of the patient's kidneys and heart will dictate how safely such rapid replacement can be given. In these cases the decision about what should be given will have to be made by the registrar or consultant.

CHILDREN

The management of babies and very small children is undertaken jointly between the surgeons and the paediatricians (see section 14.3).

ELDERLY PATIENTS

The elderly patient on intravenous fluids requires close monitoring because of the risk of precipitating left ventricular failure. It is essential that you assess any elderly patient carefully before prescribing intravenous fluids. The hydration status is best assessed by clinical signs. Ideally these patients are given a regime with less volume and no more sodium than is necessary. The following prescription may be suitable:

- 0.9% saline: 1 L + 40 mmol KCl in 12 h
- 5% dextrose: 1 L + 20 mmol KCl in 12 h.

This gives 2 L of fluid/day with 153 mmol of sodium and 60 mmol of potassium. Patients may need more fluid if they become dehydrated. Many elderly patients are on diuretics or digitalis and therefore a close eye must be kept on the electrolytes. Do not forget to change these drugs to intravenous injections if the patient does not drink.

HAEMORRHAGE

Significant blood loss will need blood transfusion, and after a certain point this is vital to maintain the oxygen-carrying capacity. With rapid losses, however, and while blood is being cross-matched, the circulating volume may be maintained with a crystalloid, colloid or even type-specific non-cross-matched blood.

ACUTE RENAL FAILURE

Here intravenous fluids must be severely restricted but must still replace the necessary constituents. The volume usually prescribed covers the daily insensible fluid loss plus the previous day's urinary output. Fluids may be written by the hour in this situation to allow closer control, e.g. 30 mL/h plus the previous hour's output. The electrolytes must be watched carefully and usually the urinary electrolyte loss is measured twice a day. Sodium is replaced in proportion to the previous day's urinary loss. Potassium must not be given as it is usually retained.

INTRAVENOUS FEEDING

Most of these patients requiring intravenous feeding are catabolic and the aim is to reverse this catabolism by giving the patient protein and energy. Sufficient energy derived from non-protein sources (e.g. carbohydrate or fat) ensures that the protein given is used for protein anabolism and is not itself broken down to provide a substrate for glycolysis. In the case of the critically ill most of the daily energy needs to be derived from fat. Fat has a lower respiratory quotient (0.7) and therefore reduces the respiratory work load. A typical surgical patient needs 12–16 g nitrogen/day (8090 g protein) and 3000 kcal.

These fluids are hypertonic and acid and need to be given through a central vein. They are given slowly as they may be toxic to the heart.

In addition to the provision of energy, total parenteral nutrition takes into account the replacement of water, electrolytes, some trace elements and vitamins. The daily requirements are often calculated by a nutrition nurse and may be provided in a ready mixed form by the hospital pharmacy.

Intravenous feeding needs to be monitored by daily measurement of the urea, electrolytes and blood sugar. The liver function tests and haemoglobin are measured every third day.

In patients with an intact intestinal tract, a better alternative to parenteral feeding is assisted enteral feeding, using a fine-bore nasogastric tube or surgical gastrostomy/jejunostomy and continuous infusion into the gut. This is easier, carries less risk of infection, has a positive effect on the immune system and reduces the risk of duodenal stress ulcers. However, it may be complicated by incomplete absorption and diarrhoea.

Monitoring the effect of infusion therapy

Whatever regime is chosen the effects must be constantly monitored. Low and high extracellular volume should be diagnosed clinically. Biochemistry tests are helpful to detect concentration and composition changes of the serum (and extracellular space). Therefore assess the following parameters.
- Cardiovascular signs: pulse, capillary refill, blood pressure, JVP.
- Central nervous signs: drowsiness, coma.
- Tissue signs: skin turgor, dry tongue and mucous membranes, oedema.
- Urine output: the minimum acceptable urine output is 0.5 mL/kg/h. It should preferably be 1 mL/kg/h. This means 35–70 mL/h or 800–1600 mL/day in a 70-kg patient.

- Fluid balance (i.e. input compared with output). Check the totals on the observation charts.
- Measurement of the urea and electrolytes: these are usually performed every 2 days.
- Central venous pressure (CVP) measurement: this gives a good indication of the degree of filling of the venous side of the circulation. It also provides information about cardiac function. A CVP line is generally required in any patient requiring intensive fluid therapy, especially those at higher risk because of reduced heart or kidney function.

OPERATION: SETTING UP A CVP LINE

The objective is to place a long intravenous cannula or catheter with its tip in the superior vena cava. A strict aseptic technique is used and the patient is placed slightly head down. It is increasingly standard practice to use ultrasound guidance. A bleb of local anaesthetic is inserted at the puncture site. Various entry points can be used as follows.

- Internal jugular vein. This vessel lies lateral to the carotid artery, beneath the apex of the triangle formed by the sternal and clavicular heads of sternocleidomastoid muscle. Turn the patient's head away, and then, feeling the carotid medially, insert the cannula at the apex of this triangle and aim for the nipple. The vein is punctured at about 2 cm depth.
- The subclavian vein beneath the clavicle. The introducing cannula is inserted at a point 1 cm below the middle of the clavicle, aiming at the centre of the suprasternal notch. The needle is kept horizontal and advanced while maintaining suction on the syringe. Blood appears in the syringe as the vein is entered.
- The basilic vein lying medially in the antecubital fossa.

A catheter is then inserted through the lumen of the introducing cannula and threaded down the correct distance.

Once in place the catheter should be fixed with a suture and adhesive tape and the entry site dressed with antiseptic spray and dry gauze. The catheter is attached to a three-way tap. One limb of the tap is attached to a manometer and the other to a saline infusion. When the manometer line is switched to the patient the meniscus should fluctuate with respiration. Switch to the saline and lower the bag below the patient to check that blood will run back down the line ('flashback'). The saline is run slowly at a rate sufficient to keep the vein open (e.g. 1 L over 16–24 h).

A chest X-ray is always taken to confirm that the catheter tip lies in the superior vena cava, and to exclude a pneumothorax.

COMPLICATIONS
- Infection of the catheter tip and septicaemia. If symptoms of septicaemia occur with no other known primary infection, the catheter should be removed and the tip cultured.
- Pneumothorax. This may follow the cannulation of internal jugular or subclavian veins by any approach. Patients should be observed for dyspnoea and chest pain following the cannulation.
- Hydrothorax. This occurs if the catheter lies in the pleural cavity.
- Haemothorax.
- Phlebothrombosis.
- Air embolus. Accidental disconnection of a CVP line in an upright patient will lead to air aspiration. Lie the patient flat whenever making connections.

MEASUREMENT OF THE CVP (Fig. 2.1.10)
The normal value for the CVP at the mid-axillary line in the supine patient is +1 to +9 cmH$_2$O. The reading is elevated if there is any right-sided cardiac failure or if the patient is being

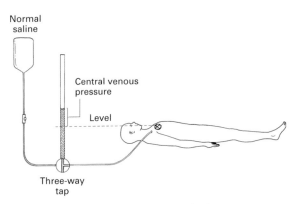

Fig. 2.1.10 Measuring the central venous pressure (CVP).

ventilated. It will be low in the hypovolaemic patient. A series of readings is more valuable than a single measurement. Due to the variation in venous tone in the normal patient, a trend will give a more accurate estimate of the venous filling of the heart and its response to therapy.

REMOVING THE LINE
Tilt the bed in the Trendelenburg position. Cut the holding suture, apply pressure over the entry point into the vein, and withdraw the line. Using a no-touch technique, cut off the tip and send it for culture if the patient is septic or septicaemia is the likely cause of the patient's symptoms.

2.2 Prescribing drugs for surgical patients

How to write a prescription

Prescribing drugs for patients is the junior surgical trainee's responsibility. It is most important that the prescription should be written clearly and correctly. You will have to prescribe both those drugs the patient was taking before coming into hospital, and also any others that are to be given during admission.

Prescriptions will generally be written on the drug chart or discharge form (TTA – to take away).

There are certain requirements that must be observed when prescribing drugs.
- Identify the patient. The prescription must be clearly labelled with the patient's name, address, hospital number and date of birth. If there are two or more patients with the same name, then extra care is needed to avoid confusion.
- Date (both start and stop dates).
- Drug. Use the approved name of the drug and not its trade name.
- Dose.
- Route.
- Rate or frequency of administration.
- Signature of a qualified doctor. This is a legal requirement.

Table 2.2.1 Abbreviations used in prescribing.

Abbreviation	Latin/meaning	Translation
Rx	recipe	take
Site		
p.o.	per os	by mouth
p.r.	per rectum	by rectal administration
i.m.	intramuscular	by intramuscular injection
i.v.	intravenous	by intravenous injection
s.c.	subcutaneous	by subcutaneous injection
s.l.	sublinguum	sublingual
Frequency		
stat.	statim	immediately
o.d.	omni die	every day (once a day)
b.d./b.i.d.	bis die/bis in die	twice a day
t.d.s	ter die sumendus	to be taken three times a day
q.d.s.	quater die sumendus	to be taken four times a day
o.m.	omne mane	every morning
o.n.	omne nocte	every evening
p.r.n.	pro re nata	occasionally, as required. Add the maximum frequency as well, e.g. p.r.n. 4-hourly (usually used for multiple doses)
Other terms		
a.c.	ante cibum	before food
p.c.	post cibum	after food
IU		international unit
tab.	tabletta/tabella	a tablet
mist.	mistura	a mixture
gtt.	guttae	drops
supp.	suppositorium	a suppository
tr./tinct.	tinctura	a tincture
ung.	unguentum	ointment
n.p.	nomen proprium	the proper name (usually means the dispenser should label the prescription with the proper name)
BNF		British National Formulary
BP		British Pharmacopoeia
BPC		British Pharmaceutical Codex

Abbreviations commonly used in prescriptions are shown in Table 2.2.1.

Controlled drugs

Drugs such as narcotic analgesics, because they are open to abuse, are controlled by the Misuse of Drugs Regulations (1973). These are known as 'controlled drugs'. The regulations state that the prescription must carry the following.

- Patient's name.
- Date.
- Prescriber's full signature in his or her own handwriting.
- Name of the drug in full.
- Form of the drug (e.g. tablets, elixir).
- Strength of the prescription.
- Total quantity of the preparation in both words and figures. Pharmacists are not allowed to dispense controlled drugs on an incomplete prescription, or on an 'and repeat' basis.

Review

Make it a rule to review the drug chart every day during the ward round. Any drugs that are no longer required should be crossed off (e.g. antibiotics). Other drugs may need changing, e.g. from intravenous to oral or from a stronger to a weaker analgesic.

Discharge

When the patient is discharged from hospital they must be given sufficient drugs to last until they can obtain more from their own doctor. Usually hospital pharmacies will supply drugs to last the patient a maximum of 2 weeks. It is important to tell the GP as soon as possible what drugs the patient has been given to take home. Point out any new drugs given for the present illness and how long they should be prescribed. Also note any change made to the patient's previous therapy. This is best done by a note sent to the GP (with the patient if this is possible) on the day of discharge.

Drug management

The following are short notes on the use of analgesics, antibiotics and sedatives in surgical practice.

Analgesics

Adequate pain relief after operation is important as it helps the patient to move and cough and thus lowers the risk of thromboembolism and pulmonary collapse. Patients will not always complain when they are in pain and you should enquire about this rather than wait for them to ask for drugs. Also ask whether the pain killers they have been given are adequate. Occasionally patients do not like to take pain killers at all and feel they should be able to do without them. They need firm reassurance that no harm will come from the drugs and indeed they will benefit from using them. If analgesia is written up 'p.r.n.' (as required) the patient should be informed of this so that they can ask for it when required.

Pain reduction can be achieved by:
- local anaesthetics
- systemic drugs.

Local anaesthetics

In modern surgical practice, with the advent of long-acting anaesthetics such as bupivacaine (marcain), local analgesia has become the method of choice for pain reduction after many surgical procedures. Excellent analgesia can be achieved for 8–10 h. It may be given as follows.

- By local infiltration of the wound at the time of surgery. This can be useful in the smaller operations such as removal of skin lumps, hernia repairs and so forth.
- By regional nerve block. Examples include intercostal nerve blocks for abdominal and thoracic operations, femoral nerve block and ring blocks of toes and fingers.
- Epidural analgesia may be used, but requires high-dependency nursing, especially if combined with epidural opiates. If regional local anaesthesia is used for day-case surgery, warn patients that they can damage the anaesthetized area without realizing it.

Systemic analgesic drugs

Systemic analgesics are chosen in a stepwise fashion depending on the severity of the pain.

ACUTE SEVERE PAIN

Opiates are the drugs of choice. These are all strong analgesics and narcotics. Morphine and pethidine are the standard drugs

Table 2.2.2 Composition of papaveretum.

Constituent	Parts
Morphine HCl	253
Papaverine HCl	23
Codeine HCl	20

in this group. Papaveretum is a mixture of opiates (Table 2.2.2). Pethidine is a weaker analgesic than morphine. All three are very effective in the short term.

- Morphine (5–15 mg i.m./i.v. 3–4-hourly). Occasionally it is useful to give a small dose (e.g. 5 mg i.v. 2–3-hourly) so as to provide analgesia but avoid the side-effects seen soon after the administration of a larger 4-hourly dose. A normal dose of morphine for a 70-kg man with an abdominal incision would be 10–15 mg i.m. 4-hourly.
- Pethidine (50–150 mg i.m./i.v. 4-hourly). The normal dose for a 70-kg man would be 100 mg i.m. 4-hourly. The i.v. dose needs to be half of the i.m. dose.
- Papaveretum (7.7–15.4 mg i.m., s.c.). The i.v. dose needs to be a quarter to half of the i.m./s.c. dose.
- Patient-controlled analgesia (PCA) systems. Intravenous infusions of opiates may give improved pain control. They are given as a basic continuous infusion with intermittent boluses on demand. For boluses the patient presses a button on the PCA. The lock-out time between boluses, the basic rate and the bolus dose can be adjusted.

Opiates have side-effects. Dependence and tolerance do develop, although this is never a problem in the patient immediately after surgery. The following, however, are of importance in the surgical patient.

- Nausea and vomiting. Prochlorperazine (Stemetil) 12.5 mg i.m. 8-hourly is the main antiemetic prophylactically prescribed, but it can, especially in children and the elderly, cause extrapyramidal dyskinesias. Metoclopramide (10 mg) is an alternative.
- Respiratory and cough suppression. Nurses are advised to check patient alertness and respiration rate before administration of every opiate dose.

- Constipation and prolonged ileus (less with pethidine). This should be treated prophylactically in patients with oral intake. A combination of a stimulant with a softening agent (e.g. codanthramer) is the most effective. Senna or lactulose are alternatives.
- Biliary tract spasm, particularly closure of the sphincter of Oddi. This occurs with all three drugs, though less so with pethidine.

Remember that these opioids cause miosis, so avoid using them for patients with a head injury. If narcotic analgesia is required in these cases, codeine phosphate should be given.

Contraindications to opiates include the following.

- Respiratory disease – narcotics may precipitate respiratory failure.
- Hepatic failure – small doses may precipitate hepatic encephalopathy.
- Hypothyroidism, hypopituitarism, Addison's disease – use of narcotics may lead to coma.
- Raised intracranial pressure – narcotics may lead to coma.
- Patients on monoamine oxidase inhibitors – these drugs potentiate narcotics.

ACUTE MODERATE PAIN

An example is somatic pain from the wound after the first 2–3 days.

- Dihydrocodeine (DF118-Forte) (25–50 mg i.m. 4–6-hourly; 30–60 mg orally 4–6-hourly). Dihydrocodeine is midway between morphine and codeine in potency and its main side-effect is constipation. With prolonged use the patient may require laxatives.
- Codeine (30–60 mg orally 4-hourly). This is an analgesic which is partly converted to morphine in the body. It has only one-quarter to one-sixth of the analgesic power of morphine and the side-effects are even less. Dependence does not usually occur, but it is very constipating.
- Diclofenac (25–50 mg orally t.d.s. or 75 mg i.m./p.r. b.d.) is a strong non-steroidal anti-inflammatory drug with good postoperative analgesic effects. It has however, the typical side-effects causing gastric erosions and ulcers and must not be given to asthmatics or to patients with renal impairment.

ACUTE MILD PAIN

Fashions vary widely in the drugs that are popular at any one time for relief of mild pain. Some suggestions follow.

- Co-proxamol (1–2 tablets 4–6-hourly). Each tablet of co-proxamol contains 32.5 mg dextropropoxyphene (related to methadone) and 325 mg paracetamol. There is a known incidence of side-effects and toxicity (respiratory and cardiac depression) due to the dextropropoxyphene and its metabolite norpropoxyphene. It is an opioid analgesic and dependence is believed to occur. Although few trials have been done there is little evidence that it is superior to paracetamol in its analgesic effect. It is contraindicated in patients with poor renal function due to the accumulation of norpropoxyphene.
- Paracetamol (0.5–1 g (1–2 tablets) 4–6-hourly). This is a good analgesic with very few in the way of side-effects.

CHRONIC PAIN

The control of chronic pain is a speciality in itself. A few points can be noted here.

- In a patient with incurable disease the aim is to prevent the pain, not to treat it once it occurs. Prevention is not only better for the patient but requires less analgesia. It is kind to leave the patient with some tablets by their bedside at night in case they wake up with pain.
- Opiates are usually required. In a terminally ill patient the danger of dependence is unimportant. However, tolerance develops, so the dose will need to be increased as time passes. The priority is to keep the patient free of pain.
- Attempt, if possible, to control pain with oral or rectal drugs to save the repeated discomfort of injections.

Hypnotics and sedatives

Surgery, however minor, is always associated with anxiety. While drugs can be no substitute for gentle reassurance and explanation by both the junior surgical trainee and nursing staff, hypnotics and sedatives do have a use. The more rested and relaxed a patient is, the better they will tolerate the operation. It is a good idea to prescribe night sedation for every patient, to be taken if required. The patient must be told that this is available. They may require reassurance that they will come to no harm by taking sleeping tablets for a few nights.

The following are short notes on some of the drugs commonly used.

- Diazepam (Valium) (2, 5 or 10 mg orally or i.m.). This drug is a benzodiazepine and is a tranquillizer and muscle relaxant. It can be used to relieve general anxiety during the day, often in small doses (e.g. 2 mg 8-hourly). It can also be used as an adjunct to pain killers for relief of pain from an abdominal wound when this pain is due to muscle spasm. It may be taken orally or intramuscularly. It is a very safe drug, although drowsiness and confusion can occur, especially in the elderly patient.
- Nitrazepam (Mogadon) (5–10 mg orally nocte). This is also a benzodiazepine and is marketed as a hypnotic. It is safe and effective although it does cause a slight 'hangover' the next day and may well cause confusion in elderly patients.
- Temazepam and flurazepam (dose temazepam 10–30 mg nocte, flurazepam 15–30 mg nocte). These are two other benzodiazepines that are used as hypnotics. Both have shorter half-lives. Temazepam, in particular, causes less 'hangover' and is suitable for the elderly.
- All benzodiazepines can cause respiratory depression and are contraindicated in patients with chronic respiratory disease.
- Zopiclone (3.75–7.5 mg orally nocte). This is a non-benzodiazepine hypnotic which acts on the same receptor as benzodiazepines. It has a short duration of action and is not licensed for long-term use. Avoid in the cases of myasthenia gravis, respiratory failure, severe sleep apnoea, severe hepatic impairment, pregnancy and breast-feeding.

Antibiotics

Antibiotics are used either for prophylaxis or for treatment.

Antibiotic prophylaxis

Prophylactic antibiotics are designed to prevent wound infection and timed to be present in wound fluids when the patient is most at risk from infection. Generally this means the peroperative period and the antibiotics are given just before the operation. The choice of drug is usually made by the consultant as part of routine management. Some suggestions are shown in Table 2.2.3, although it

Table 2.2.3 Prophylactic antibiotics.

Procedure	Organism	Prophylaxis	Alternatives
Large bowel surgery*	Anaerobes, coliforms, *Streptococcus milleri*	Gentamicin 120 mg i.v. plus metronidazole 500 mg i.v.	Cefuroxime 1.5 g, i.v. plus metronidazole 500 mg i.v.
Appendicitis	Anaerobes	Cefuroxime 1.5 g, i.v. plus metronidazole 1 g p.r. 2–3 h preoperatively	
Biliary surgery	Coliforms	Ciprofloxacin 200 mg i.v./oral	Gentamicin 120 mg i.v.
Arterial surgery	*Streptococcus* or *Staphylococcus*	Co-amoxiclav 1.2 g i.v. at induction, continue for 24 h every 8 h.	Gentamicin 120 mg and flucloxacillin 500 mg i.v. at induction, continue for 3 doses with 80 mg gentamicin
Amputations	*Clostridium* (gas gangrene in stump)	Benzylpenicillin 1.2 g i.v. at induction	
Insertion of orthopaedic metal implants	*Staphylococcus aureus*, *Staphylococcus epidermidis*	Cefuroxime 1.5 g, i.v. at induction, continue 750 mg i.v. for two–three further doses	Flucloxacillin 1 g i.v. at induction
Urinary tract surgery	*Escherichia coli*, *Proteus*, faecal *Streptococcus*, *Pseudomonas*, *Klebsiella*, enterobacter	Ciprofloxacin 500–750 mg oral/i.v.	Gentamicin 120 mg i.v. at induction.

*If faecal contamination has occurred then continue a 2–5 day course of medication. The dose of gentamicin is then 80 mg t.d.s.

Table 2.2.4 Antibiotics for acute infections.

Condition	Likely organism	Initial antibiotic therapy
Wound infection		
Indurated, localized, white pus*	? Staphylococcus	Flucloxacillin 500 mg–1 g q.d.s. p.o.
Indurated, spreading cellulitis*	? Streptococcus	Phenoxymethylpenicillin 500 mg q.d.s. p.o.
Foul-smelling pus	? Anaerobes	Metronidazole (e.g. 400 mg t.d.s. p.o. or 1 g supp. t.d.s. p.r.)
Infected drip site	Staphylococcus	Flucloxacillin 500 mg q.d.s. p.o.
Chest infection		
Pneumonia at admission (community acquired)	Pneumococcus	Benzylpenicillin 1.2 g q.d.s. i.v.
Pneumonia postoperatively (hospital acquired)	Haemophilus influenzae	Cefotaxime 1 g b.d. i.v., if severe add gentamicin 80 mg t.d.s. i.v.
Pneumonia after aspiration	Gram-negative rods and anaerobes	Cefotaxime, 1 g b.d. i.v. and metronidazole 500 mg t.d.s. i.v.
Urinary tract infection		
Uncomplicated		Norfloxacin 400 mg b.d. p.o.
Severe, i.e. fever over 38.5°C, rigors, acute pyelonephritis		Benzylpenicillin 1.2 g i.v., and gentamicin 80 mg 8-hourly i.m. or i.v. initially (24 h), then norfloxacin 400 mg p.o. b.d.
With indwelling catheter (no symptoms, positive culture only)		No treatment

*Often wound infection is treated by both penicillin and flucloxacillin.

is realized that these will rapidly become out of date. The reader may then wish to fill in the drugs that are at presently in local use for future reference.

Patients on gentamicin are at risk from damage to kidneys and the acoustic nerve if levels rise too high. Levels should be measured before and after the third dose and then twice weekly. Acceptable levels are less than 2 mg/L before, and 6–10 mg/L 1 h after, injection (nomograms are available to adjust the dose according to the weight, age and creatinine clearance).

Antibiotics for acute infections

The antibiotic used will depend on the suspected site of infection and thus on the predicted organism. Confirmation of the causative organism and its antibiotic sensitivity will be obtained when a bacteriological culture has been performed. It is useful to send appropriate specimens (urine, swabs, sputum, blood culture) before starting treatment.

In Table 2.2.4 some common sites of perioperative infections are shown, together with the possible initial antibiotics to use. Specific surgical infections (e.g. acute cholecystitis) are discussed in the appropriate section.

Anticoagulants

The usual drugs used for anticoagulation are heparin, low molecular weight heparins and warfarin.

Heparin

PROPHYLAXIS OF DEEP VEIN THROMBOSIS

Heparin (5000 units s.c., b.d.) and its low molecular variants (e.g. Enoxaparin, 20 mg s.c. daily) reduce the risk of deep vein thrombosis, especially in patients who are obese, on bed rest, are elderly, have lower limb surgery or have a debilitating disease such as sepsis or cancer. Do not forget to institute physical means of prophylaxis such as compression stockings, leg exercises and raising the foot of the bed.

TREATMENT OF DEEP VEIN THROMBOSIS

Anticoagulation for established deep vein thrombosis has a less proven benefit on survival or later complications than prophylaxis, but is generally used. Initial treatment is with heparin given intravenously in a dose of 5000 units immediately, followed by an intravenous infusion of 15–25 units/kg/h. The level of anticoagulation should be monitored with daily partial thromboplastin times (PTT) and these should be kept at 1.5–2.5 times the normal level by adjusting the rate of the infusion. For uncomplicated deep vein thromboses subcutaneous tinzaparin (175 units/kg body weight s.c. daily) can be used, which avoids having to check the prothrombin time.

Warfarin

Long-term anticoagulation may be maintained with warfarin. It is commenced as soon as the diagnosis is made. This drug takes 48–72 h to take effect and therefore a loading dose is given while the patient is still on heparin. A suitable regime is as follows.

- Prescribe a loading dose of warfarin. This is usually 10 mg/day orally given at 6 p.m. for 2 consecutive days. A lower dose may be required for patients with a low body weight, the elderly or those with hepatic disease.
- On the morning of day 3, test the coagulation times. The prothrombin time is used to assess the effect of warfarin and expressed as the international normalized ratio (INR). The INR times should be 2–3. Less than 2 denotes underanticoagulation and more than 3 over-anticoagulation. If the INR is in the expected range stop the heparin.
- Prescribe further warfarin on the basis of this test and recheck the clotting values 1–2 days later. The dose to be given is adjusted according to the value of the INR. The blood tests are taken in the morning and the warfarin is prescribed in the evening. Continue to check the INR until it is in a therapeutic range with constant warfarin doses.

The main side-effect of over-anticoagulation is haemorrhage. Table 2.2.5 summarizes the management of over anticoagulation.

Many drugs and conditions affect the activity of warfarin and the INR must be reviewed regularly after changes in the concurrent drug therapy.

- Some drugs displace warfarin from plasma proteins, increasing the anticoagulation effect, e.g. aspirin, phenylbutazone and clofibrate.

Table 2.2.5 The management of high international normalized ratio (INR) due to over-anticoagulation. FFP, fresh frozen plasma.

INR/complication	Management
Major bleeding	Stop warfarin Vitamin K1 5 mg slow i.v. Prothrombine complex concentrate (factors II, VII, IX, X) 50 u/kg or FFP 15 mL/kg
INR > 8, no bleeding or minor bleeding	Stop warfarin Restart when INR < 5 If risk factor for bleeding, vitamin K1 0.5 mg slow i.v. or 5 mg oral
INR 6–8, no bleeding or minor bleeding	Stop warfarin Restart when INR < 5
INR < 6 but > 0.5 above target	Reduce or stop warfarin Restart when INR < 5

- Liver disease potentiates warfarin activity.
- Liver enzyme induction (e.g. by chronic alcoholism or phenobarbitone therapy) increases the rate of metabolism of warfarin and a higher dose is required. The dose must be reduced when the inducing agent is withdrawn.

Anticoagulation is contraindicated if there is a recent history of haematemesis, peptic ulceration, ulcerative colitis, haematuria, cerebral haemorrhage or hypertension, and in women in the first trimester or last 4 weeks of pregnancy. These contraindications are not absolute and the risks must be balanced against the benefits.

Thrombolytic therapy

Thrombi, once formed, may be dissolved using thrombolytic agents such as streptokinase or tissue plasminogen activator (TPA). These are dealt with on p. 515.

Bowel preparation

The aim of preparing the bowel before abdominal surgery is to clear the colon of exogenous material and lower the number of infective organisms. Numerous studies including meta-analyses have shown that this is of no value in reducing any type of complication relating to open elective colonic surgery. Many surgeons, however, believe that it may be of value in laparoscopic procedures or in operations involving the rectum.

If there is a colostomy or ileostomy planned or any chance of this being required, the patient must be seen by a stoma nurse who will explain the handling of the stoma to the patient and mark the most convenient site.

EMPTYING THE BOWEL FOR LEFT-SIDED LESIONS
The patient is started on a low-residue diet 2 days before the operation. The day before operation they may have clear fluids. The usual drug given to empty the bowel is Picolax (one sachet at 8 a.m. and at 2 p.m., orally). This causes severe diarrhoea, so advise the patient to drink 2–3 L for rehydration that day.

HAEMORRHOIDECTOMY AND MINOR ANAL PROCEDURES
The rectum is emptied with phosphate enemas given 4–6 h before theatre. Do not give enemas to patients immediately before an operation, for example in day surgery. Liquid faeces may contaminate the operating field.

2.3 Sutures, staples and drains

Sutures

It is useful to be familiar with the various types of suture, their uses and their effect on the management of wounds. Generally, a suture may be either absorbable or non-absorbable, and has either a braided, twisted or monofilament structure. It can be made from natural or synthetic material.

Types of suture
Absorbable sutures are broken down in the body tissues over a varying number of days either by enzymes or by hydrolysis by the

tissue fluid. It is important to differentiate between the times of loss of tensile strength and of disappearance of the material as these are not necessarily the same. An increasing range of suture materials with planned absorption times is becoming available.

Non-absorbable sutures remain in place for some years unless they are removed.

Braided sutures (where the strands are plaited together) and twisted sutures (where the separate strands are twisted round each other) are very flexible and therefore easy to handle and knot. The knots usually hold and are secure. The disadvantage of these types of suture is that fluid can seep between the strands (capillarity) and micro-organisms can get into the interstices of the yarn, giving rise to long-term infections. Most braided sutures are proofed or coated in an attempt to prevent this.

Conversely, monofilament sutures consist of only one strand of material. They tend to be less flexible and more 'slippery'. They are therefore less easy to handle and knot, and the knots need more throws to be secure. However the only nidus provided for infection is within the interstices of a knot.

Absorbable sutures

Absorbable sutures are used if no permanent support is required, especially if the knot as a foreign body could lead to complications.

- Tying off small arteries and veins near the skin (knot could erode skin).
- Stitches in the ureter, urinary tract, or biliary tract (where permanent sutures form a focus for stone formation).
- Closing off tissue spaces.
- For closing the skin when it is an advantage not to have to remove the stitches (children, day surgery, scrotum).
- In gastrointestinal anastomosis (non-absorbable sutures in the stomach can cause long-term ulceration).

The most common types of absorbable suture are listed in Table 2.3.1.

Non-absorbable sutures

If the loss of strength of a suture might have severe consequences (as in vascular anastomoses, heart valve replacements, ligation of major vessels or closure of the abdominal wall), non-absorbable

Table 2.3.1 Absorbable sutures sorted by time until loss of 50% strength.

Material	50% loss of strength (days)	Other features
Poliglecaprone 25	7	New development, monofilament
Polyglactin 910	14	Braided, good knotting properties, minimal tissue reaction, most commonly used
Polyglycolic acid	20	Braided, similar to polyglactin
Polydioxanone	28	Monofilament, very little tissue reaction, absorbed by hydrolysis beginning to replace nylon for closure of abdominal wounds
Polyglyconate	35	Similar to polydioxanone, monofilament

Table 2.3.2 Non-absorbable sutures.

Material	Features
Nylon	Monofilament, very slowly degraded, minimal scarring
Polypropylene	Monofilament, strong, most permanent suture reaction
Silk	Braided or twisted, loses 80% strength in 80 days
Polyester fibre	Braided, particularly strong, well tolerated by tissues
Polyester with polybutylate coating	As above, braided, slides better through tissues because of coating
Expanded PTFE	Strong, specially designed for knot security and used for vascular anastomoses
Stainless steel	Extremely strong, does fragment over period of years, used in orthopaedics and in cardiothoracic surgery for closure of sternum

sutures are generally used. Non-absorbable material is also often used in tissues that heal slowly like tendons and ligaments. The materials commonly used are reviewed in Table 2.3.2.

Sizes of sutures

The size of the suture refers (non-linear) to the diameter and therefore to its strength. During the operation the choice of size depends on the necessary strength. To give a few examples:

- Vicryl size 2/0 and 3/0 provides the standard ties for blood vessels
- skin is generally closed with size 3/0 or 4/0, face with 5/0 and 6/0 in plastic surgery
- size 5/0 and 6/0 are fine sutures used in arterial surgery
- size 10/0 is only just visible to the naked eye and is used in microvascular surgery and nerve repairs.

Suture removal

The time of suture removal depends on the site of the incision and the general state of the patient.

- Head and neck. Wounds in the head and neck heal rapidly. A cosmetic result is also needed and therefore early suture removal is an advantage. Sutures in this area are generally removed within 3–5 days, e.g. thyroid scar 3 days, face scar 4 days.
- Abdomen and thorax. Transverse or oblique incisions 5–7 days. Vertical incisions 7–10 days.
- In patients who are cachectic, i.e. those with carcinomatosis, on steroid therapy, with severe infection, or with hepatic or renal failure, the tissue healing can be delayed and therefore the sutures must be left longer (10–14 days or longer).

Needles

All modern surgical needles are eyeless. The suture material is swaged onto the needle so that the diameter of the needle and suture is virtually identical. See Table 2.3.3.

Staples

Staples are widely used inside the body and to approximate skin.

A variety of instruments exist for internal use to close or anastomose structures. They are widely used in gastrointestinal surgery. The staples are made from titanium. This is stronger than steel, causes less artefact on a CT scan and is non-magnetic (so is safe in an MR scanner). Irrespective of design, two or more rows of interlocking staples close in a B-shape. Appropriate sized staples are made for different tissue thicknesses. Instruments that place only two rows of staples are generally not haemostatic and bleeding from an anastomotic staple line can occur, usually

Table 2.3.3 Needles.

Curved	Small – used with needle holders
Straight	Large – hand needles
Atraumatic	The suture material is built into the end of the needle and the needle puncture therefore causes only a minimally larger hole than the suture itself
Round-bodied	The needle has a round shape and is only sharp at its tip. Used for suturing bowel, liver, etc.
Taper-cut	The needle also has a round shape but is sharpened on several sides towards the tip, giving it cutting properties. This type of needle is useful for passage through tough tissues where it important to keep the needle track size to a minimum
With cutting edge	These are flattened and 'sword-like' and cut through the tissues as they are passed. They can be used on tough fibrous tissue (e.g. breast) or the skin. They may cause haemorrhage by cutting neighbouring blood vessels
With blunt taper point	This type of needle was developed to reduce the risk of needle-stick injuries. It is used to suture the abdominal wall, but does not penetrate skin

into the GI tract. You should be aware of this possibility after surgery.

Skin staplers are made of stainless steel and form a simple C-shape. Steel is cheaper than titanium. They are removed at the same time as conventional skin sutures.

Drains

Drains are put in by the surgeon to allow any fluid or air collecting at the operation site or in the wound to drain to the surface while allowing the main wound to heal. Their use is highly idiosyncratic. Remember that the presence of a specific fluid in a drain may be highly informative, but the reverse is not. The absence of fluid in a drain might indicate blockage. Blood and leaks from the GI tract are not guaranteed to appear in a drain.

Drains may be:
- superficial
  - in the wound
  - in an abscess cavity
- deep
  - intraperitoneal, to limit fluid accumulation in a recess e.g. the pelvis
  - in a hollow organ or duct, e.g. a T-tube in the bile duct
  - in an abnormal channel, e.g. a fistula
  - to drain a deep cavity, e.g. an abscess or haematoma
  - to create a fistula if there should be a leak e.g. to the duodenal stump after gastrectomy.

Types of drains and their uses

Virtually all drains used in modern surgical practice are of the closed type, where the collection system is not open to the air. Most drains are made from inert plastics that do not excite a strong tissue reaction. Conversely drainage tubes made from latex rubber form a strong track over a 10-day period, and these may be specifically used when the surgeon wishes to divert fluid from within the gastrointestinal tract to the surface such as a biliary T-tube (see p. 323).

Closed systems can be:
- on free drainage, e.g. drainage of ascites by gravity
- on suction, e.g. Redivac drains
- controlled by a one-way valve, e.g. an underwater seal or chest drains (see p. 250).

A variety of types are in common use.
- Redivac drain. This is a fine tube, with many holes at the end, which is attached to an evacuated glass bottle providing continuous suction. It is used to drain blood beneath the skin, e.g. after mastectomy or thyroidectomy, or from deep spaces, e.g. around a vascular anastomosis.
- 'Shirley' wound drainage or sump drain. This is a suction drain with an intake tube supplying air to the bottom of the main tube. This allows continuous suction and the flow of air prevents the tube getting blocked.
- Silastic tube drain. Silastic is a polymeric silicone and incites little tissue inflammation. Therefore, once this type of drain is

removed the track closes rapidly. A Silastic tube can be used to drain any dependent space or cavity.

- Red rubber tube drain. This causes an intense tissue reaction and fibrosis. The track will therefore persist for some time after the drain is removed. This feature can be useful for drainage of chronic abscess cavities such as an empyema.
- T-tube drains. After bile duct surgery a latex rubber T-tube is inserted in the bile duct, which allows bile to drain externally. T-tubes are made from a variety of materials and surgeons vary in the design they prefer.

Removal of drains

A drain is removed as soon as it is no longer required. Hence it is necessary to know the purpose for which it was inserted and you should ascertain this from the surgeon at the time of operation. If fluid is still draining the drain is serving a purpose. Check the drainage chart and consider carefully before removing it. The following are general guidelines:

- Drains put in to cover perioperative bleeding and haematoma formation can come out after 24–48 h.
- Drains put in to cover serous collections can come out after 3–5 days.
- Where a drain has been put in because the wound may later become infected, it should be left for 1–5 days.
- A T-tube should not be removed before 10 days.
- Chest drains – see management of thoracotomy (p. 252).

2.4 Relatives, discharge, death and documents

Dealing with relatives

It is an important part of the junior surgical trainee's job to answer enquiries from relatives as to the nature of the disease, the type of operation that is intended and the prognosis. The relatives will view any operation as a very major undertaking and will often be dreading the outcome. Keeping them informed is not just a humanitarian exercise. If the relatives are happy about a patient's management, they will pass on this confidence to the patient and this can be a great help to you as their doctor. Conversely many patient complaints are based on a lack of communication and misunderstanding. It is worthwhile setting aside two periods a week when you will be available on the ward for any relatives to come and see you. Tell the nursing staff when these will be.

The personal touch

It is better if one person coordinates this communication with the relatives, otherwise misunderstandings may arise. This is difficult to achieve in a full shift rota system with cross-cover, when the on-call junior surgical trainee looks after patients on other wards as well. Continuity is important because only you know what you have already told the relatives. It is best to do this with an experienced nurse present and if this is not possible then always tell the nurse in charge what you have said. If you know that the family are visiting one evening, stay on the ward until you have seen them. This often takes less time than repairing the damage caused by an interview with someone who does not know the case.

If you are asked to see the relatives of a patient on another ward about whom you know nothing, start by asking them what they have been told so far and apologise that the doctor they normally see is not available. Ask the nursing staff for any background information. Before the interview look at the notes, not only to find out about the case, but also to see if any record has been made of previous conversations.

Documentation

It is important that all interviews with patients and relatives should be clearly documented. The entry should be signed with the date and time. You should include your contact details. After you have spoken to a patient or relatives about a situation or diagnosis that may cause concern, let the nursing staff know what was said and write this down in the notes, commenting on any difficulty or reaction from those listening. For example, 'Mrs James told that her son has a malignant growth on the leg. Very upset. Has requested that the son should not be told yet. She is coming tomorrow with husband and would like to be seen again. Would also like an appointment with the consultant in the next clinic.' Tell the senior members of your surgical unit about the interview.

Patient discharge

When discharging a patient you must give them instructions on the following.
- Stitches. When and how stitches are to be removed if this has not been done already.
- Activity. How active can they be in the postoperative period? When can they drive? Return to work depends on the nature of the job.
- Drugs. The patient should usually be given the drugs which they were on when they came into hospital together with any others which may be necessary as part of their present treatment. They should be told clearly how long they need to take these. Their GP must be informed of the therapy as soon as the patient is discharged from hospital. This is best done by giving them a note to take home.
- Follow-up. When is the patient to be seen again?

Discharge summary

A summary of the patient's admission should be completed as soon as possible after the time of discharge and sent to the patient's GP. This can be produced from data entered into a computer and sent by fax. A copy is filed in the notes. The letter should carry a printed legible name and contact telephone number and should include concise relevant information under the following headings.
- Patient details (name, registry number, GP, address, date of birth).
- Admission details (ward, date, emergency/elective, consultant, etc.).
- Reason for admission.

- Investigations (summary of inpatient results).
- Diagnosis.
- Operation details (very brief).
- Non-operative treatment.
- Postoperative details (problems, complications).
- Information given to patient/relatives – very important, especially if the prognosis is grave.
- Method of discharge (e.g. home, transferred, died).
- Drugs and other discharge treatment.
- Follow-up arrangements – does the patient know when they will be seen, or how they can find out?
- Other comments.

Dealing with death

The junior surgical trainee often has the task of telling relatives that a patient is going to die or has died. You are also responsible for the care of these terminally ill patients. This is a delicate job and each individual doctor will develop their own methods. Below are written some ideas, aimed to help you formulate your own approach.

Informing the relatives that a patient is going to die

The relatives will need to be told if the patient is likely to die. This is best done by taking them into a quiet room and explaining that nothing further can be done usefully to prolong life. Arrange not to be disturbed. This includes leaving your bleep elsewhere.

It is often best to start by asking the relatives what they feel is going to happen. Using this as a guide, the patient's situation must be explained honestly, clearly and slowly. Generally it is important to be absolutely truthful. Try to be positive, rather than negative, emphasizing what you can still do to help the patient. Often the one comfort that you can give is to say that their relative will be given sufficient analgesia to stay free of pain. Point out what the relatives can do themselves to help the patient through this inevitable period of life.

A situation has become increasingly common where there are the means to keep a patient 'alive' although this would clearly be inappropriate (i.e. in cases of brain death). This may be difficult to explain to relatives. You may have to explain the hopelessness of the situation and the loss of dignity that keeping a patient with brain death 'alive' entails. Usually the relatives will understand and agree that the right thing to do is what is suggested. When the relatives remain worried and further guidance is needed, arrange for them to see your consultant. In this situation he or she is likely to wish to see them anyway.

Care of the terminally ill patient

A terminally ill patient also needs to know what is going on. They are often completely aware of what is happening to them.

Choose a time to talk privately. Patients are not always ready to face the prospect of death and may have to be brought gently round to this over several interviews. A few patients make it clear that they never wish to discuss the possibility of death and you must be sensitive to this and respect their wishes.

Once the patient has accepted that death is imminent, they will often ask, 'How long do I have, doctor?' It is best to be truthful and tell them that you do not know. Discuss this with your seniors. You may decide to talk in terms of 'a matter of days, weeks or months' as seems appropriate. You will usually be wrong.

The everyday care of a dying patient is a nursing speciality, requiring great sensitivity and skill. You must make certain that the pain relief is adequate. Added sedation at night is often necessary. Otherwise the purpose of treatment is the control of symptoms with the minimum of discomfort. The patient should still be seen regularly, especially when he or she is dying. Most patients know the situation and could take a lack of visits by the junior surgical trainee as evidence that they have been forgotten and are already regarded as deceased. Remember too their spiritual welfare. Many people have deep questions. A hospital chaplain is available, and can be very helpful.

Confirming death

A doctor is required to verify death. The four signs are as follows.
- No pulse.
- No heart sounds.
- No breath sounds.
- Pupils fixed and dilated.

Sufficient time must be spent listening for heart and breath sounds to confidently exclude a very slow cardiac rate or intermittent breathing. Be particularly careful if the patient has taken an overdose or has been on sedative drugs. This is a diagnostic process that is done with complete respect for the person who has just died. It is dignified, and needs protected time.

As you leave the patient and are approached by the relatives, you must be absolutely certain whether or not death has occurred.

Informing the relatives of a patient who has died

The death may be expected or unexpected. Telling relatives about an expected death is usually easier. Giving information about an unexpected death often results in great distress and is a difficult situation to handle.

Privacy is important when talking to the relatives. Leave your bleep outside and ask not to be disturbed. Find a place with seats, a phone and some refreshment available. Speak clearly, slowly and truthfully. How are they prepared? Always ask someone else to come with you. Usually a nurse colleague has already met the relatives. However much the surgical team may have done for the patient, at that moment the relative sees you as the conveyor of bad news, and there may come a point when it is best to leave the relative in the company of a nurse who can sit, talk quietly and comfort them.

Usually the best line to take is to tell them of the death early and then talk about the reasons why and how it happened. They have been called in unexpectedly and know there's trouble. Offer comfort where possible, saying, for example, that the patient died peacefully and was not in pain. Relatives will usually want to know why the death has occurred. They may ask 'What has gone wrong?' Do not be defensive about the care the patient has received and make the seriousness of the patient's illness clear. Emphasize that prolonged suffering has been avoided, if this is the case. After that it is useful to sit briefly in silence allowing the relatives to take it all in. Where appropriate, physical contact like grasping a hand does more good than several minutes of talking. Offer to call for spiritual care. You may not know the faith of the person and hospital chaplains are trained in inclusive care. If the death has just happened encourage them to see the body. A warm hand is part of the goodbye.

The postmortem

Postmortems are performed for two reasons.

- All cases referred to the coroner undergo a postmortem unless they are fully satisfied about the cause of death. This is done as a routine and is a legal requirement.
- Postmortems are performed to obtain information about a death, which may be of value in treating other patients later. An autopsy should ideally be performed on all surgical patients dying in hospital, though this is now difficult to achieve. Such a postmortem is requested by the consultant responsible for the case and requires the permission of the relatives. You may have to obtain this. Most relatives understand the need but they do not wish to discuss details at a time of great distress. They also wish to be reassured that the funeral arrangements will not be delayed.

Death certificates, the coroner and cremation forms

When one of your patients dies, you are legally required to fill in a death certificate and send this to the Registrar of Births and Deaths. The information is used to prepare national statistics about causes of death.

You can only fill in the death certificate if you attended the deceased before death. If you see the body for the first time after death you are not qualified to sign the certificate. It cannot be signed by someone else on your behalf either. Any medical practitioner who signs a death certificate must be registered. Provisional registration entitles a junior surgical trainee to sign death certificates only in cases arising out of his or her duties in an approved hospital while working for a fully registered practitioner.

Ideally a certificate should be issued for all deaths, even those that are also being referred to the coroner. In this case Box A on the back of the certificate must be initialled informing the registrar that he or she must wait for the coroner's decision before allowing the body to be buried or cremated.

In addition, a separate form must be signed and given to the informant saying that the death certificate has been issued. The informant, usually a relative of the deceased (other persons entitled to perform this role are listed on the back of the death certificate), is legally required to take the death certificate sealed in an envelope to the registrar within 5 days (8 days in Scotland).

The informant will also be required to state certain particulars relating to the deceased's life. A counterfoil is filled in to be kept by the hospital.

The death certificate starts by stating the patient's particulars. There then follows a section where the junior surgical trainee is required to state whether he or she saw the body after death. This is not a legal requirement, although it is a sensible thing to do in order to avoid cases of mistaken identity.

The statement of cause of death is in two parts.

- Part I records the sequence of conditions and diseases that led to the patient's death. This is written in sequential order, starting with the condition that actually caused death, and going on to the underlying disease. This sequence must be causally linked. Each condition entered at the top of the list should occur as a consequence of the condition written immediately below it, eventually ending up with the underlying cause. For example, a patient with chronic peptic ulceration who dies of peritonitis a few days after an operation for perforation of a duodenal ulcer would be entered as follows:
  - Ia   Peritonitis, due to
  - Ib   Perforation of duodenal ulcer [operation and date], due to
  - Ic   Peptic ulcer of the duodenum.

  The terms used must be precise. Words like 'pulmonary oedema' or 'coma' are not accurate enough. Words like 'cirrhosis' imply alcohol toxicity and, whether or not this is true, the registrar will refer the case to the coroner. If the condition was infectious, the site, causal organism and duration of infection must be stated. If a tumour occurs in the list, state the histology and whether it was malignant or benign, the anatomical site, and whether it was primary or secondary. If it was a secondary tumour, indicate the site of the primary and whether this had been removed or not.

- Part II records other conditions that may have contributed to the death, but are not related to the causal sequence of disease described in part 1. For example, the above patient's form might be completed with 'Part II: Chronic bronchitis'.

On the back of the death certificate there are two boxes. Box A has already been described. Box B is a box that must be initialled by the practitioner if they are still awaiting results of laboratory tests which may aid the diagnosis that they have put on the certificate.

It is most important that this death certificate is filled in legibly and correctly. Otherwise it will be rejected by the registrar and delay the arrangements for burial or cremation. There is no significant variation in the form of death certificate in Scotland, Wales or Northern Ireland. If you feel that the patient's death is unexplained, you cannot sign the death certificate and the case must be referred to the coroner.

Referral to the coroner

The role of the coroner is to investigate death. He or she does this in order to ensure that the cause of death was natural and to identify deaths where further enquiry is necessary. Such deaths include those where a crime may have been committed, where there is an accusation of negligence on behalf of the police authorities or medical profession, or where claims for compensation might follow. All the facts necessary to answer any such enquiry must be available before the disposal of the body.

Circumstances in which a death should be reported to the coroner are as follows.

- Where the cause of death is unknown.
- Where no doctor has treated the deceased in their terminal illness, or where the deceased's medical practitioner did not attend the patient within 14 days of death.
- Where death is associated with medical treatment, e.g. deaths occurring during an operation or during recovery from a general anaesthetic. Generally, any death occurring in the 24 h after an anaesthetic is reportable, although there is some variation with different coroners. Also, cases where any form of medical treatment, including drug therapy, has contributed to a patient's death should be reported.
- Sudden, unexplained or suspicious death. This includes death occurring within 24 h of emergency admission to hospital.
- Death from industrial accident or disease, road traffic accidents, domestic accidents (e.g. death following a fall causing fractured neck of femur), deaths from violence or neglect, death following abortion, death from poisoning (including alcohol), and cases of suicide.

- Any case where, following death, there is a definite or suspected claim for negligence against either the doctors or nursing staff. In such a case medical practitioners must not only inform the coroner but also inform their defence union immediately and give no verbal or written statement to the injured party until this is done.
- Death while a patient was in legal custody. For instance, you might be involved in treating a person who has been brought in from police custody, having been found unconscious.
- In cases where you are uncertain whether or not you ought to report the case to the coroner, always telephone them or their officer and discuss it. After hearing your story they may well give permission for you to write a death certificate.

The coroner has three courses of action in dealing with the case.

- They may, after considering the facts, be satisfied that the cause of death was natural and no postmortem is required. They will then allow a death certificate to be issued.
- They may require that a postmortem be carried out, usually by a coroner's pathologist. If the result shows that the death was from natural causes then there is no need for an inquest and the death certificate can be issued.
- They may feel, following a postmortem, that an inquest should be held. This includes all criminal cases, suicides, death from accidents or industrial mishap, deaths in custody and deaths where claims of negligence have been put forward. In cases where negligence is claimed against a medical practitioner, they must be legally represented by their defence society.

The system in Scotland and Northern Ireland is broadly similar, although in Scotland the role of the coroner is performed by the procurator-fiscal.

Ethical issues in surgery

There is increasing dialogue between clinical practice and medical ethics. This is for a number of reasons.
- What used to be assumed as good practice now needs to be defined in an ethical framework for educational and governance purposes.

- Other pressures within healthcare are a potential threat to the good practice of 'putting patients first'. These include rationing of resources, and measures of clinical performance.
- As medical research continues to advance what could become possible may not be deemed desirable. Genetic engineering and reproductive cloning are examples of this.
- End of life decisions and the appropriateness of surgery is a further area that bears discussion.

Clearly, doctors should strive at all times to adhere to the highest clinical and ethical standards. Two areas deserve specific mention as they have seen a change in attitude over the last few years.

Obtaining a patient's informed consent

Consent is now far more than a 'tick-box formality'. Much greater emphasis is placed on informed consent. This is to protect the doctor performing any intervention from three possible legal wrongs:

- trespass of the person (a civil wrong)
- negligence (a civil wrong)
- assault or battery (a criminal wrong).

Moreover, the ethical foundation is one of recognising and respecting a patient's autonomy. There are two possible defences that a doctor has.

- The patient provided a valid consent.
- The doctor acted out of necessity. i.e. in the 'best interests' of the patient (e.g. to save life).

If the patient is deemed competent and the consent is adequately informed and provided voluntarily, then the doctor is not legally liable (assuming of course that any intervention is competently performed).

The assessment of the patient's mental competence is based on a set of questions ascertaining whether the patient is able to make a decision. Specific issues include whether the patient can comprehend and retain information given, use the information given, and communicate their decision (in some way).

The requirement for informed consent means that the patient should be informed about significant risks, have their questions answered, and be given such information that responsible surgeons would impart to a patient in that situation. This basically means that consent should be obtained by a doctor capable of explaining the procedure and answering questions about it. Ideally this should be the surgeon performing the procedure. This may be delegated to someone else as long as that person is suitably trained and qualified and has sufficient knowledge of the proposed investigation or treatment.

Therefore, it is unlikely that the consent will be obtained by a newly qualified doctor. However, it is still your responsibility to ensure that the appropriate person has indeed signed the consent form with the patient before theatre.

Intimate examinations

Rectal or vaginal examinations, defined as 'intimate examinations', must be performed with absolute care to safeguard a patient's autonomy. This will include considerations of consent, privacy and dignity, and may require the use of a chaperone (where relevant).

There has recently been serious debate in the medical and ethical literature about the practice of medical students performing intimate examination for their training. It is no longer appropriate to suggest that medical students (who may be very keen to learn) should prepare to perform intimate examinations on anaesthetized patients in theatre irrespective of whether explicit consent has been obtained.

However, one role of any surgical unit is to train medical students and junior doctors. Competence in performing intimate examination is an important skill in diagnosis and management. This skill is acquired in a number of ways, including now the use of mannequins prior to patient examination. Where the patient under your care has a clinical sign that trainees should elicit by intimate examination then it is appropriate for informed consent to be obtained, both for the examination and for its performance by trainees. This may then be done during anaesthesia. It is good practice to indicate in the patient notes that this (advance) informed consent has been obtained.

3 Head and neck surgery

3.1 Lumps in the head and neck

An important early step in the diagnosis of lumps in the head and neck is to decide whether the lump is in the skin or deep to the skin.

Lumps in the skin include those peculiar to this area, such as cervical auricle (see below), and others common anywhere in the skin such as sebaceous cysts, dermoids, lipomas, fibromas, basal cell carcinomas and squamous cell carcinomas. The latter are dealt with in chapter 13.

If the lump is deep to the skin you will have to decide in which anatomical region it belongs and particularly whether it is behind, beneath or in front of the sternomastoid muscle. The important anatomical regions are the parotid region, the submandibular region, the pretracheal area, and the anterior and posterior triangles of the neck (see Fig. 3.1.1). Lumps in these regions are dealt with on the following pages.

- Cervical auricle (p. 127).
- Lumps in the parotid region (p. 128).
- Lumps in the submandibular region (p. 132).
- Lumps in the anterior triangle:
  - branchial sinus (p. 135)
  - branchial cyst (p. 137)
  - carotid body tumour (p. 139)
  - pharyngeal pouch (p. 140).
- Lumps in the posterior triangle:
  - cervical rib (p. 142).
- Pretracheal area:
  - thyroid (section 4.1)
  - parathyroid (section 4.2).

Surgery: Diagnosis and Management, 4th edition. Edited by N. Rawlinson and D. Alderson. © 2009 Blackwell Publishing, ISBN: 978-1-4051-2921-3

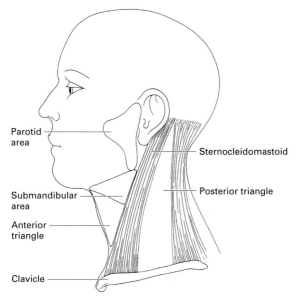

Fig. 3.1.1 Some important anatomical areas in the head and neck.

- All areas:
  ○ cervical lymphadenopathy (p. 144)
  ○ malignant lymphoma (p. 147)
  ○ cystic hygroma (p. 149).

Cervical auricle

This is an accessory ear lobe and is situated low in the neck anterior to the sternomastoid. It consists of a cartilaginous skeleton covered with skin, and is easy to diagnose providing the clinician is familiar with it.

Treatment is by cosmetic removal.

Lumps in the parotid region

You must be familiar with the normal extent of the parotid gland (see Fig. 3.1.1). If the swelling is in this area and deep to the skin, then it is in the parotid gland until proved otherwise. Swellings of the parotid are of two kinds.
• Generalized, involving the whole gland.
• Localized lumps within the gland.

Generalized enlargement of the parotid

The parotid is enlarged secondary to either inflammatory disease or obstruction of the main parotid duct.

Viral parotitis – mumps

This disease is common in children and causes bilateral parotid swelling. Occasionally it may affect only one side. The parotid duct opening looks inflamed, but there is no pus. There is usually a history of contact with the disease about 3 weeks previously. Check whether the patient has had mumps in the past as second attacks are very rare. The virus may also cause orchitis, pancreatitis and submandibular sialadenitis. In doubtful cases, two mumps virus antibody titres taken 1 week apart may be helpful. No specific treatment is required and the swelling usually resolves over 7–10 days.

Bacterial parotitis

Acute bacterial parotitis used to be common in surgical wards, particularly in debilitated patients, secondary to dehydration and reduced salivary flow. The condition is usually secondary to obstruction of the duct by viscid secretions. (Embolization during septicaemia has also been implicated.) The condition is now much rarer but may be seen occasionally. The usual organisms are staphylococcus, streptococcus, pneumococcus or anaerobes.

Recognizing the pattern

It occurs in dehydrated patients postoperatively, particularly in the elderly and in ambulatory patients with xerostomia such as Sjögren's syndrome. The history is of a dull throbbing pain and swelling on the side of the face. The pain is worse on speaking or eating. Examination of the inside of the mouth may show pus extruding from the opening of the parotid duct. The whole gland becomes acutely inflamed and very tender and the patient looks toxic and ill.

Management
A pus swab is taken for culture and antibiotic sensitivity. The treatment is with antibiotics (ampicillin and flucloxacillin). The patient must be adequately rehydrated, and the mouth kept clean. Occasionally an abscess forms and may require drainage.

Autoimmune parotitis
Autoimmune disease usually affects the major salivary glands and the lachrymal glands, causing symmetrical, painless progressive enlargement. Primary Sjögren's is enlargement of the salivary glands and lachrymal glands associated with a dry mouth and dry eyes. Secondary Sjögren's disease is similar, but the syndrome also includes dry eyes and arthritis and other connective tissue diseases. The diagnosis and management of these conditions are beyond the scope of this book.

Obstruction of the parotid duct
Obstruction of the parotid duct due to stones is unusual as the parotid secretion is watery and the duct is wide. It is more often due to stenosis of the opening of the parotid duct. This may occur due to trauma of the inside of the cheek secondary to ill-fitting dentures. Often the duct has an irregular pattern similar to bronchiectasis, described as sialectasis. This results in sludging of secretions and obstruction, with secondary infection.

Recognizing the pattern
The patient is usually adult and complains of painful swelling of the parotid gland during meals. Inspection of the opening of the duct opposite the second upper molar tooth may reveal the stenosis.

Proving the diagnosis
A sialogram may be helpful in excluding the presence of stones and may also show 'sialectasis'. This is dilatation of the ducts

within the gland due to chronic obstruction and previous inflammatory episodes.

Management

This is usually conservative and the patient is taught to 'milk' the duct contents forward by massaging the cheek and thus preventing stasis in the duct. If the stenosis is severe, it may be dilated using lachrymal duct dilators under a local anaesthetic. Antibiotics are given if infection is present.

Localized lumps in the parotid

Seventy-five per cent of parotid neoplasms eventually prove to be benign mixed tumours (pleomorphic adenomas, see below). An adenolymphoma (also called Warthin's tumour) is benign but may be bilateral or multiple. This tumour accounts for 10% of parotid neoplasms. The tumour is soft and may feel cystic.

The 15% of neoplasms that are malignant include the mucoepidermoid tumour and acinic cell carcinoma. Both of these usually have a benign histological appearance but may recur locally and occasionally metastasize. The adenoid cystic carcinoma (cylindroma) is a malignant lesion and has a tendency to spread along nerve sheaths. Squamous cell carcinoma of the parotid is a highly malignant lesion which may arise from a mixed cell tumour. By the time it presents there may already be extensive local infiltration with or without nerve paralysis.

The most common non-neoplastic solitary nodule is a cyst.

Mixed tumours of the parotid

Mixed tumours are so called because they contain adenoma cells surrounded by pools of mucin, which look like cartilage on histological sections. These tumours are benign but have an incomplete capsule and consequently have a high rate of local recurrence if incompletely removed. There is also a risk of malignant change in the long term. Because of these factors it is very important to excise the tumour by performing a formal parotidectomy.

Recognizing the pattern

The history is of a slowly growing painless swelling on the side of the face. The patient may be of any age beyond the teens. There is a firm, smooth lump in the parotid area, usually in the lower anterior part of the gland just above the angle of the jaw. This may appear to be quite superficial, but careful examination will show that the skin moves over it. Establish that the lump is indeed in the parotid gland and not attached deeply to bone or muscle. Look for extensions inside the mouth or pharynx, and check whether the facial nerve is involved by observing facial movements. Look for involved lymph nodes on both sides of the neck. If any of these are found the lesion may be malignant.

Proving the diagnosis

The diagnosis is proved by fine-needle aspiration cytology. Deep lobe involvement and spread to the parapharyngeal space can be assessed by CT or MRI scanning.

Management

A suspected mixed tumour of the superficial lobe of the parotid should be removed by superficial parotidectomy.

The patient should be warned of the possibility of a facial weakness postoperatively, although this is usually transient. Loss of sensation in the distribution of the greater auricular nerve (earlobe region) and Frey's syndrome or 'gustatory sweating' should also be discussed. A nerve stimulator may be required during the operation and theatre should be informed of this.

OPERATION: SUPERFICIAL PAROTIDECTOMY

An incision is made anterior to the ear, extending behind the ear into the upper neck. The facial nerve trunk is firstly identified and its branches are then traced forwards in the parotid gland and all tissue superficial to them excised together with the tumour. If the tumour is deep to the facial nerve it can be excised by displacing the nerve branches. The wound is usually drained using a suction drain.

Procedure profile

Blood requirement	0
Anaesthetic	GA
Operation time	2–3 hours
Hospital stay	3–5 days
Return to normal activity	2–3 weeks

Postoperatively check and record the movements of the facial muscles supplied by each individual branch of the facial nerve, i.e. temporal, zygomatic, buccal, mandibular and cervical. If there is any weakness, note whether it is partial, when full recovery is likely. If it is complete, recovery is also likely (in 6–8 weeks), unless a nerve is known to have been divided at operation.

If the tumour is malignant, radiotherapy will probably be given. Occasionally radiotherapy is also given to benign mixed tumours of the parotid, particularly if the surgery is being done for recurrent disease or where tumour spillage has occurred. With mixed tumours of the parotid, regular follow-up is advisable.

Management of other parotid lumps

Because of the possibility of neoplasia, these lumps will usually be excised to establish an exact diagnosis. However, fine-needle aspiration cytology should be performed before any form of open biopsy. If the lump is obviously malignant then excision and radiotherapy may be the only possible treatment. For lesions of unknown aetiology, however, biopsy alone is not advisable as it may result in local implantation of a neoplasm. Most lesions of the parotid are therefore removed by superficial parotidectomy, although adenolymphoma can be safely enucleated.

Lumps in the submandibular region

The submandibular salivary gland measures about 4×3 cm and is situated beneath the angle of the jaw. Its superficial portion is in the neck outside the mylohyoid muscle and its deep portion

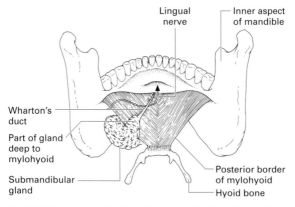

Fig. 3.1.2 The anatomy of the submandibular gland. The floor of the mouth viewed from behind (tongue removed).

lies in the floor of the mouth deep to the mylohyoid. Its duct drains from the deep part of the gland forwards to the floor of the mouth beneath the tip of the tongue (Fig. 3.1.2).

Enlargement is either generalized or localized. Generalized enlargement of the gland is commonly secondary to stone formation. It also occurs in autoimmune syndromes (as in the parotid gland). Localized enlargements are of the same aetiology as those already described for the parotid gland (p. 130), although a greater proportion (approximately 30%) are malignant.

Submandibular stones

The secretion of this gland is more viscous than that of the parotid and the duct is narrower, so stone formation and obstruction are relatively common. Secondary infection (usually with staphylococcus, streptococcus or pneumococcus) is dangerous because of the risk of swelling and oedema in the floor of the mouth and consequent respiratory obstruction (Ludwig's angina).

Recognizing the pattern

The condition can occur at any age and is common in young adults. The history is of intermittent painful swelling beneath the jaw occurring with meals. The patient may also have noticed 'gravel' in the mouth. The gland is palpable and tender during these episodes. A stone may be palpable in the duct in the floor of the mouth beneath the tongue.

Proving the diagnosis
Most stones are radio-opaque and may be seen on a plain X-ray of the floor of the mouth. A submandibular duct sialogram will also confirm the presence of the stone, and detect any sialectasis within the gland (p. 129). The stone may be palpable.

Management
In a few patients the stone will pass spontaneously. If it has been giving symptoms for 3 or 4 weeks, it can be removed from the duct using a local anaesthetic. Where the condition has become chronic, where stones are recurrent, or where the stone is situated in the gland itself, removal of the submandibular gland is preferable.

OPERATION: REMOVAL OF STONE FROM SUBMANDIBULAR DUCT
Local anaesthetic is infiltrated in the floor of the mouth and a suture temporarily passed around the duct proximal to the stone. This prevents the stone slipping back into the main gland. The buccal mucosa and the duct are incised over the stone and the stone removed. The wound in the floor of the mouth is not sutured to prevent ligation of the duct.

Procedure profile

Blood requirement	0
Anaesthetic	LA (GA if stone is small and hard to find)
Operation time	30 minutes
Hospital stay	Day case
Return to normal activity	1 day

Postoperative mouthwashes should be given as required.

No special preparation is necessary before removal of the gland. Warn the patient of possible transient weakness of the corner of the mouth (see below). A nerve stimulator can be useful at operation but it is not essential. Lingual nerve paraesthesia is possible.

OPERATION: REMOVAL OF SUBMANDIBULAR GLAND
An incision is made 2.5 cm below the angle of the jaw over the gland. The mandibular branch of the facial nerve curves up over the jaw at this point, lying on the facial artery. It can be damaged if the incision is too high. It can also be damaged by retraction. This damage results in weakness of the corner of the mouth and care should be taken to avoid this. When the deep portion of the gland is removed, care is taken not to damage the lingual or hypoglossal nerves which lie deep to it. The wound is drained.

Procedure profile

Blood requirement	0
Anaesthetic	GA or LA
Operation time	1–2 hours
Hospital stay	48 hours
Return to normal activity	1 week

Lumps in the anterior triangle of the neck

These include the following:
- branchial sinus
- branchial cyst
- carotid body tumour
- pharyngeal pouch.

Branchial sinus
During fetal life the second arch skin grows over the branchial clefts closing them off. If this closure is incomplete a fistula, sinus

or cyst may result along the tract. A branchial sinus usually opens as a tiny hole in the lower part of the neck. Although the external opening may seem very small there is frequently a track running up the neck, which may go as high as the posterior pillar of the fauces in the pharynx (forming a fistula).

Recognizing the pattern
The patient is almost always a child, often in the first year of life. The sinus has usually been present from birth and the mother notices the discharge. On examination the opening is situated in front of the anterior border of the sternomastoid, one-third of the way up from the origin of the muscle. It discharges 'glairy' fluid intermittently.

Proving the diagnosis
The above history and signs are quite characteristic and no further investigation is necessary.

Management
The treatment is surgical removal of the whole sinus or fistula. The operation is best performed early in life before the child's neck grows. In a baby it is often possible to excise even a long tract through one incision. The optimum time for operation is between the ages of 6 months and a year.

With an older child the mother should be warned that more than one incision may be necessary to remove the whole tract. She will be surprised to hear this as the external lesion looks so insignificant.

OPERATION: REMOVAL OF BRANCHIAL FISTULA/SINUS
The external opening is mobilized with an ellipse of skin. The tract is followed up in the neck using a lachrymal probe in its lumen as a guide. Some surgeons use methylene blue to outline the tract. The tract is dissected out as high as possible and then, if necessary, a second transverse incision is made, usually at about the level of the hyoid bone. The tract is then followed up between the internal and external carotid arteries, until it reaches the pharyngeal epithelium. Frequently it peters out before this. The wound is usually drained.

Procedure profile

Blood requirement	Group and save
Anaesthetic	GA
Operation time	30–90 minutes depending on extent
Hospital stay	24–48 hours
Return to normal activity	10 days

Branchial cyst

A branchial cyst (Fig. 3.1.3) is thought to be formed by squamous cell inclusions within cervical lymph nodes, or less frequently from an isolated remnant of a branchial cleft in the neck. Its wall contains lymphoid tissue and it may become inflamed in any generalized lymphadenopathy in the neck. Not infrequently the cyst contents become purulent and it may present as a cervical abscess.

Recognizing the pattern

The cyst usually makes its appearance in childhood or early adult life. It frequently appears as a swelling during an upper respiratory tract infection. It may be painful. The swelling persists once the infection has subsided. Abscess formation causes severe pain, which is worse on moving the head. On examination it is usually about 5–10 cm in diameter and lies deep to the sternomastoid muscle, appearing beneath its anterior border. It is frequently related to the upper third of this muscle behind the angle of the jaw (see Fig. 3.1.3). It fluctuates, but does not transilluminate as its contents are opaque.

Proving the diagnosis

The diagnosis is made on the history and the site of the swelling and confirmed by MRI scan. Fine-needle cytology can be helpful.

Management

OPERATION: REMOVAL OF BRANCHIAL CYST

A transverse incision is made over the lump and deepened until the cyst is encountered. It is then excised. Care is taken to avoid

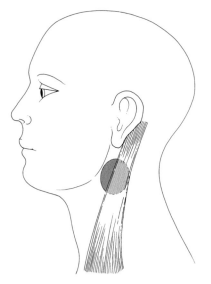

Fig. 3.1.3 A branchial cyst.

damage to the carotid vessels, internal jugular vein and hypo-glossal nerve which usually lie deep to the swelling.

Procedure profile

Blood requirement	0
Anaesthetic	GA
Operation time	30–60 minutes
Hospital stay	24 hours
Return to normal activity	3–7 days

Carotid body tumour

This tumour is a chemodectoma arising from the cells in the carotid body. It grows very slowly over many years. Histologically it is a non-chromaffin paraganglionoma.

Recognizing the pattern

Patients are usually aged over 50, although the condition can present earlier. They may notice the lump themselves or it may be found at a routine medical examination. The lump is firm but compressible and transmits pulsation rather than being pulsatile itself. It is situated at the carotid bifurcation and appears as a tumour beneath the anterior border of the sternomastoid. It is mobile from side to side but not up and down. Despite the location and origin, they are rarely symptomatic.

Proving the diagnosis

MRI will usually define the extent of the tumour, delineate its exact relationship to the carotid arteries and establish that there is an adequate collateral through the opposite carotid artery.

Management

The tumour is usually removed. It can, however, be safely watched for many years and this course may be preferable in the elderly, frail patient.

OPERATION: REMOVAL OF CAROTID BODY TUMOUR

A vertical incision anterior to the sternomastoid is usually employed. The lesion is carefully dissected from the carotid artery (this can be a very haemorrhagic procedure). Some surgeons may require the use of a carotid shunt (see p. 522). Alternatively, it can be excised and a graft placed between the common and internal carotid arteries. A suction drain is used. The wound is closed with clips or sutures.

Procedure profile

Blood requirement	4
Anaesthetic	GA
Operation time	3–4 hours
Hospital stay	5–7 days
Return to normal activity	3–4 weeks

Postoperatively the care is the same as after carotid artery surgery (p. 522). The blood pressure should be monitored regularly and may tend to fall lower than preoperatively.

Pharyngeal pouch

A pharyngeal pouch is a pulsion diverticulum of the pharyngeal mucosa, probably arising as a result of a relative obstruction at the level of the cricopharyngeus muscle or as a consequence of loss of coordination in the pharyngeal phase of swallowing where the upper sphincter fails to relax in response to contraction of the pharyngeal constrictor muscles. There is frequently a previous history of heartburn and reflux due to hiatus hernia and it has been suggested that the obstruction is due to hypertrophy in an attempt to prevent overspill of refluxing gastro-oesophageal contents into the larynx. The mucosa protrudes through Killian's dehiscence (Fig. 3.1.4).

Recognizing the pattern

The condition occurs in elderly patients and it is more common in males. Initially the patient may experience symptoms of coughing or choking related to loss of coordination in the conscious phase of swallowing. As the pouch enlarges, food enters it as well as the oesophagus and characteristically the first mouthful is easily swallowed but thereafter the pouch fills up with food and obstructs the upper oesophagus. The patient is then unable to swallow further food and will regurgitate the contents of the pouch. Inhalation of regurgitated contents, especially at night, causes fits of coughing and episodes of pulmonary infection.

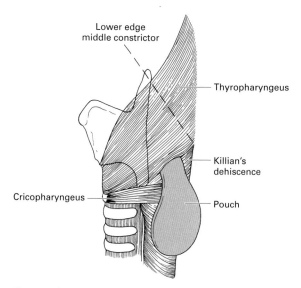

Fig. 3.1.4 The anatomy of a pharyngeal pouch.

Proving the diagnosis
The pouch is easily demonstrated on a barium swallow. Ask the radiologist to look specifically in the upper neck.

Management
The management is to prevent the pouch from filling and relieve the cricopharyngeal obstruction. This can be achieved by endoscopic or open surgical techniques. Both are highly effective. The patient should be put on fluids only for 24 h preoperatively. For open surgery the patient is warned about risk of pharyngeal perforation and damage to the recurrent laryngeal nerves.

In the endoscopic procedure a stapled communication is made between the posterior wall of the oesophagus and the anterior wall of the pouch. It is the procedure of choice for relatively small pouches. In open surgery the pouch may be excised or simply mobilized and suspended so that the fundus of the diverticulum lies superiorly (diverticulopexy). The key feature, however, is division of the transverse fibres of the cricopharyngeus muscle.

OPERATION: EXCISION OF PHARYNGEAL POUCH
An incision is made at the level of the hyoid bone, usually on the left side. The mucosal pouch is found and excised and the mucosal defect closed. The cricopharyngeus muscle is divided longitudinally (myotomy). The wound is drained and a nasogastric tube is passed down into the stomach. The endoscopic technique usually results in a shorter hospital stay and recovery period.

Procedure profile

Blood requirement	0
Anaesthetic	GA
Operation time	1–2 hours
Hospital stay	3–5 days (open), day case (endoscopic)
Return to normal activity	2 weeks

Postoperatively the patient is fed through a nasogastric tube and most surgeons carry out a contrast swallow between 3 and 5 days after surgery. If this shows no leakage, normal feeding can be instituted. If leakage is demonstrated feeding continues with a nasogastric tube until a repeat barium swallow shows the pharyngeal wound has healed.

Lumps in the posterior triangle

Cervical rib (thoracic outlet syndrome)
In approximately 1 in 200 people the costal element of the seventh cervical vertebra overdevelops to a varying degree. The result is a cervical rib which, when fully formed, is bony and attached to the first normal rib. It may, however, be nothing more than a fibrous strand. In half the cases the condition is unilateral, usually on the right side. The subclavian artery and first

thoracic nerve pass over the cervical rib to gain access to the upper limb. The artery may be narrowed over the rib and dilated distally. In the latter case mural thrombus may form and give rise to distal emboli. The first thoracic nerve can also be damaged by direct pressure. Very often a thin fibrous strand causes more symptoms than a fully formed cervical rib.

Recognizing the pattern

The condition may occur in either sex and symptoms usually begin in the late teens when the neck extends and the shoulders droop. The patient may notice a swelling or tenderness in the neck on the affected side. There may be pain due to vascular insufficiency. This is worse on exercise, especially if the arm is elevated. There may be distal ischaemia with a cold pale hand and occasional numbness or even trophic changes in the fingers. Raynaud's phenomenon is not unusual. Some patients may complain of neurological symptoms, which include numbness and paraesthesiae in the forearm and weakness of the hands but it is important not to assume that these symptoms are due to a thoracic outlet problem just because a radiological abnormality is present. Most patients with neurological upper limb symptoms have degenerative disease in the cervical spine. Palpation of the neck may reveal the abnormal rib. There may be signs of ischaemia or emboli in the hand. The radial pulse may disappear if the arm is fully elevated. Look for wasting in the hypothenar or thenar muscles and motor and sensory changes in the first thoracic nerve distribution. There may be a bruit over the subclavian artery.

Proving the diagnosis

An X-ray of the cervical spine will demonstrate the presence of a bony cervical rib or an enlarged anterior tubercle of the seventh cervical vertebra (associated with a fibrous band). Angiography may demonstrate a constriction and poststenotic dilatation in the region of the cervical rib, especially if taken with the arm elevated.

Management

A cervical rib causing neurological symptoms may be managed conservatively with physiotherapy to improve the muscles that elevate and support the upper limb girdle. A cervical rib causing vascular problems or well-marked neurological problems should be treated surgically.

OPERATION: REMOVAL OF A CERVICAL RIB
The cervical rib is approached through a skin crease incision and removed, including its periosteal covering. If this covering is not removed there is a danger of recurrence. A fibrous band may also be excised. In some cases it is only necessary to split the scalenus anterior to relieve the pressure.

Procedure profile

Blood requirement	2
Anaesthetic	GA
Operation time	1–2 hours
Hospital stay	3–5 days
Return to normal activity	2–3 weeks

The postoperative course is usually uncomplicated. The patient should have a chest X-ray in the first few hours to exclude a pneumothorax.

3.2 Cervical lymphadenopathy

Enlarged lymph nodes and lymphatic conditions

Enlarged cervical lymph nodes are the most common palpable lumps in the head and neck. The nodes may be enlarged due to either inflammatory or neoplastic processes and the precise node involved depends on the site of the primary pathology. It is therefore important to know which areas of the head and neck drain to the various lymph nodes (Fig. 3.2.1 and Table 3.2.1).

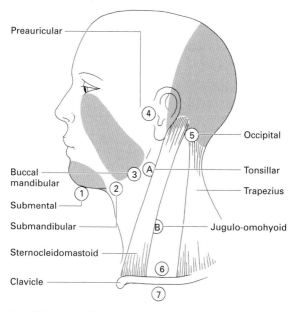

Fig. 3.2.1 The cervical lymph nodes and their areas of drainage.
See Table 3.2.1 for key.

Inflammatory causes of enlarged lymph nodes may be acute or chronic. Acute inflammations are common in children and may be due to viruses or bacteria. The latter may progress to pus formation and present as a cervical abscess.

A typical chronic inflammatory cause of cervical lymphadenopathy is tuberculosis. These lymph nodes become very indurated and tend to give rise to sinuses.

Neoplasms producing enlarged cervical lymph nodes include primary disease of the lymphatic system and secondary metastases from head and neck squamous carcinomas or thoracic or abdominal carcinomas. Hodgkin's disease is a primary lymphoma commonly presenting in the neck.

Sarcoidosis may also present as cervical lymphadenopathy.

Table 3.2.1 The cervical lymph nodes and their areas of drainage.

Name	Area of drainage
Submental group	Tip of tongue, anterior end of lower lip, floor of mouth and lower gum, bilateral drainage
Submandibular group	Submental group, centre of forehead, nose, paranasal sinuses, front of neck, lips, anterior two-thirds of tongue
Buccal and mandibular group	Cheek, lower eyelid
Preauricular group	Temple, vertex, eyelids, orbit, external acoustic meatus
Occipital group	Back of scalp, posterior edge of pinna
Supraclavicular group	Occipital nodes, axillary nodes, breast, body wall
Infraclavicular group	Lower neck, preaxial border of upper limb, body wall, breast
Jugulodigastric node	Subcutaneous nodes, tonsil
Jugulo-omohyoid node (posteroinferior deep cervical node)	Submental group, submandibular group, posterior third of the tongue. These nodes therefore receive all the lymph drainage from the tongue

Recognizing the pattern

Consider the patient's age, whether the lymphadenopathy is localized or generalized, the texture of the nodes – hard, soft, rubbery – and the duration of the enlargement. It is important to look for the possible primary sites of disease. Look inside the mouth, including the fauces, tonsils, tongue and teeth. A full ear, nose and throat (ENT) examination should be carried out. Nodes low down in the neck may arise from intrathoracic or intra-abdominal pathology (Virchow's node). Look for enlarged nodes elsewhere and hepatosplenomegaly.

Proving the diagnosis and management

Screening tests indicated in any lymphadenopathy include a full blood count, erythrocyte sedimentation rate (ESR), virology screen including infectious mononucleosis and chest X-ray.

Open biopsy is only done after repeated fine-needle aspiration and a formal panendoscopy have excluded a primary squamous carcinoma of the upper digestive tract.

OPERATION: BIOPSY OF CERVICAL LYMPH NODE
An incision is made over the enlarged node and it is removed. Remember to send part of the node for bacteriological culture, including tuberculosis, as well as for histological examination. Beware of the accessory nerve in the posterior triangle.

Procedure profile

Blood requirement	0
Anaesthetic	LA or GA
Operation time	15–45 minutes, depending on site and adherence of node
Hospital stay	Depends on cause
Return to normal activity	Variable

Postoperatively the cause of the lymphadenopathy will have to be treated.

Acute inflammatory lymphadenopathy
The correct treatment in the first 24 h is antibiotics, but once pus formation occurs (after 48 h) drainage becomes necessary. Treating a cervical abscess with antibiotics leads to a chronic swelling (antibioma).

Tuberculous lymphadenitis
Modern treatment is with antituberculous therapy and excision of lymph nodes if they fail to settle.

Malignant lymphoma
Lymphomas are malignant neoplasms of lymphoid tissue. They are divided on a histological basis into Hodgkin's disease and non-Hodgkin's lymphoma. Further subdivisions of lymphomas are made on histological and immunological criteria. These

subgroups have different prognoses and may require different approaches to treatment.

A lymphoma typically presents with asymptomatic lymphadenopathy which may or may not be localized. Some patients (type B) have systemic symptoms which may include fever, weight loss and night sweats. Other symptoms include malaise, pruritus and alcohol-induced pain. The diagnosis is confirmed by biopsy of an enlarged node. It is essential to send fresh unfixed material to the laboratory.

Proving the diagnosis
STAGING THE DISEASE

Once the diagnosis has been made, further investigation is performed to stage the disease. This is done to determine what type of treatment is required and to predict the prognosis. The staging is as follows.

- Stage I: a single group of nodes involved.
- Stage IE: a single extralymphatic organ or site, e.g. skin (rare).
- Stage II: two or more lymph node sites are involved on the same side of the diaphragm.
- Stage III: lymph node sites are involved on both sides of the diaphragm. This includes involvement of the spleen.
- Stage IV: extralymphatic organ involvement (e.g. liver, bone marrow or lung).

Each stage is subdivided into A or B depending on the absence (type A) or presence (type B) of symptoms. The patients are usually worked up on a medical or haematological unit. The investigations may include the following.

- Full blood count, erythrocyte sedimentation rate (ESR), liver function tests and plasma proteins.
- Chest X-ray.
- CT of the chest and abdomen.
- Bone marrow biopsy.
- Lymphangiogram – this is now rarely used.
- Bone scan and/or liver and spleen scan.
- Liver biopsy. This is done if there is significant hepatomegaly (more than 3.5 cm). A positive result means stage IV disease and makes laparotomy unnecessary.
- Staging laparotomy. This is occasionally required to obtain histological evidence of the extent of disease.

- MRI scanning may be useful for imaging glands in the high cervical region and assessing node involvement.

Management

Lymphomas may be treated by radiotherapy, combination chemotherapy or both, the choice depending on the stage of the disease and histological subtype, and whether the patient has significant symptoms.

Radiotherapy may be given either to the group of involved nodes (involved field) or to wider areas (extended field, e.g. 'mantle' or 'inverted Y').

Chemotherapy is given systemically either with a single drug or more usually with a combination of drugs. The choice depends on the stage of the disease, the patient's age, the ESR, the bulk of the disease and the histological grading. The present principles of treatment are outlined below.

- Stages IA and IIA of Hodgkin's disease are treated with radiotherapy (involved field or extended field). Adjuvant chemotherapy is increasingly used, even in limited stage disease.
- All other stages are treated with combination chemotherapy.
- Non-Hodgkin's lymphomas are treated on similar lines, although chemotherapy is introduced at an earlier stage, with combination chemotherapy for the higher histological grades and single agents for lower grade lymphomas.
- Radiation may be used to control local sites of disease.

Cystic hygroma

This is a congenital lesion made up of lymph-filled spaces which arise from an embryonic remnant of the jugular lymph sac. Its correct name is a cavernous lymphangioma. It occurs in the base of the neck, both in the posterior triangle and anteriorly. It may extend up to the jaw, over the anterior chest wall, and down into the axilla. Very occasionally it may occur in the axilla alone.

Recognizing the pattern

The lesion occurs in young children and is often noticed at birth. On examination there is a soft, cystic and compressible lump just beneath the skin, superficial to the neck muscles. It transilluminates brilliantly, tends to vary in size and may have a lobular surface.

Management

The lesion is best treated by surgical excision. Sclerosants have been used.

Preoperatively the patient or parent should be warned of the slight possibility of damage to branches of the brachial plexus and that some of the lesion may have to be left behind in order to avoid this. If this is the case, there will be a possibility of recurrence.

OPERATION: EXCISION CYSTIC HYGROMA

Removal of a large lesion can be tedious as it may ramify amongst the branches of the brachial plexus. It should be removed completely if possible, or it will recur. Occasionally a cystic hygroma extends into the axilla and in that case a separate incision is needed to remove it.

Procedure profile

Blood requirement	1 unit in babies, otherwise group and save
Anaesthetic	GA
Operation time	Depends on extent – 1 or 2 hours
Hospital stay	2–5 days
Return to normal activity	Variable

Postoperative care is usually uncomplicated. The main problem is that fluid and blood tend to collect at the site of the cystic hygroma and the suction drains therefore need to be left for a long time. If fluid continues to collect after they are removed, it will have to be aspirated until the cavity heals completely. The length of hospital stay depends on the extent of the lesion.

Solitary lymph cyst

This is a variant of the cystic hygroma in which only one cyst is present. It is treated by simple excision.

3.3 Conditions of the mouth

Those conditions of the mouth to be considered include the following.
- Cleft lip and palate.
- Cysts in the mouth (p. 152).
- Benign tumours of the mouth (p. 157).
- Malignant tumours of the mouth (p. 158).
  Conditions of the tongue are considered in section 3.4.

Cleft lip and palate

One of the most common developmental abnormalities are cleft lip and palate (1 in 700 births). These occur when there is failure of fusion of the processes contributing to facial development (Fig. 3.3.1). 12% of cases are familial. The left side is more commonly affected than the right. Of those babies with abnormalities, 25% have a cleft lip alone and 25% have a cleft palate alone. The other 50% have both lesions. Fifteen per cent of cleft lips are bilateral.

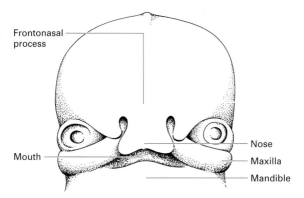

Fig. 3.3.1 Cleft lip and palate. The facial processes during development (7 weeks of gestation).

Recognizing the pattern

All but the most minor abnormalities are seen at birth. The main problem is with sucking and therefore feeding. Speech and dentition are also affected when there is a cleft palate, while a cleft lip on its own leads to an abnormality of facial development. Fifty per cent of patients with cleft palates have some hearing loss due to oedema around the eustachian tube.

On examination note:
- whether the condition is unilateral or bilateral
- whether the palate is involved
- how extensive the palatal lesion is.

A thorough general examination should be undertaken as 10% of cases have other abnormalities.

Management

Treatment is surgical repair and is undertaken by a specialist plastic surgeon. In a cleft lip alone feeding is unimpaired and the lesion may be repaired at about the age of 2–3 months so that normal facial development may occur.

A cleft palate is associated with feeding problems and the baby will need to be either spoon-fed or fed with liquid dripped into the mouth. The lesion is usually repaired between 1 and 2 years of age to avoid significant speech impairment and dentition problems.

When both abnormalities exist together, the cleft lip is often repaired at the age of 8 weeks and the cleft palate at the age of 1 year.

Cysts in the mouth

Mucous retention cysts

When the duct of a mucous gland becomes blocked, mucus collects under the epithelium of the lip. Although these cysts may occur anywhere where there are mucous glands, they are usually on the lower lip or inside the buccal mucosa (Fig. 3.3.2).

Recognizing the pattern

The patient may be of any age and complains of a slowly growing lump which is painless. It may be accidentally bitten. On

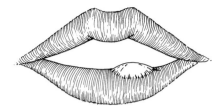

Fig. 3.3.2 A mucous retention cyst.

examination the cyst is a pale pink or blue colour with a 'glairy' appearance. It usually measures between 0.5 and 2.0 cm in diameter and is not fixed to the underlying muscle.

Management
OPERATION: REMOVAL OF MUCOUS RETENTION CYST
Although the operation may be carried out under a general anaesthetic (in a particularly nervous patient or in a child), it is usually done with local anaesthetic infiltration (e.g. 1% xylocaine with 1/200 000 adrenaline). The lip is incised and the cyst enucleated or deroofed.

Procedure profile

Blood requirement	0
Anaesthetic	LA (or GA if nervous)
Operation time	15–30 minutes
Hospital stay	Day case
Return to normal activity	2–3 hours

Ranula
Ranula is Latin for a small frog. The term is used to describe a unilateral cystic swelling in the floor of the mouth formed either from a blocked mucous gland or from an accessory salivary gland.

Recognizing the pattern

The patient is usually a child or young adult of either sex who presents with a history of a swelling in the floor of the mouth. This develops over a few weeks and may fluctuate in size. There may be a past history of similar swellings. The lump is painless.

On examination the swelling lies on one side of the floor of the mouth between the tongue and mandible. It is semitransparent, grey and up to 5 cm in diameter. It is smooth, spherical and cystic. It transilluminates. Rarely a ranula may possess a deep extension into the neck (possibly developing from the cervical sinus). The ranula is not attached to the overlying mucosa, mylohyoid or muscle of the tongue. The submandibular duct either overlies the lesion or is displaced to one side.

Management

Management is excision or marsupialization.

OPERATION: EXCISION/MARSUPIALIZATION OF RANULA

Ideally the cyst is completely excised. This is occasionally difficult and in that case it may be marsupialized, the remains of the cyst now becoming the floor of the mouth. If there is deep extension of the ranula below the mylohyoid, the cyst must be completely removed. This needs an approach from the neck as opposed to the floor of the mouth. Care has to be taken to avoid the submandibular duct and the lingual nerve.

Procedure profile

Blood requirement	0
Anaesthetic	GA
Operation time	Depends on extent and depth
Hospital stay	2–5 days
Return to normal activity	Variable

There is a risk of postoperative bleeding.

Dermoid cyst

This is a midline swelling in the floor of the mouth, originating during development by entrapment of ectoderm beneath the skin during fusion of the mandibular processes. It may be above or below the mylohyoid.

Recognizing the pattern

A patient of either sex usually presents between the ages of 10 and 25 years complaining of a painless swelling under the floor of the mouth. This may cause a double chin appearance. It may occasionally become infected. On examination the swelling is in the midline in the floor of the mouth or beneath the chin. It is 2–5 cm in diameter and is spherical, smooth and cystic or 'putty-like'. The contents are opaque and it will not transilluminate.

Management

OPERATION: EXCISION OF DERMOID CYST IN THE MOUTH

The cyst may be approached from an external incision beneath the mandible or a small one can be removed from within the mouth.

Procedure profile

Blood requirement	0
Anaesthetic	GA
Operation time	30 minutes
Hospital stay	Day case
Return to normal activity	1–2 weeks

Developmental cyst

This is a cyst that forms in the same way as a dermoid cyst but occurs within bone. The commonest is the globular maxillary cyst, which occurs in the upper jaw between the premaxilla and the maxilla, i.e. between the incisor and canine. Management is excision.

Dental cyst

This is a cyst around the root of an erupted but decayed or infected tooth, which develops from epithelial cells of the enamel organ.

Recognizing the pattern

The patient may be of any age or sex and presents with a diagnosis of painless swelling, usually of the upper jaw. There is a history of dental caries. The cyst may become infected and therefore painful.

Proving the diagnosis

The diagnosis is confirmed by X-ray.

Management

Treatment of dental cysts requires complete excision of the epithelial lining and is undertaken by an orodental surgeon. Obviously existing dental caries must also be treated.

Dentigerous cyst

This is a cyst containing an unerupted tooth and usually develops around the upper or lower third molar.

Recognizing the pattern

The patient is usually a young adult who presents with a painful swelling. On examination there is swelling of the jaw, usually near the upper or lower third molar, and this may have damaged the outer table of the bone. There will be one tooth missing.

Proving the diagnosis

The diagnosis is confirmed by X-ray.

Management

The cyst is excised by a dental surgeon (as under dental cyst above).

Alveolar abscess

This is an abscess formed around the root of a decaying tooth, often in a previous dental cyst. Under pressure the pus tracks out, usually through the thinner lateral plate of the jaw, to form an abscess beneath the cheek or mandible.

Recognizing the pattern

The patient is usually a child or young adult and presents with a dull, throbbing ache and swelling of the jaw. They may be generally unwell with a past history of dental caries. On examination the patient is pyrexial with a hot, tender, red swelling of the jaw, spreading to either the labial or buccal margin. When the patient still has their first dentition, either the upper or lower jaw may be affected. There is evidence of dental caries and there may be cervical lymphadenopathy.

Proving the diagnosis

The diagnosis is proved by X-ray.

Management

This consists of drainage and antibiotics. Advanced cases may be complicated by severe swelling of the floor of the mouth and the danger of incipient respiratory obstruction.

Benign tumours of the mouth

Epulis

An epulis is a localized swelling of the gum.

Fibrous epulis

This is a fibroma developing from the periodontal membrane and presenting as a localized lesion between the gum and the tooth. Malignant change may occur, forming a friable, bleeding mass.

The management is removal. Histology should be requested.

Bony epulis

This is an osteoclastoma causing the overlying gum to become locally hyperaemic and oedematous. It is also called a giant cell tumour. Depending on its size, it may be curetted out or may require excision of a large amount of mandible and bone grafting.

Granulomatous epulis

This is a mass of granulomatous tissue forming around a chronically infected or carious tooth or ill-fitting denture. The treatment is tooth extraction and curettage of the granulomatous tissue, which should be sent for histology.

Mixed salivary tumour (accessory pleomorphic adenoma)

There are accessory salivary glands in the oral cavity, particularly lining the hard palate, where salivary tumours can arise. As in the parotid gland, a mixed salivary tumour is benign but has an incomplete capsule. This may result in recurrence after simple enucleation. Malignant change is more common in accessory salivary glands than in the parotid.

Recognizing the pattern

The patient may be of either sex and is usually elderly. The lesion presents as a slowly growing but progressively enlarging painless lump in the palate. Eventually it may interfere with eating and speaking. On examination there is a smooth, hard lump beneath the mucous membrane. The mucosa is usually mobile over it. Initially the lump is also mobile over the mandible but it may later become attached. Alteration or a rapid increase in size suggests malignant change.

Proving the diagnosis

The diagnosis is proved by excision biopsy.

Management

Management is by excision with a margin of normal mucosa. It is unusual to have to remove palatal bone.

Malignant tumours of the mouth

Ameloblastoma

This is a locally invasive tumour of epithelial cells derived from the enamel organ and it resembles a basal cell carcinoma in both histological appearance and behaviour. It usually forms multi-loculated cysts.

Recognizing the pattern

The patient is usually a schoolchild or young adult, more commonly of African or Asian origin, who presents with a painless swelling of the jaw. There may be a past history of excision and recurrence. On examination there is swelling, usually of the molar region or the mandible, which may cause eggshell cracking of the overlying bone.

Proving the diagnosis

The X-ray appearances are characteristic. There are large loculi in the bone, which has a honeycomb appearance. This differentiates it from the cysts described above.

Management

Local curettage is inadequate as the condition will recur. The tumour must be excised with a margin of normal bone either side and bone graft may be required postoperatively.

Carcinoma of the lip

This carcinoma is often called 'countryman's lip'. Histologically it is a keratinizing squamous cell carcinoma. Aetiological factors include pipe-smoking and long exposure to sunlight or severe weather.

Of the lesions, 93% occur in the lower lip, 5% in the upper lip and 2% at the angle of the mouth. The lymphatic drainage is to the submental nodes if the lesion is in the lower lip and to the submandibular nodes if the lesion is in the upper lip. Blood-borne spread to the liver and lungs is late and rare. Lesions in the angle of the mouth have a worse prognosis due to the involvement of two lymph fields.

Recognizing the pattern

Ninety per cent occur in men aged over 65 years. Most have led an active outdoor life or have been pipe-smokers. The history is of a chronic ulcer of the lip which enlarges and fails to heal.

It may present as a warty growth or a fissure. More advanced lesions may be painful, become infected and disturb eating. On examination the ulcer usually has a characteristic raised rolled edge with bloodstained slough in the base.

Proving the diagnosis
This is done by biopsy.

Management
An early lesion may be treated by either surgery or radiotherapy. There is a 75% 5-year survival with either form of treatment. Some of these lesions are small and can be treated as an out-patient procedure under a local anaesthetic. A larger lesion will require resection and plastic reconstruction of the lip.

OPERATION: WEDGE EXCISION OF CARCINOMA OF THE LIP

A simple wedge resection is performed (Fig. 3.3.3). There is marked bleeding from the marginal artery of the lip and this can be controlled by pressure on the lip while a suture is inserted. It is important to remove an adequate margin of normal tissue on either side. The cosmetic result is very satisfactory.

Procedure profile

Blood requirement	0
Anaesthetic	GA or LA
Operation time	30–60 minutes
Hospital stay	Day case
Return to normal activity	3 days – 2 weeks

Squamous cell carcinoma
Squamous cell carcinoma or anaplastic variants of it can occur at any site in the mouth where there is stratified squamous epithelium. Carcinoma of the tongue is an example (p. 166). The presentation and management of lesions elsewhere depends on the precise site and extent of the lesion. The mainstay of treatment is

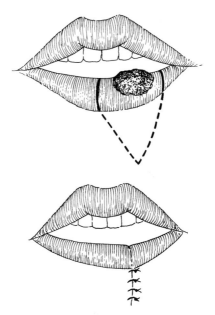

Fig. 3.3.3 Wedge excision of carcinoma of lip.

either radiotherapy or excision with or without reconstructive surgery.

Malignant melanoma

Malignant melanoma can rarely occur in any part of the lining of the mouth. Its treatment is considered in the section on skin conditions (p. 554).

Tumours of the jaw

These may be either primary or secondary and both are rare.

Carcinoma of the maxillary antrum

The maxillary antrum is lined by respiratory epithelium. The usual type of carcinoma occurring in this site is a squamous cell carcinoma, although adenocarcinomas are also seen. Carcinoma in the nasal sinuses occurs in woodworkers after a long latent period.

Recognizing the pattern
The patient is usually male and elderly. The primary is usually undetected whilst it remains within the sinus and only becomes evident when it has invaded the surrounding structures including either the orbit, the nasal cavity or the hard palate and upper jaw. In these situations it presents as a mass or an ulcerated lesion. On examination the tumour is then fixed to bone.

Proving the diagnosis
The diagnosis is confirmed by CT scanning and MRI.

Management
This consists of either radiotherapy, or excision and reconstruction. Combined therapy with radiotherapy and surgery is often used.

Malignant disease of the tonsil
Malignant disease of the tonsil is usually due to squamous cell carcinoma (85%) or a lymphosarcoma. The lymphoid tissue may also be involved in a more generalized lymphoma. A carcinoma of the tonsil spreads to adjacent structures such as the palate and base of the tongue and thence on to the deep cervical nodes.

Recognizing the pattern
The patient with squamous cell carcinoma is usually over the age of 60 years and presents with pain in the throat which radiates to the ear. There is progressive enlargement of the tonsil causing dysphagia and 'thickening' of the speech. Eventually the growth ulcerates, causing bleeding and marked fetor oris.

In contrast, lymphosarcoma occurs in slightly younger patients between the ages of 50 and 65 years and the enlargement is usually painless. Ulceration and bleeding occur very late.

The ipsilateral deep cervical nodes may be enlarged due to secondary growth or due to infection secondary to a malignant ulcer.

Proving the diagnosis
The diagnosis is proved by biopsy of the enlarged tonsil.

Management
Both types of tumour are treated by radiotherapy to the affected tonsil and the ipsilateral side of the neck. Large squamous cell tumours are occasionally treated by surgical resection combined with radiotherapy. Metastases in the cervical nodes may be treated by dissection of the neck (see p. 169).

3.4 Conditions of the tongue

Glossitis

Glossitis is frequently associated with anaemia – particularly iron deficiency and pernicious anaemia. It also occurs with candidiasis and riboflavin deficiency. Lichen planus may also cause a smooth tongue.

Recognizing the pattern
Glossitis associated with anaemia is more common in females. The tongue is smooth, red and usually sore. Glossitis associated with candidiasis is also red, smooth and sore and often associated with antibiotic usage and the patient may have angular stomatitis. Lichen planus may result in a smooth tongue but if it is not ulcerated then it is not usually sore. There may be a whitish layer on the surface of the tongue.

Management
Haematological abnormalities must be investigated including mean corpuscular volume (MCV) and serum iron, ferritin, B12 and folate and treated appropriately. Candidiasis should be swabbed for identification. Masses of hyphae can be seen on a Gram-stained smear. Treatment is with oral antifungal agents. Lichen planus is diagnosed by biopsy and is treated symptomatically.

Tongue ulcers

Tongue ulcers may be:
- traumatic
- aphthous
- tuberculous
- syphilitic
- chronic non-specific
- carcinomatous.

Traumatic ulceration
This is an ulcer on the side of the tongue caused by a sharp tooth or ill-fitting denture.

Recognizing the pattern
The patient is of any age and complains of a painful ulcer on the side of the tongue. On examination there is a chronic infected ulcer close to a cause such as a cracked tooth or an ill-fitting denture.

Management
When the cause is removed or remedied, the ulcer heals over a few days.

Aphthous ulceration
The aetiology of these small ulcers is unknown and includes haematological deficiencies, infections, gastrointestinal disease, immunological and genetic factors.

Recognizing the pattern
The patient is usually an adolescent or young adult and the condition is more common in women than men. The ulcers are very painful. On examination there is a small, round, white ulcer on the tongue, gums or inner aspect of the lips. The ulcers may be multiple.

Management
The patient should be reassured that the condition is not serious. The ulcer will heal on its own over a period of about 10 days. Healing can be hastened by topical hydrocortisone tablets. Oral

salicylate gel gives symptomatic relief. If the ulcer fails to heal, then the diagnosis should be reviewed and if necessary a biopsy performed.

Tuberculous ulcer
This is now a rare cause of tongue ulceration. It occurs in undiagnosed advanced pulmonary tuberculosis.

Recognizing the pattern
Multiple, very painful ulcers with undermined edges occur along the edges of the tongue.

Proving the diagnosis
The diagnosis of tuberculosis is proved on chest X-rays, sputum culture and microscopy.

Management
Treatment is antituberculous therapy.

Syphilitic ulcer
The typical lesions of the tongue are the chancre of primary syphilis, snail-track ulcers, Hutchinson's wart of secondary syphilis and the gumma of tertiary syphilis.

Treatment is with antibiotics (penicillin).

Chronic non-specific ulcer
This is a chronic ulcer which is usually situated on the anterior two-thirds of the tongue. No predisposing factor can be found. The lesion is usually painful. Syphilis and tuberculosis are excluded by investigation. The diagnosis is confirmed and the lesion cured by excision biopsy.

Neoplasms of the tongue

These may be either benign or malignant. Most benign neoplasms of the tongue are rare. The following may occur:
- papilloma
- haemangiomas

- lingual thyroid
- neurofibroma
- lipoma.

These are treated by excision. In the case of a lingual thyroid, it is important to be sure that there is other thyroid tissue lower down in the neck. A thyroid isotope scan will give this information.

Carcinoma of the tongue

This is usually a squamous cell carcinoma. Tobacco and alcohol are the most important causes of squamous cell carcinoma. The prognosis becomes worse the further back the lesion is on the tongue. Overall the 5-year survival is 25%.

Recognizing the pattern

The patient usually presents between the ages of 60 and 70 years. Carcinoma of the tongue used to be much more common in men, although changes in the epidemiology of smoking are leading to an increased incidence in women. More advanced carcinomas cause pain in the tongue, which may be referred to the ear. There may also be excessive salivation and defective tongue movement or difficulty with speech due to spread into the floor of the mouth. If the lesion becomes infected, fetor oris results. On examination the lesion may be one of the following.

- An exophytic growth with a broad firm base and surrounding induration.
- An ulcer with typical everted rolled edge and infected bleeding slough in the base.
- A hard indistinct nodule.

The patient may have had a pad of cotton wool in their ear for the pain and there may be evidence of secondary lymph node involvement. The extent of secondary spread must be assessed. The tip of the tongue and the posterior third have bilateral lymphatic drainage (Fig. 3.4.1) so examine both sides of the neck. Blood spread occurs late and almost always from carcinoma on the posterior third of the tongue.

Proving the diagnosis

The diagnosis is confirmed by biopsy. The differential diagnosis includes that of other ulcers of the tongue (see p. 164) and other solid lesions of the tongue (see p. 165).

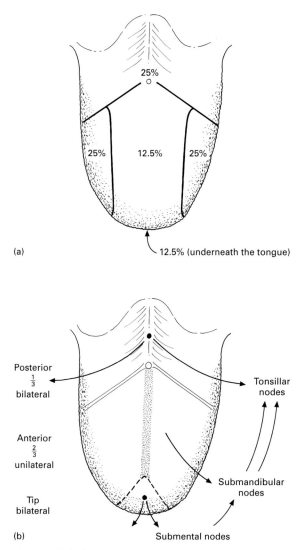

Fig. 3.4.1 (a) The distribution of sites of malignancy of the tongue. (b) The lymphatic drainage of the tongue.

Other investigations should include the following.
- Full blood count and ESR.
- Chest X-ray.
- CT or MRI scan of the head and neck and X-rays of the mandible if tumour extent and bone invasion are to be assessed.

Management

Treatment is by excision and/or radiotherapy. The latter can be administered either as external beam or by radioactive implants. The choice of type of therapy depends on the extent of the lesion.

A small lesion less than 1 cm in diameter may be excised locally. With larger lesions surgery is extensive and consists of either a partial glossectomy, a hemiglossectomy or subtotal glossectomy (see below). If lymph nodes are involved, a dissection of the neck lymph nodes will be required.

Preoperative mouthwashes may help to clean up an infected lesion.

OPERATION: PARTIAL GLOSSECTOMY FOR CARCINOMA OF THE TONGUE

The amount of tissue removed depends on the size of the lesion and an adequate margin is necessary (at least 1 cm). Bleeding may be profuse and the assistant can help to control this by compressing one side of the tongue posteriorly to compress the lingual artery.

Procedure profile

Blood requirement	Group and save
Anaesthetic	GA
Operation time	1 hour
Hospital stay	3–5 days
Return to normal activity	1 month

Postoperatively regular daily mouthwashes are given.

OPERATION: HEMIGLOSSECTOMY

In this operation half the tongue is removed. It is performed for lesions of the lateral border of the tongue that are clear of the mandible. A neck dissection is required if lymphadenopathy is present. In a clinically unaffected neck, a selective neck dissection may still be required to identify vessels for microvascular reconstruction of the tongue with a free flap (see below) or to clear microscopic disease.

Procedure profile

Blood requirement	2
Anaesthetic	GA
Operation time	1–3 hours
Hospital stay	10–14 days
Return to normal activity	4–6 weeks

OPERATION: NECK DISSECTION

This operation is undertaken as part of an attempted radical cure of any lesion which has spread to the cervical lymph nodes. A variety of neck dissections can be performed, the most common being a radical neck dissection of the lymph nodes in continuity with the internal jugular vein and the sternomastoid muscle.

Procedure profile

Blood requirement	2
Anaesthetic	GA
Operation time	3–5 hours
Hospital stay	7–10 days
Return to normal activity	4–6 weeks

OPERATION: COMPOSITE RESECTION

In this procedure an extensive dissection of the neck, mouth and pharynx is carried out, including a segment of the body or ramus of the mandible. The intraoral defect is repaired, using a vascularized skin flap. The symphysis menti, geniohyoid and genioglossus muscles are disrupted, and the airway is in danger as the tongue is liable to fall back. Elective tracheostomy is required. A fine-bore nasogastric tube is used for feeding purposes.

Procedure profile

Blood requirement	4
Anaesthetic	GA
Operation time	6–8 hours
Hospital stay	3–4 weeks
Return to normal activity	3 months

4 Endocrine surgery

4.1 Swellings of the thyroid gland

Assessment

Faced with a swelling in the pretracheal region of the neck, you have to decide on the following.
- Is it in the thyroid?
- Is it solitary or generalized?
- Is the patient euthyroid or not?
- Which investigations will be needed?

Is the swelling in the thyroid gland?

The term 'goitre' applies to any swelling in the thyroid and is not a diagnostic term.

The thyroid gland is situated behind the pretracheal fascia and, as this fascia is attached to the larynx, the gland moves up and down on swallowing. This feature makes the diagnosis of thyroid swellings easy. The clinician first observes the lump from in front and then feels it standing behind the patient. The patient is asked to swallow from a glass of water and the movement of the lump is noted.

Is it solitary or generalized?

Is the enlargement:
- diffuse, involving the whole gland? This is dealt with on p. 173
- a nodule within the gland (solitary nodule)? This is dealt with on p. 178.

Is the patient euthyroid or not?

The patient may be:
- thyrotoxic

Surgery: Diagnosis and Management, 4th edition. Edited by N. Rawlinson and D. Alderson. © 2009 Blackwell Publishing, ISBN: 978-1-4051-2921-3

- euthyroid, i.e. normal
- hypothyroid.

Patients with thyrotoxicosis have an overactive thyroid gland causing symptoms of tiredness, weight loss, anxiety, tremor, palpitations and amenorrhoea, and tend to prefer cold to hot weather. On examination there is nervousness and agitation, a tachycardia of over 100, fine tremor of the fingers and lid lag. There may also be exophthalmos. A bruit is occasionally audible over a toxic goitre.

Hypothyroid patients are slow in thought, speech and movement, are overweight, have thickened skin and tend to lose their hair. They have a slow pulse rate. They prefer warm weather.

Investigations for thyroid swellings

The following tests are used to investigate thyroid swellings.

- Serum tri-iodothyronine and tetra-iodothyronine (T3 and T4). These are raised in thyrotoxicosis.
- Thyroid-stimulating hormone (TSH). This gives an indication of the activity of the pituitary in stimulating the thyroid. There is a feedback mechanism whereby TSH is raised when the thyroid hormone level is below normal. An elevated TSH therefore confirms hypothyroidism. In hyperthyroidism it is depressed. The sensitive immunoradiometric assay (IRMA) for TSH is very accurate in detecting hypo- and hyperthyroidism.
- Thyrotrophin-releasing hormone test (TRH test). In this test TSH levels are measured after a dose of TRH (200 μg in 2 mL i.v.). Normally this produces a rise in TSH by 20 min and levels fall again by 60 min after the injection. No such rise occurs in thyrotoxicosis because the pituitary is suppressed by the high T4 level. The rise is exaggerated in primary hypothyroidism.
- Thyroid antibody estimation (see Hashimoto's disease, p. 174).
- CT scan of neck and upper mediastinum. The important points to look for are whether the trachea is deviated and whether it is narrow in either its anteroposterior or lateral diameter.
- Fine-needle aspiration cytology. This has largely superseded radioactive scans in the investigation of thyroid disease.
- Thyroid scan. The patient is given radioactive iodine to drink and the uptake in the thyroid gland is plotted. A toxic gland shows a markedly increased uptake of radioactive tracer over

the normal. This increased uptake may be generalized as in Graves' disease, or focal (a 'hot nodule') as in a toxic autonomous nodule. A cold (inactive) nodule suggests possible malignancy.

- Ultrasound scan. This shows if the lump is solid or cystic and may show if it is solitary or part of a multinodular goitre.

Diffuse goitres

There are four main types:
- physiological
- nodular
- inflammatory
- toxic.

Physiological goitre
A physiological goitre occurs at puberty, during pregnancy and in conditions of iodine deficiency. Apart from the latter state, no treatment is necessary.

Nodular goitre
A nodular goitre can be a benign or malignant enlargement of the thyroid gland with areas of hyperplasia and involution. Treatment is necessary when:
- the patient becomes thyrotoxic
- there is compression of other neck structures, resulting in dyspnoea or dysphagia
- the patient is particularly worried by the cosmetic appearance of the goitre
- a focal increase in size or the development of hoarseness (due to recurrent laryngeal nerve palsy) suggests malignant change.

   In any of these cases thyroidectomy may be indicated (see below).

Inflammatory goitre
The usual causes of diffuse inflammation of the thyroid gland are Hashimoto's disease and De Quervain's thyroiditis. Riedel's thyroiditis is very rare.

Hashimoto's disease

In this condition antibodies are produced against thyroglobulin and microsomes.

Recognizing the pattern

The patient is usually a middle-aged female who presents with a goitre and is usually at first thyrotoxic and later hypothyroid. The gland is diffusely enlarged initially, but later becomes replaced by a small fibrotic remnant with a characteristic bosse-lated firm surface.

Proving the diagnosis

The diagnosis is proved by finding thyroid antibodies in the serum, and a characteristic picture on fine-needle biopsy.

Management

Patients should be warned that they may eventually require thyroid hormone replacement. If they are already myxoedematous, this should be instituted (T4 50–200 μg/day). Thyroidectomy is occasionally required to relieve pressure symptoms, for cosmetic reasons or to establish a diagnosis (see p. 177).

De Quervain's thyroiditis

This is a non-suppurative inflammation of the gland due to a viral infection. The usual infective agent is the coxsackie virus.

Recognizing the pattern

A patient of either sex (more commonly female) presents with an acutely swollen, tender gland, often preceded by a sore throat and mild constitutional upset. The patient becomes pyrexial and transiently thyrotoxic. Hypothyroidism is very unlikely in the long term.

Proving the diagnosis

There may be a lymphocytosis and a raised erythrocyte sedimentation rate (ESR). Typically the T4 may be elevated in the acute state. There are no thyroid antibodies in the serum.

Management

Mild analgesia is usually sufficient. More severe cases may be treated with courses of prednisolone (10–20 mg/day). The condition settles spontaneously but may recur.

Riedel's thyroiditis

Riedel's thyroiditis is a rare condition of the thyroid in which the gland becomes hard and enlarged with infiltration of scar tissue, which then involves the surrounding tissues. It results in hypothyroidism and sometimes recurrent laryngeal nerve palsy and stridor. Because of these features, it mimics carcinoma of the thyroid. It often has to be biopsied in order to establish the diagnosis. The management, once the diagnosis is established, is to leave well alone and treat with T4 if the patient becomes hypothyroid.

Toxic goitre (thyrotoxicosis or Graves' disease)

Thyroid hormones regulate the basal metabolic rate. Their own level is controlled by TSH, released by the pituitary. Graves' thyrotoxicosis is an autoimmune disease. Autoantibodies against the TSH receptor on thyroid membrane stimulate the gland. The TSH levels are abnormally low.

The condition has a familial incidence, and there is an association between it and other autoimmune diseases (e.g. myasthenia gravis, pernicious anaemia, Addison's disease). There is diffuse enlargement of the gland with hyperplasia and hypertrophy. There may be a lymphocyte and plasma cell infiltration. In approximately 25% of patients the disease is self-limiting.

Recognizing the pattern

Females are more often affected than males and the disease usually occurs between the ages of 15 and 45 years. Thyrotoxicosis may, however, occur in both younger and older patients. The symptoms of toxicity are described on p. 172.

In a toxic goitre the gland is smoothly enlarged and the patient shows signs of thyrotoxicosis. The skin over the gland may be warm and there is often a systolic bruit. Thyrotoxicosis may also be associated with exophthalmos or pretibial myxoedema.

Proving the diagnosis
The investigations are described above.

Management
There are three possible forms of management available for the thyrotoxic patient.
- Medical treatment. This is the first-line treatment of Graves' disease in patients younger than 50, providing the goitre is not too large.
  ◦ The production of thyroid hormones can be blocked using drugs such as carbimazole (5–10 mg 8-hourly) or propylthiouracil (100 mg 8–hourly). The drugs are stopped after 18–24 months. If the patient relapses, then surgery should be considered.
  ◦ Propranolol gives symptomatic relief, particularly of tachycardia, palpitations, tremor, sweating and nervousness. The usual dose is 80–120 mg/day in divided doses. It is used in the preoperative preparation of the patient (see below) and in the control of a 'thyroid crisis'.
- Radioactive iodine treatment. This is used for patients over 50 and after the child-bearing years. It is used for recurrent thyrotoxicosis. The patient drinks radioactive iodine, which is concentrated in the thyroid, which thus undergoes self-destruction. A variable dose is required and it takes about 3 months to take effect. In that time propranolol is used to control symptoms. A second dose of radioactive iodine may be needed. Regular follow-up is required and at least 40% of patients become hypothyroid within 10 years, requiring replacement therapy.
- Surgical treatment by thyroidectomy is indicated for patients:
  ◦ with large goitres that are causing pressure symptoms or are unsightly
  ◦ who relapse after one or two courses of drugs
  ◦ with nodular goitre
  ◦ who do not want the inconvenience of prolonged medical treatment
  ◦ who are young. These patients have a high relapse rate and many physicians refer patients under the age of 25 years for surgery as soon as they become euthyroid, rather than undertaking a trial of medical therapy

◦ who are planning a pregnancy or have a young family where radioiodine use would require segregation from the children for some weeks.

OPERATION: SUBTOTAL THYROIDECTOMY

(Total thyroidectomy is also used to treat thyrotoxicosis – see later.)

It is dangerous to operate on a patient who is actively thyrotoxic. Manipulation of the gland during operation produces considerably raised blood levels of T4 and this can result in a 'thyroid crisis' (see p. 178). A crisis is prevented by adequate preoperative preparation. The patient is made euthyroid by using carbimazole or some other antithyroid agent that blocks the production of T4. Thyroxine is prescribed as replacement therapy once the patient is no longer thyrotoxic.

The patient's serum must also be checked for antibodies as thyrotoxicity is not uncommon early in Hashimoto's disease and thyroidectomy may be contraindicated in this condition. Take blood to check the calcium level.

The thyroid is exposed by a 'collar' incision. Care is taken to avoid damage to the recurrent laryngeal nerves and also the parathyroid glands. Seven-eighths of the thyroid gland is removed, leaving remnants posteriorly on both sides of the trachea. The wound is drained with suction.

Procedure profile

Blood requirement	Group and save
Anaesthetic	GA
Operation time	90–120 minutes
Hospital stay	2–3 days
Return to normal activity	3–4 weeks

Postoperative observation must be close. Rarely the neck swells up rapidly due to haemorrhage, and there is a danger of compression of the trachea. In this case the wound may have to be reopened in the ward to avoid asphyxia. Wound clip removers must accompany the patient. When the neck has been decompressed, the patient is returned to theatre to restore haemostasis.

Postoperative stridor may be due to laryngeal oedema and unconnected with contained haemorrhage. The patient must be returned to theatre and re-intubated by an experienced anaesthetist. Failure to reinsert the tube will necessitate tracheostomy. The intubated patient is nursed in intensive care for 12 h, given hydrocortisone or dexamethasone and can usually be extubated without problem.

The vocal cords should be routinely checked to ensure that the recurrent nerves have not been damaged. Hypocalcaemia is an occasional complication of operations for thyrotoxicosis. This may be due to accidental damage to parathyroid glands but is more often due to temporary ischaemia. If the serum calcium does fall, tetany may occur (see p. 192), if not treated promptly. Routine postoperative calcium levels should be checked in all patients.

Long term the patient should be reviewed regularly for signs of developing myxoedema. The serum T3, T4 and TSH are measured regularly.

Management of thyroid crisis

This is caused by a sudden surge of T4 and may occur if surgery is performed on inadequately prepared patients. Signs include delirium, anxiety, tachycardia, cardiac failure, hyperpyrexia, abdominal pain and diarrhoea. It may result in adrenal failure and coma.

It is treated by a slow infusion of propranolol (5–15 mg) followed by oral administration of 40 mg 8-hourly. Intravenous fluids may be required and steroids may be given to cover adrenal failure.

Solitary thyroid nodule

Lesions presenting as solitary thyroid nodules can be classified as follows.
- Benign:
  - cyst
  - adenoma
  - a dominant nodule in a nodular goitre.

- Malignant, primary:
  - thyroid adenocarcinoma
  - malignant lymphoma
  - medullary carcinoma.
- Malignant, secondary:
  - breast
  - colon
  - kidney
  - lung.

Recognizing the pattern

Having decided that the swelling is in the thyroid, determine whether the opposite lobe of the thyroid is also palpable and whether it is nodular. In this way you may be able to determine whether the nodule is truly solitary or part of a nodular goitre. The patient should also be fully examined to determine their thyroid status (as on p. 171).

Proving the diagnosis

All solitary nodules should be investigated by the following.

- Fine-needle aspiration cytology. A fine-bore needle is positioned in the tumour and cells aspirated. The smear produced is interpreted by a cytopathologist.
- Thyroid hormones (T3, T4, TSH). These determine the patient's thyroid status.
- Thyroid antibodies. To look for evidence of thyroiditis.

Management

Cystic lesions may be aspirated. Some solitary solid thyroid nodules will require surgical removal and histological examination in order to exclude thyroid malignancy. This usually involves a thyroid lobectomy +/– full thyroidectomy. This will first be described, followed by some notes on the individual lesions presenting as a solitary thyroid nodule.

Preoperatively the patient is warned of the slight danger of a husky voice following the operation.

OPERATION: THYROID LOBECTOMY

The thyroid gland is explored through a 'collar' incision. The involved lobe is exposed and excised completely. In order to do

this the recurrent laryngeal nerve must be exposed, and both
parathyroids preserved.

There are differing views as to what to do once the lobe has
been removed. Some surgeons send it for frozen-section histology and may proceed to a full total thyroidectomy at the same
operation if the lesion is malignant. Others will leave the contralateral lobe strictly alone and be prepared to come back and
remove the other lobe later if necessary (see under management
of individual thyroid carcinomas). Frozen-section histology of
thyroid tumours is not easy.

Procedure profile

Blood requirement	Group and save
Anaesthetic	GA
Operation time	40–60 minutes
Hospital stay	Day case or overnight
Return to normal activity	2 weeks

Postoperative care is as for subtotal thyroidectomy and is
described on p. 177. Hypocalcaemia and hypothyroidism are not
a problem if the other lobe has been left intact.

OPERATION: TOTAL THYROIDECTOMY
In this procedure both lobes of the gland are removed. There is
an increased danger of parathyroid deficiency postoperatively.
Transient hypocalcaemia occurs in up to 15% of patients.

Procedure profile

Blood requirement	Group and save
Anaesthetic	GA
Operation time	1–2 hours
Hospital stay	2–3 days
Return to normal activity	2 weeks

Postoperatively the serum calcium is monitored daily and any hypoparathyroidism treated as on p. 192. The patient will require thyroid replacement therapy (150 μg/day of T4).

In the unlikely event of both recurrent laryngeal nerves being damaged at operation, the patient will develop severe stridor or complete airway obstruction. Emergency re-intubation is required and a tracheostomy may be necessary.

Cysts and adenomas

Thyroid cyst

This is usually a degenerative part of a nodular goitre although true thyroid cysts do occur. A common complication is haemorrhage into the cyst. When this occurs, there is rapid enlargement and the lump may be painful. There is a possibility that such rapid enlargement may compress the trachea.

Recognizing the pattern

The patient is of any age and is euthyroid. There may be a history of rapid enlargement and pain.

Proving the diagnosis

The lump may be shown to be cystic on fine-needle aspiration.

Management

If the swelling is thought to be cystic and the rest of the gland is normal treatment will be to simply aspirate the cyst. Some carcinomas have cystic areas in them but cytology should identify these. Excise the cyst if malignancy is suspected or if the cyst repeatedly refills.

Thyroid adenomas

There are four types of thyroid adenoma. The names refer to the histological appearance. They are:
- papillary
- follicular
- embryonal
- Hurthle cell.

Recognizing the pattern
A few adenomas are functioning and may even produce thyrotoxicosis (solitary hot nodule). Occasionally haemorrhage may
occur into the tumour causing a rapid increase in size. A solitary
nodule often turns out to be the dominant nodule in a multinodular goitre and not truly solitary. However, this should be
detected by an ultrasound scan preoperatively.

Management
The distinction from a carcinoma can only be made on histological examination in the case of follicular adenomas. For this
reason all follicular adenomas are excised by thyroid lobectomy.

Carcinoma of the thyroid

There are five types of primary thyroid malignancy:
- papillary adenocarcinoma
- follicular adenocarcinoma
- anaplastic carcinoma
- medullary carcinoma
- lymphoma.

Recognizing the pattern
Each has a characteristic pattern of behaviour and management
plan.

PAPILLARY CARCINOMA
This is of low-grade malignancy and rarely fatal. It occurs in the
younger age group, usually in children or young adults, and is
more common in females. On histology there is hyperplastic
epithelium in the follicles with very little colloid. The disease may
be multifocal. It tends to spread to lymph nodes and these may
appear before the primary growth is palpable. This was described
in the past as a 'lateral aberrant thyroid'. There is an association
with irradiation of the neck in childhood.

Management
Papillary carcinomas are hormone sensitive. Following thyroid

lobectomy the patient is started on T4 and maintained on this therapy for life. Some surgeons perform a total thyroidectomy for this lesion because of its multifocal nature. Others adopt a 'wait and see' policy and remove the other lobe of the thyroid gland if there is evidence of further disease. Direct suppression is achieved with T4 100 µg/day. Radioiodine is used to treat metastases.

FOLLICULAR CARCINOMA

This tends to occur in slightly older patients, often middle aged. Females are more affected than males. The growth spreads through the bloodstream and bony secondaries are common. The lesion may arise in a pre-existing nodular goitre. The tumour is radiosensitive.

Management

Total thyroidectomy is the operation of choice. Radioactive iodine is the treatment of choice for secondary disease. Metastases will not, however, take up the iodine if the rest of the thyroid is present and the gland has to be ablated by radioactive iodine or excised before they can be treated. Metastases can then be detected and treated by further radioactive iodine. Patients with follicular carcinoma are also maintained on T4 suppression therapy.

ANAPLASTIC CARCINOMA

This is an aggressive neoplasm that occurs in elderly patients, particularly in women. It grows rapidly and infiltrates the tissues in the neck. Compression of the trachea is common. Cervical lymphadenopathy and recurrent nerve paresis are often apparent when the patient is first seen.

Management

Many anaplastic carcinomas are sensitive to external-beam radiotherapy and this is the treatment of choice, although there are special problems when the airway is compromised, as it frequently is. Treatment with radiotherapy causes further swelling of the gland and this can prove fatal. A tracheostomy may be required. This can sometimes be carried out at the initial biopsy operation.

MEDULLARY CARCINOMA

This arises in the parafollicular C cells. It is of moderate malignancy and spreads to lymph nodes. It secretes calcitonin which can then be used as a tumour marker. There is a familial incidence and an association with adenomas elsewhere (see p. 192). Genetic screening is now available to detect the affected relatives of the index case. The patient may be of any age and the tumour has an equal sex incidence. In these respects it is different from other thyroid carcinomas. It is also much less common.

Management

Medullary carcinoma is treated by total thyroidectomy and central dissection of lymph nodes. Calcitonin can be regularly measured postoperatively to detect metastases.

MALIGNANT LYMPHOMA

This arises in lymphatic tissue in the thyroid gland. They may also occur as secondaries from other sites. Lymphomas may occur in patients with Hashimoto's thyroiditis.

Management

They are treated in the same way as lymphomas elsewhere, by chemo- or radiotherapy and apart from biopsy, surgery has little role to play.

Thyroglossal cyst

The thyroid develops from the floor of the mouth. It migrates down from the foramen caecum of the tongue, passing anterior to, and then behind, the hyoid bone, to eventually lie in the pretracheal space. As it descends it leaves a small canal connected to the tongue called the thyroglossal duct (Fig. 4.1.1a). Remnants of this duct may persist and give rise to a thyroglossal cyst.

The cyst lies in the midline anywhere between the chin and the thyroid isthmus; 50% lie over the hyoid bone. It may be connected to the tongue or the thyroid by fibrous remnants of the thyroglossal duct. Very occasionally these remain patent, forming either a sinus or a thyroglossal fistula.

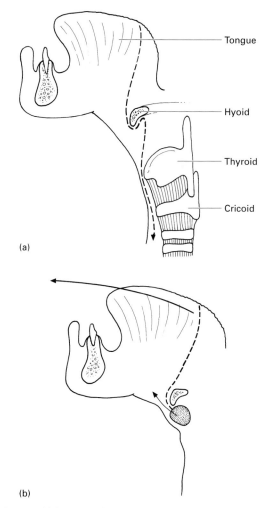

Tongue

Hyoid

Thyroid

Cricoid

(a)

(b)

Fig. 4.1.1 (a) The descent of the thyroid – the track forms the thyroglossal duct. (b) As the tongue is protruded a thyroglossal cyst moves upward.

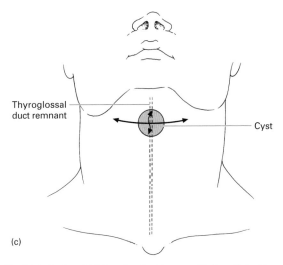

Thyroglossal duct remnant

Cyst

(c)

Fig. 4.1.1 *Continued* (c) A thyroglossal cyst is more mobile from side to side than up and down.

Recognizing the pattern

The patient may be of any age, although the condition is commoner between the ages of 15 and 30 years. Women are more often affected.

The patient notices a painless lump in the neck. It may become infected, in which case it presents as a localized abscess which points to the skin.

On examination there is a smooth, round, 1–3 cm diameter swelling lying in the midline of the neck, often near the hyoid bone. The skin moves over it unless it has been fixed by scarring following an episode of inflammation. The lump is of firm consistency and may fluctuate and transilluminate.

Ask the patient to open the mouth, steady the jaw and then protrude the tongue. Characteristically the cyst will move upwards (Fig. 4.1.1b). This may be easier to feel than see and is due to traction on the fibrous remnant of the thyroglossal duct. The cyst is more mobile from side to side than up and down (Fig. 4.1.1c). It may also move on swallowing, due to its attachment to the hyoid bone.

Palpate the base of the tongue for any thyroid tissue and look for any sinus opening to the skin (usually just above the thyroid isthmus).

Management

The treatment is to excise the cyst and any remnant of the thyroglossal duct. Because of the latter, the operation is more extensive than the patient will expect and they should be informed of this preoperatively.

OPERATION: EXCISION OF THYROGLOSSAL CYST
A transverse elliptical incision is made over the lump and the cyst is dissected out. The fibrous track running up towards the tongue is also excised and this should include removing the central portion of the body of the hyoid bone. Similarly any downward extensions are also removed.

Procedure profile

Blood requirement	Group and save
Anaesthetic	GA
Operation time	30–60 minutes
Hospital stay	Day case or overnight
Return to normal activity	2 weeks

The postoperative care is usually uncomplicated. If remnants of the track have been left behind, however, recurrent sepsis can occur.

4.2 Parathyroids

Hyperparathyroidism

The diagnosis and management of hyperparathyroidism rests on an understanding of the nature and physiology of the parathyroid glands and their secretion, parathormone. There are two glands on each side of the neck and they lie behind the thyroid gland. Each measures about $4 \times 2 \times 2$ mm. They consist of one main cell type, the 'chief cell', which has a 'water clear' appearance on microscopy when it is active.

Parathormone is an amino acid peptide hormone which regulates calcium metabolism. Its secretion is controlled by the serum calcium level, being increased in hypocalcaemic states. It has effects on the kidney, bone and gastrointestinal tract.

- In the kidney it increases the reabsorption of filtered calcium. It also stimulates the production of the active metabolite of vitamin D.
- In bone parathormone increases the number and osteolytic activity of osteoclasts and osteocytes, thereby mobilizing both calcium and phosphate. Vitamin D metabolites are necessary for this process.
- In the gut parathormone indirectly increases calcium absorption by increasing the production of 1,25-dihydroxycholecalciferol (the active metabolite of vitamin D).

Hyperparathyroidism may be primary, secondary or tertiary. Primary hyperparathyroidism occurs when the parathyroid glands may become overactive and secrete excess parathormone causing hypercalcaemia. Secondary hyperparathyroidism occurs as a physiological response to chronic hypocalcaemia (e.g. chronic renal failure). Occasionally one of the glands involved in secondary hyperparathyroidism may develop an autonomous adenoma. This is tertiary hyperparathyroidism.

Primary hyperparathyroidism

This is due to one of the following.

- A solitary benign adenoma (in 90% of cases of hyperparathyroidism).
- More than one adenoma (2%).
- Generalized hyperplasia of all four glands (6%).
- Carcinoma (2%): this is locally invasive and may metastasize via the bloodstream. Recurrence after removal is common.

Recognizing the pattern

Primary hyperparathyroidism is more common in women than men and is usually seen after the age of 40 years. There may be a familial history of multiple endocrine neoplasia (see p. 192). The majority of cases diagnosed are asymptomatic and discovered incidentally on biochemical analysis. When present the clinical features are varied.

- Renal stones. The patient presents with ureteric colic, haematuria or urinary tract infection; 3% of those with stones are shown to have primary hyperparathyroidism.
- Renal disease. The kidneys are damaged by nephrocalcinosis, which predisposes to pyelonephritis and eventually chronic renal failure.
- Bone involvement. This can cause vague bone and joint pains. Pathological fracture is rare.
- Hypercalcaemic symptoms, e.g. anorexia, weight loss, dyspepsia, polydipsia, polyuria, muscle weakness and tiredness. Hypertension and dyspnoea can occur.
- Pancreatitis. There is a raised incidence of this condition with parathyroid overactivity.
- Duodenal ulceration. This can occur in hyperparathyroidism and the latter is diagnosed when a serum calcium is measured as part of the general work-up.

On examination there is rarely anything to find. There may be corneal calcification adjacent to the corneoscleral margin. Bone disease can cause tenderness and swelling. It is very rare to feel an adenoma in the neck.

Proving the diagnosis

- Serum calcium. The specimen must be taken from a fasting patient with no cuff on the arm. 50% of the calcium is bound to albumin so a correction must be made if the albumin is low. The range of normality (which may vary slightly between laboratories) is 2.25–2.55 mmol/L.
- Serum phosphate. This is low in primary disease but may be increased if there is any renal impairment.
- Alkaline phosphatase. This is raised if there is significant bony disease.
- Urinary calcium and phosphate clearance. The 24-h clearances of both calcium and phosphate are usually elevated.
- Parathormone assay. Parathormone can be measured by an immunoradioactive assay of intact parathormone (normal

range 0.9–5.4 pmol/L). Patients with primary hyperparathyroidism occasionally have normal levels of parathormone, but this is still inappropriate in the presence of their high calcium levels. Hypercalcaemia from other causes will suppress parathormone production and the levels will be undetectable.

- Radiology. There are characteristic bone changes due to excess of parathormone, particularly seen in the skull and hands. X-rays also help in the differential diagnosis, e.g. carcinoma of the bronchus seen on chest X-ray or myeloma seen on a skull X-ray.
- Localization of an adenoma. Ultrasound of the neck and isotope (sestamibi) scanning are the most reliable methods. It is possible to cannulate the thyroid veins selectively and measure the parathormone levels, a technique reserved for patients who have had a failed cervical exploration. CT and MRI can also be used where other methods have failed.

OTHER CAUSES OF HYPERCALCAEMIA
Once hypercalcaemia has been detected, other causes of hypercalcaemia must be excluded. These include:

- carcinoma (bone metastases causing mobilization of calcium, or production of parathormone by a tumour)
- myeloma
- vitamin D intoxication (due to excess intake of vitamin D-containing foods)
- milk–alkali syndrome (due to ingestion of milk and alkalis for indigestion)
- thyrotoxicosis
- sarcoidosis
- Addison's disease
- Paget's disease of bone or osteoporosis (where the patient is immobilized).

Management
The management of hyperparathyroidism is surgical. There are important preoperative preparations.

In acute hyperparathyroidism the calcium level exceeds 3.75 mmol/L. The patient is dehydrated due to vomiting and polyuria and complains of headache, weakness and thirst. There may be tachycardia and low blood pressure, and eventually coma.

An electrocardiogram (ECG) may show a short QT interval and evidence of dysrhythmia.

This condition must be treated before operation can be undertaken, primarily by correcting dehydration. A saline infusion is given and potassium may be required. Intravenous therapy should be monitored by central venous pressure measurement as the mortality is high. If the calcium level still remains very high after rehydration, dialysis should be considered.

Immediate histology by frozen section may be required during operation if there is doubt identifying parathyroid tissue.

It is worthwhile warning the laboratory that serial calcium estimations will be required postoperatively.

OPERATION: EXPLORATION OF THE NECK FOR PARATHYROID ADENOMA

The neck is opened with a transverse skin crease incision and the thyroid is exposed as in thyroidectomy. The thyroid lobes are mobilized and retracted forwards. A methodical search is made for each parathyroid gland. If an adenoma is found it is removed and the diagnosis confirmed on frozen section. Further adenomas must also be excluded. Minimally invasive parathyroidectomy using a focused approach to the preoperatively identified gland is increasingly popular.

When all four glands are hyperplastic as in secondary hyperparathyroidism it is usual to remove three and a half glands, possibly re-implanting a remnant into a forearm muscle for ease of subsequent access. The other three removed glands may also be stored by cryopreservation.

If carcinoma is found, a radical local excision is performed, to include the thyroid lobe on that side.

Procedure profile

Blood requirement	0
Anaesthetic	GA
Operation time	1 hour
Hospital stay	1–2 days
Return to normal activity	1–3 weeks

Hypocalcaemia happens in 20% of cases in the first 48 h after operation. Serum calcium levels must be taken each day after operation. The clinical features of hypocalcaemia are tingling of the lips, fingers and toes, followed by the development of spasm of the hands and feet (tetany). Incipient tetany can be demonstrated by Trousseau's sign (if the patent is hypocalcaemic, carpal spasm develops within 2 min of inflating a blood pressure cuff on the arm above systolic pressure) or Chvostek's sign (tapping of the facial nerve in the cheek causes a twitch of the corner of the mouth and side of the nose). Overt tetany is shown by carpopedal spasm, when the hand is flexed at the metacarpophalangeal joints with straight fingers and the thumb strongly adducted. The foot and toes are plantar flexed.

Treatment of acute hypocalcaemia in the short term is with slow intravenous boluses or infusions of calcium gluconate (10 mL of 10%). If the calcium level does not return to normal over the next few days, with oral calcium, treatment with vitamin D is required. Control can be difficult and often the levels need to be checked repeatedly and therapy altered until stable calcium levels are achieved.

Multiple endocrine neoplasia

Parathyroid neoplasia (adenomas/hyperplasia) may be associated with neoplasia of other endocrine tissues that are characterized by the presence of amine precursor uptake and decarboxylation (APUD) cells. The most frequently encountered endocrine tumours linked in this way are medullary carcinoma of the thyroid, phaeochromocytoma, and parathyroid adenoma (multiple endocrine neoplasia type IIA/Sipple's syndrome). The other principal syndrome is multiple endocrine neoplasia type 1 in which tumours may arise in APUD cells of the pituitary (e.g. prolactinoma), pancreas (insulinoma) and gastroduodenum (gastrinoma).

4.3 Adrenal and benign pancreatic tumours

Adrenal tumours

The adrenal gland consists of an inner medulla and an outer cortex. The medulla originates from neuroectoderm and secretes catecholamines. The cortex develops from mesoderm and produces glucocorticoids, mineralocorticoids and some androgens and estrogens.

Primary tumours may arise in both parts of the gland and can be benign or malignant. The adrenal gland is also occasionally a site for metastases, particularly from carcinoma of the breast or bronchus, or melanoma.

If the tumour is actively secreting hormones, specific treatment may be required before surgery can safely be undertaken. Most functional tumours are relatively small and amenable to minimally invasive surgery. This section outlines the management of four conditions.

- Phaeochromocytoma.
- Cushing's syndrome due to adrenal adenoma or carcinoma.
- Conn's syndrome due to adrenal adenoma or carcinoma.
- Adrenal carcinoma.

Phaeochromocytoma

This is a tumour of chromaffin cells which secrete noradrenaline, dopamine and adrenaline. There is a familial incidence and an association with medullary carcinoma of the thyroid and parathyroid adenomas (multiple endocrine neoplasia type II A/B). It usually occurs as a single benign tumour in the adrenal gland. It is useful to remember that 10% are bilateral, 10% are malignant and 10% arise outside the adrenal gland. Tumours arising from chromaffin cells outside the adrenal gland only secrete noradrenaline. There is also an association with neurofibromatosis.

The tumour causes hypertension which may be persistent or paroxysmal.

The patient may present with attacks of sweating, pallor, palpitations, angina, nausea and vomiting, abdominal pain, headache and nervousness.

Proving the diagnosis

The diagnosis is proved by finding high concentrations of catecholamine metabolites in the urine (metanephrine, normetanephrine and vanilylmandelic acid, VMA).

Various methods of tumour localization are used. CT scanning is most frequently used to define tumour site and size. I^{131} MIBG (*m*-iodo benzyl guanidine) scintigraphy can locate active chromaffin tissue, especially in secondary and ectopic phaeochromocytomas. T_2-weighted MRI is also helpful.

Management

The tumour is treated by surgical removal. This can be by open operation through a laparotomy. Endoscopic removal using a trans- or retroperitoneal route results in a quicker and less painful recovery.

Preoperatively there is usually a degree of hypovolaemia in these patients due to prolonged vasoconstriction. A sudden drop in catecholamine levels as the tumour is removed may cause severe hypotension. The patient should be given α-blockers in an attempt to reverse vasoconstriction and restore blood volume. Phenoxybenzamine and phentolamine are suitable and once started, β-blockers such as propranolol may be needed to stop tachycardia.

The preoperative management must be discussed with the anaesthetist.

OPERATION: OPEN EXCISION OF AN ADRENAL PHAEOCHROMOCYTOMA

During operation there are two potential problems.

- α- and β-blockade inhibits the sympathetic response to hypovolaemia and so a central venous pressure (CVP) line is needed. A cardiac monitor and arterial line are also used.
- Handling the tumour may cause a sudden surge in catecholamine levels which, despite the preoperative blockade, may cause a hypertensive crisis. A short-acting α-blocker, phentolamine (5 mg i.v.), must be available to treat this. Propranolol (0.5–1 mg i.v.) or sodium nitroprusside (0.5–1.5 µg/kg/min i.v.) may also be used.

The tumour is usually approached transabdominally and the whole adrenal gland removed, after the adrenal vein and arteries are secured. This can be a difficult procedure, particularly in an obese patient. The sophistication and accuracy of preoperative investigation alerts the surgeon to possible bilateral or ectopic adrenal disease, which may also have to be removed.

Procedure profile

Blood requirement	4–6
Anaesthetic	GA
Operation time	1–2 hours
Hospital stay	1 week
Return to normal activity	3–4 weeks

Postoperatively a close watch must be kept on the urine output to detect any hypovolaemia. Volume loading to anticipate vascular dilatation secondary to the sudden withdrawal of catecholamines is essential. This is more appropriate than the use of pressor agents. Hypoglycaemia can also occur as a result of catecholamine withdrawal.

OPERATION: LAPAROSCOPIC ADRENALECTOMY

The gland may be approached transperitoneally or through the retroperitoneal tissues. A retroperitoneal space can be formed by placing cannulae in the flank and expanding the space using a balloon. The perirenal fascia is exposed and followed upwards to find the adrenal within its fascia. This is then mobilized and its vessels clipped and divided. The gland is removed.

Procedure profile

Blood requirement	4–6
Anaesthetic	GA
Operation time	1 hour
Hospital stay	1–2 days
Return to normal activity	2 weeks

Postoperative care is as for the open operation but the patient has less pain and is therefore somewhat easier to manage. Recovery is quicker.

Cushing's syndrome due to adrenal tumour

Cushing's syndrome is due to excess production of glucocorticoids. This is most commonly secondary to an abnormally high adrenocorticotrophic hormone (ACTH) level, itself produced either by a pituitary adenoma or from an ectopic site (e.g. carcinoma of the bronchus). In 20% of patients with Cushing's syndrome there is a primary lesion in the adrenal gland, either an adenoma or a carcinoma. Adenomas may be bilateral.

The patient characteristically gains weight and develops a bloated appearance. The syndrome also consists of hypertension, hyperglycaemia and glycosuria, increased protein catabolism and a predisposition to infection.

Proving the diagnosis

The diagnosis is proved by finding an elevated serum cortisol with loss of the normal diurnal variation. There are increased levels of cortisol metabolites in the urine. An adrenal primary lesion is characterized by markedly depressed serum ACTH levels. The tumour can be localized and assessed by CT scanning. MRI scanning may identify vascular invasion indicating malignancy and possible inoperability.

Management

The tumour is removed surgically.

The production of adrenal hormones by tissue other than the tumour will be suppressed and the patient will be unable to respond to the stress of operation by increasing steroid secretion. Supplemental therapy must therefore be prescribed starting at the time of premedication. The usual dose is hydrocortisone 100 mg intravenously.

OPERATION: ADRENALECTOMY FOR CUSHING'S'
SYNDROME
(See phaeochromocytoma.)

Cushingoid patients are more susceptible to postoperative

complications such as poor wound healing, wound infection or haemorrhage, which is a compelling reason to consider the less traumatic endoscopic removal.

Conn's syndrome

This is due to excessive production of aldosterone by an adenoma of the zona glomerulosa cells of the adrenal gland. Occasionally it is due to bilateral hyperplasia. Carcinoma is a rare cause.

The syndrome is characterized by hypertension, hypokalaemic alkalosis and muscle weakness.

Proving the diagnosis

Investigations show a high urinary potassium content despite a low serum potassium and a high serum bicarbonate. The serum aldosterone level is elevated, and renin levels are low.

Localization of the tumour is difficult as it is often small and may be multiple and bilateral. Radionucleotide imaging using radiolabelled cholesterol during dexamethasone suppression identifies functioning adrenocortical tissue and can detect tumours as small as 5 mm in diameter. CT and MRI are also invaluable.

Management

Surgery is advised to avoid long-term antihypertensive medications with their side-effects.

Preoperatively the body is potassium-depleted and this should be corrected before operation with spironolactone (200–400 mg/day).

OPERATION: ADRENALECTOMY FOR CONN'S SYNDROME
As for phaeochromocytoma.

Adrenal carcinoma

Carcinoma may occasionally present with no evidence of endocrine disturbance. It is usually fast growing with rapid invasion and early metastases. It presents with loin discomfort, weight loss and possibly a palpable mass. It is localized with the aid of CT, ultrasound or MRI scan.

Management
Surgery is the only hope of cure. Some inoperable or recurrent disease responds to chemotherapy using mitotane (*o,p*'-DDD, a derivative of the insecticide DDT).

Benign endocrine tumours of the pancreas

Benign tumours of the pancreas are derived from the islet cells. These are part of the APUD system (see p. 192). An insulinoma is a tumour derived from the β cells of the islets. It produces an excess of insulin and causes hypoglycaemia. A gastrinoma is derived from non-β cells and produces an excess of gastrin. The latter results in gastric hyperacidity and severe duodenal ulceration (Zollinger–Ellison syndrome).

Other tumours may secrete vasoactive intestinal peptide (VIP), causing diarrhoea and hypoglycaemia (Verner–Morrison syndrome), or glucagon, causing mild diabetes. Most of these tumours are benign and for convenience both benign and malignant forms are described here. They may be associated with other lesions in the APUD system.

Insulinoma

Ten per cent of β-cell tumours are multiple and 10% are malignant. Over 90% are situated in the pancreas, the remaining few being found in ectopic pancreatic tissue. The tumour is frequently less than 2 cm in diameter.

The patient is usually between the ages of 20 and 40 years. The excessive insulin production results in marked hypoglycaemia and the patient suffers from attacks of unconsciousness or strange behaviour and may become intensely hungry. He or she may gain a lot of weight.

Proving the diagnosis
This may be difficult. Patients are frequently misdiagnosed as having epilepsy or psychiatric disease. Whipple's triad is helpful when trying to make the diagnosis and states the following.
• The 'attacks' are induced by starvation or exercise.

- Hypoglycaemia is present during an attack (blood glucose less than 2 mmol/L).
- The episode is relieved by giving sugar orally or intravenously.

Once the possibility of this condition has been recognized the diagnosis can be confirmed by measuring the plasma insulin and proinsulin levels by radioimmunoassay. The levels are inappropriately elevated in the presence of hypoglycaemia.

The tumour may be identified by the following.

- Abdominal CT scan, ultrasound or MRI (detection rate 40–50%).
- Selective coeliac axis arteriography. An abnormal tumour 'blush' is seen in 60–70% of cases.
- Venous sampling. The portal vein is cannulated transhepatically and blood is sampled from various sites around the pancreas. The level of insulin is measured and can give an indication of the site of a tumour. The technique is not without hazard.
- Endoscopic ultrasound.
- Intraoperative ultrasound.

Management

The tumour is excised. Medical treatment can be used when the tumour is not localized or if there is a malignant tumour with metastases. Diazoxide (5 mg/kg daily in divided doses) suppresses insulin release and is effective in 50% of patients. Streptozotocin (1 g/m^2 body surface) can be used for malignant insulinomas. It is selectively toxic to islet cells.

Preoperatively set up an intravenous infusion of 5–10% dextrose 12 h before the operation to maintain the blood sugar during the preoperative fast.

OPERATION: EXCISION OF AN INSULINOMA

A laparotomy is usually performed. Some tumours may be amenable to laparoscopic excision. The pancreas and surrounding tissues are inspected and scanned with intraoperative ultrasound, to search for the tumour. When it is found, it is excised. The rest of the pancreas must be examined to exclude multiple adenomas. Blood sugar may be measured after enucleation. Persistent hypoglycaemia suggests that a second tumour is present.

Procedure profile

Blood requirement	2–4
Anaesthetic	GA
Operation time	1–2 hours
Hospital stay	4–7 days
Return to normal activity	4 weeks

Postoperatively the remaining β cells may be suppressed by the chronic hypoglycaemia. When the tumour is removed, rebound hyperglycaemia may develop in the first 4–5 days and insulin therapy may be needed for a short period. There is also a danger of postoperative pancreatitis, and pancreatic sepsis and fistula formation are not uncommon. If a pancreatic fistula develops, the skin must be protected from autodigestion, using a barrier cream. The fistula will usually heal spontaneously.

Zollinger–Ellison syndrome

In this condition there is excessive production of gastrin by a non-β-cell adenoma, often situated in the head of the pancreas or the duodenal wall The patient develops severe duodenal and gastric ulceration and their life may be threatened by recurrent haemorrhage or perforation. Thirty per cent of such tumours are malignant and 80% are multiple in the familial form (multiple endocrine neoplasia type I); 60% are malignant and solitary in the sporadic form.

Recognizing the pattern

The usual age at presentation is around 40 years and the condition is slightly more common in males. The symptoms and signs are those of an aggressive duodenal ulcer which is difficult to control. The condition should always be considered in patients who develop recurrent ulcers on adequate treatment.

Proving the diagnosis

- Serum gastrin levels are high in spite of a low gastric pH (which normally inhibits gastrin secretion).

- The gastric function tests show a raised basal acid output (e.g. over 15 mmol/h).
- Endoscopy shows extensive ulceration and scarring.
- Secretin or calcium administration produces an abnormal rise in serum gastrin. This rise is not seen with simple hyperplasia of the antral cells.
- Methods of localizing the tumour are the same as those described above for insulinoma.

Management

This may be medical or surgical, and is still controversial. Symptoms may be relieved by proton-pump inhibitors (omeprazole 20–180 mg/day). This may be used either for short-term treatment before operation or in the long term.

Tumour enucleation or excision (pancreatic resection – see p. 345) is performed, and a careful search made in the duodenum for submucosal gastrinomas. Total gastrectomy is rarely used nowadays due to the effectiveness of PPI therapy in controlling symptoms.

5 Breast surgery

5.1 Breast lumps and benign breast conditions

Most women presenting to hospital breast clinics have benign breast conditions, complaining of lumps, lumpiness, pain or nipple discharge.

Normal breast

Normal breast tissue is in continual change in response to the varying hormonal profiles during adult life (including pregnancy) and the menstrual cycle. Each breast comprises 15–20 lobes. The functional unit of the breast is the terminal duct lobular unit or lobule. The lobule drains via a branching duct system towards the nipple. Between the lobules and lobes is a supporting connective tissue of fat, fibrous septa (Coopers ligaments), blood vessels and lymphatics. The separation of the breast lobes is not as orderly as the spokes of a wheel and the ducts do not travel in a strict radial pattern towards the nipple. Most benign breast conditions and almost all breast cancers arise from the tissues of the terminal duct lobular unit (Fig. 5.1.1).

Normal breast and the menstrual cycle

The breast undergoes minor changes during the menstrual cycle. The lobular stroma becomes oedematous under the influence of estrogens. There is mild proliferation of the acinar epithelium in the second half of the menstrual cycle, with programmed cell death (apoptosis) when hormone levels fall at the onset of the menstrual bleed.

Surgery: Diagnosis and Management, 4th edition. Edited by N. Rawlinson and D. Alderson. © 2009 Blackwell Publishing, ISBN: 978-1-4051-2921-3

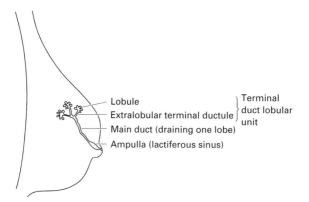

Fig. 5.1.1 A schematic diagram of the anatomy of a breast lobe – see text for a detailed description.

Changes in the breast with age

The prepubertal breast is a simple bud of tissue beneath the immature nipple. At this stage the male and female breasts are identical. Breast development begins at the telarche which often precedes the onset of menstruation (menarche) by 18 months to 2 years. After the menarche the breast develops rapidly but often does not reach maturity until the late teenage years or even early twenties. Initially the development may be asymmetrical and any parental concerns at this stage should be allayed.

Following maturation during the teenage years, the female breast is composed of very variable proportions of fat and glandular tissue, contributing to considerable variations in size, shape and consistency. Varying degrees of asymmetry between left and right breast are not uncommon, the left often larger than the right. The breast varies in consistency from softness to considerable nodularity, particularly palpable in the upper outer quadrants of the breast.

The proportion of fatty tissue and glandular tissue varies with age, a process that is often accelerated following childbirth and breast-feeding. This brings the underlying glandular tissue and natural lumpiness into greater prominence, particularly in women in their 30s and 40s. Although this is an entirely normal process the woman notices a change and, therefore, may present to a symptomatic breast clinic concerned she may have developed breast cancer.

The responsiveness of the breast to the fluctuating endocrine environment often changes considerably in the late 30s and 40s, with mastalgia (breast pain) becoming much more common. Involutional and ageing changes also make breast cysts very common between 35 and 50 years. These cysts can sometimes be multifocal and very large (even over 100 mL).

The increasing use of hormone replacement therapy has altered the pattern of ageing of the breast in some women and the pattern of presentation of benign breast disorders. For example, there may be a prolongation of the age range over which breast cysts and mastalgia may persist.

Assessment of symptomatic breast disorders

Objectives
- To reach an accurate diagnosis as rapidly and cost-effectively as possible, so as to be able to reassure the patient with a benign breast lump or disorder.
- To initiate treatment as rapidly as possible where malignancy is confirmed.
- To avoid surgery as far as possible for benign breast disorders.
- To use 'triple assessment' with the diagnostic triad wherever appropriate. This combines the skills of clinicians, radiologists and pathologists comprising:
  - clinical history and examination
  - imaging (ultrasound scan and/or mammography)
  - tissue diagnosis: cytological or histological examination, usually from fine-needle aspiration (FNA) cytology, or from devices to obtain cores of tissue – wide-bore needle (WBN) biopsy.

Many breast units score each component of the triad on a scale of 1–5, such that the higher the score, the stronger the indication for definitive treatment, thus:
- completely normal
- abnormal, definitely benign

- abnormal, uncertain
- probably malignant
- definitely malignant.

With adequate organization and resources, it is often possible to achieve these objectives within a single hospital visit. This has become popularized as the 'one stop' clinic concept.

History

The following points may be helpful in reaching the diagnosis.

- Age. Fibroadenomas and benign lumpiness/nodularity are common below the age of 30 years, but cancers are rare. Cysts are common in 40s and 50s but so too are cancers.
- Length of history. Determine how long the lump has been noticed. What was the relationship of its appearance to the menstrual cycle? Has it changed in size? Cysts often develop quickly.
- Pain. Was the lump painful and is it painful now? Cysts are often uncomfortable at first. Cancers are rarely painful.
- Menstrual history. Remember that a premenopausal woman who has had a hysterectomy with ovarian conservation may still experience cyclical breast symptoms.
- The lump. Has it changed? Does it vary in size? Lumps which decrease in size after the menstrual period are usually benign.
- Nipple discharge (colour, volume, pattern, duration, frequency). Is it bloodstained or not? Does it come from both nipples or just one, or from one duct or several.
- Pregnancy and breast-feeding. Has she had children and if so how old are they? This will tell you how old she was when she conceived them. There is some evidence to suggest that pregnancy in early life protects against malignancy. Were any children breast-fed or not and if so for how long?
- Family history. A detailed family history will be helpful for epidemiological purposes and for risk assessment, in conjunction with specialist advice on screening and follow-up. Many breast units now run a family history clinic. Current information suggests that 5–10% of breast cancer cases may have a genetic or familial component, with a predisposition to other epithelial and ovarian carcinomas. Since breast cancer is a very common disease, many women will have a relative who has had breast

cancer. Her risk is increased if several relatives (particularly first-degree relatives) have been affected and in particular at an early age (< 40 years).
- Medication, particularly whether she has been on the pill or hormone replacement therapy. What is the form of administration (e.g. depot, oral)?

Examination

The patient must be examined in a good light, as changes in the contour of the breast are helpful in making a diagnosis.
- Ask the patient to sit up first and observe both breasts looking for masses or dimpling of the skin. Ask her to indicate any lump.
- Ask the patient to raise both arms high in the air. Skin tethering due to a tumour may become visible. Attachment to the pectoral fascia is assessed by asking the patient to place her hand on her hip. Pressure on the hip causes contraction of the pectoral muscle and this will increase fixity of the lump if it is attached deeply.
- Observe for breast erythema and oedema, and for arm lymphoedema.
- Sit the patient comfortably at between 20–45 degrees. Palpate each quadrant of each breast systematically. Start with the normal breast. Palpate with straight fingers, and avoid digging into the breast with the fingertips.
- If a lump is found, determine its:
  ◦ shape
  ◦ size
  ◦ surface
  ◦ edge
  ◦ consistency
  ◦ fixity, and attachments.
- Look for evidence suggestive of metastatic spread. Make no assumptions! Palpable axillary nodes are sometimes reactive and not malignant. Examine the axillary, infraclavicular and supraclavicular lymph nodes (Fig. 5.1.2), the chest (for an effusion) and the abdomen (for hepatomegaly). The liver may be enlarged for many reasons other than metastatic breast cancer.

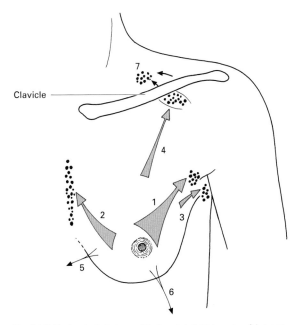

Clavicle

Fig. 5.1.2 The lymphatic drainage of the breast. 1, 2: Main routes of drainage, to the anterior axillary nodes and internal mammary nodes. 3, 4: Minor routes; the axillary tail can drain to the posterior axillary nodes. Rarely, the upper and outer quadrant drains directly to the infraclavicular nodes. 5, 6: Potential routes of drainage, to the opposite breast, axilla and the extraperitoneal lymphatics of the anterior abdominal wall. 7: Routes 1, 3 and 4 drain ultimately to the supraclavicular nodes. Medial tumours do not necessarily drain via the internal mammary nodes and may drain via the axillary lymph nodes.

Self-examination and breast awareness

Often the examination on presentation will be normal. Point out the relevant features to the woman and encourage her to assess her own breasts and report any new lumps that persist beyond menstruation, or change in character (breast awareness).

Breast imaging

Ultrasound scanning

Ultrasound examination of lumps and nodularity is an essential part of the assessment of breast disorders in women under the age of 40 years and it has a useful adjunctive role in older women. It can be used to guide FNA or WBN sampling. The accuracy of breast ultrasound depends on the skill of the radiologist performing the examination. In trained hands it can be confidently used to distinguish cysts, tumours and benign nodularity. As the natural density of glandular tissue in the under 40s significantly reduces the sensitivity of mammography, ultrasound is usually the imaging investigation of choice in this age group.

X-ray mammography

X-ray mammography is useful in the assessment of breast symptoms and in screening of asymptomatic women for the earliest (presymptomatic) signs of breast cancer. It is particularly useful in women over 40 years of age but can be used with caution in women of 35–40 also. Biplanar views (oblique and craniocaudal) are usually selected. The false-negative rate is significant (up to 10%), and some obviously palpable tumours do not show up on X-rays. It should thus not be used in isolation from FNA and skilled examination. It is only one part of the triple assessment of a woman with breast symptoms.

The features on a mammogram suggestive of cancer are as follows.
- An asymmetrical density particularly with spiculate margins.
- Distortion of surrounding structures (skin contour, underlying muscle)
- Microcalcification within the substance of a mass or alone. Microcalcification often has a branching appearance as it is within the microscopic ductules and indicates the presence of ductal carcinoma in situ (DCIS).
- Thickening of the skin over the lesion due to early oedema.

There is a small false-negative and false-positive rate since not all spiculate distortions or microcalcifications indicate cancer. The combination of malignant appearances on mammography, ultrasound and biopsy combined are needed for an accurate diagnosis to be made.

Breast screening

The introduction of a nationwide breast-screening programme in the late 1980s has had a major impact on the organization and provision of breast services in the UK. It allows for community-based mammographic screening of all women between the ages of 50 and 69 years at 3-yearly intervals, and sets strict criteria to ensure quality and cost-effectiveness. Patients with lesions diagnosed on screening are further assessed and treated in specialist referral centres. Women whose cancers are detected through mammographic screening before they become symptomatic usually have an improved prognosis.

FNA cytology

Where a lump is present, fine-needle aspiration biopsy (FNA) will commonly be performed. Trained cytopathologists can interpret FNA samples with considerable accuracy when sufficient sample is provided. FNA may be undertaken immediately before or often after imaging. Tissue distortion induced by bruising, a relatively common event, may mislead the radiologist if imaging is not performed immediately after biopsy. Cell samples may be 'hot reported' from slide smears immediately, or stored in fixative solutions for later study. The accuracy of this method depends on the experience of the cytologist and the clinician's ability to produce an adequate sample.

To perform FNA, the lump is fixed between the thumb and forefinger. A 21-gauge (blue) needle attached to a 20-mL syringe is passed several times through the centre of the mass slightly varying the direction of passage, while maintaining full suction. Suction is released before withdrawing the needle thus preserving the aspirate in the needle hub for subsequent preparation of cytological smears. The consistency of the lump to the needle may, identify the 'gritty' feel of a carcinoma or the rubbery feel of normal glandular tissue. A cyst may immediately yield fluid.

Wide-bore needle (WBN) breast biopsy

A guiding principle of modern breast surgical practice is the avoidance of open surgery without a definitive diagnosis. Where FNA sampling is uninformative WBN biopsies may be helpful.

With this technique a small cylinder of the lesion is excised using a special needle on a spring-loaded gun. There is no good evidence to suggest that either fine-needle aspiration or WBN biopsy causes local spread of cancer. While FNA biopsy can be performed without anaesthetic, local infiltration anaesthesia is required for WBN biopsy.

Open surgical biopsy
Open surgical biopsy is occasionally necessary for symptomatic lumps, and for screen-detected lesions where FNA or WBN biopsy is non-diagnostic.

OPERATION: BIOPSY OF BREAST LUMP
Open biopsies are usually undertaken under general anaesthesia. The lump must be marked preoperatively by the surgeon undertaking the procedure and confirmed by the patient. A periareolar incision often provides good access and excellent cosmesis. Good haemostasis within the biopsy cavity is necessary. The wound may also be vacuum drained, though this is usually unnecessary.

Procedure profile

Blood requirement	0
Anaesthetic	GA (LA for some superficial lesions)
Operation time	15–30 minutes
Hospital stay	Day case
Return to normal activity	Less than a week

An early outpatient appointment should be made for the discussion of results.

Pathological examination of tissue
Biopsy samples may be studied in two ways.
- Paraffin section. The tissue is first fixed in formaldehyde solution, embedded in paraffin wax and allowed to set before sections are cut and stained. The process takes about 2–3 days.

- Frozen section. The fresh tissue is rapidly frozen, cut and stained immediately. A histological diagnosis is usually available in about 15–20 min. The quality of such sections is inferior to paraffin sections, and false-positive results have been obtained with disastrous results both clinically and medico-legally. Requests for frozen-section diagnoses at the time of breast surgery, therefore, are becoming increasingly uncommon. They do not allow informed planning with the patient of the treatment options in advance of surgery.

No therapeutic surgical procedure for breast cancer should be performed without a positive tissue diagnosis of malignancy.

Figure 5.1.3 summarises the diagnostic management of a breast lump.

Benign mammary disorders

Terminology about benign breast disorders has in the past been very confusing. Most symptoms, even when severe, are simple manifestations of normal physiological change and occur in the absence of any pathology. Nodularity and mastalgia are separate conditions that can coexist. The inappropriate use of terms like mastitis (strictly implying infection or inflammation), or dysplasia (strictly implying premalignant change) can be misleading. Most benign breast disorders are usefully described as an 'aberration of normal (breast) development and involution' (ANDI).

Benign mammary nodularity

This is the normal, nodular variant of glandular breast tissue previously described as fibrocystic change. It represents a variation of the normal changes of hyperplasia and involution. It is often asymmetrical and unilateral. It is most often prominent in the upper, outer quadrant of the breast. It may or may not be associated with mastalgia (pain) and/or cyst development. It becomes more prominent in the 35–50 age group, as the glandular and supporting tissue that gives the breast its fullness undergoes patchy involution.

Various terms are used to describe the changes that occur in the breast. Fibroadenosis is an old-fashioned term from the days

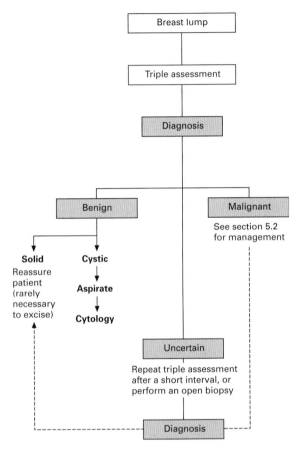

Fig. 5.1.3 Summary of the diagnostic management of a breast lump.

when innocent lumps were regularly removed and examined histologically. In some the ductal epithelium can become hyperplastic (usual or regular ductal hyperplasia). Occasionally atypical cells are seen in the hyperplastic ductal epithelium and these appearances can be a precursor of breast cancer.

Women with marked nodularity are particularly difficult to assess by clinical examination, and may need to be followed up in a specialist clinic. Regular self-examination is helpful since the woman becomes gradually more 'breast aware' and can pick out the abnormal from the normal.

Recognizing the pattern

The patient has diffuse nodularity, particularly in the upper outer quadrant. This may be either unilateral or bilateral, and may or may not be associated with breast cysts or mastalgia. Women between 16 and 60 years of age may be affected. The nodularity may change with the menstrual cycle. There may be an associated history of premenstrual breast pain. There may be one or several areas of thickening in either or both breasts. The nodularity is diffuse and its edge is difficult to define. It is not fixed and there is no skin puckering. It may be tender.

Proving the diagnosis

This is achieved by conventional triple assessment with skilled clinical examination, breast imaging and needle biopsy (FNA or WBN) of areas of more discrete lumpiness or radiological uncertainty.

Management

Modern practice in the UK is conservative. It is geared towards the exclusion of malignancy, reassurance and avoidance of surgery. Scar nodularity can give rise to further anxiety later in life and subsequent difficulties interpreting clinical and mammographic findings. Once it is appreciated that these conditions essentially represent normal breast change it can be understood why surgical treatment is both unnecessary and inappropriate.

Fibroadenoma

Fibroadenomas are a distinct benign tumour and may present throughout adult life but almost certainly develop during breast growth and maturation (before 30). They present most commonly in the early adult years. They may be discrete, rounded or lobulated, and occur in a range of sizes, from a few millimetres to several centimetres. They usually remain static or undergo spontaneous involution but occasionally can increase in size, sometimes spontaneously or in response to pregnancy or other hormonal change (e.g. the oral contraceptive pill). Histologically two forms are described, although clinically the difference is of no relevance.

- In intracanalicular fibroadenomas, the stroma predominates and projects into the lumen of the ducts within the adenoma.
- In pericanalicular fibroadenomas, small, rounded islands of glands are encircled by whorls of stroma.

A phyllodes tumour is a distinct pathological entity separate from large or giant fibroadenoma which has histological features identical to the more common and small fibroadenoma. The phyllodes tumour has a much more cellular stroma histologically and has characteristic leaf-like glandular structures giving it its name (phyllodes = leaf like). These tumours are much less common than fibroadenomas and can grow to enormous sizes. Most are entirely benign, but some exhibit a low-grade malignant behaviour with a tendency to local recurrence after surgical excision (borderline lesions). Very rarely phyllodes tumours can behave in a frankly malignant way but their pattern of metastasis is sarcoma-like with haematogenous spread (usually to the lungs). The pathologist will often differentiate between grades of phyllodes tumour on the basis of a mitotic count within the cellular stroma. Tumours with a mitotic count of greater than 10 per high power field are conventionally regarded to have significant malignant potential. In these women a chest X-ray should be arranged (to exclude pulmonary metastases) and if clear a total mastectomy advised (lymph node dissection not required and often immediate reconstruction possible). Women who have had borderline lesions excised should probably be followed for up to 3 years to watch for local recurrence.

Recognizing the pattern

The patient complains of a discrete lump, which may have gradually enlarged. In fibroadenomas pain is not usually a feature. On examination the lump is firm, discrete or lobulated and mobile beneath the examining fingers (a 'breast mouse').

Proving the diagnosis

Clinical examination, FNA cytology and ultrasound scan usually form the triple assessment in this predominantly young age group. Mammography may help in equivocal cases, particularly in women 35–40 years old.

Management

Once the diagnosis has been made with confidence modern practice is to avoid surgery. True fibroadenomas have no malignant potential. Triple assessment has dramatically reduced the benign biopsy rate in specialist breast units in recent years. However, some women will still require surgical removal of the fibroadenoma. Larger lesions, particularly in the smaller breast, may be uncomfortable and surgical removal is therefore indicated. All surgically removed lesions should be examined histologically.

Breast cysts

Breast cysts are a very common feature of breast involution and usually occur from the mid-30s until after the menopause. Acini dilate, fill with fluid and form cysts. The degenerating epithelial cells draw in fluid due to osmosis and quite large cysts may form rapidly. They cause considerable anxiety as they occur in an age group when breast cancer is rising in incidence.

Cysts may be various diameters from a few millimetres to several centimetres, with volumes of 0.5 to over 100 mL. The majority contain less than 15 mL fluid when aspirated. They usually present as a palpable lump, sometimes painful. The cyst fluid may be straw coloured, greenish or brownish. Blood in the cyst fluid is usually iatrogenic, although it may occasionally indicate a coexisting tumour. It is usually straightforward to aspirate cysts to dryness. Incidental small cysts noted on screening mammography can safely be left alone.

Recognizing the pattern

Breast cysts can occur at any age before, and within 2–3 years of, the menopause. They may be recurrent, multiple and unilateral or bilateral. The lump usually appears and enlarges rapidly. It may be painful. Some cysts may regress spontaneously.

On examination cysts are usually discrete, tense, smooth and rounded. The cyst may arise deep within the breast and may then be less well defined and be mistaken for a possible cancer.

Proving the diagnosis

Triple assessment is appropriate where there is doubt. FNA proves the diagnosis. Cytological examination of cyst fluid is not necessary provided the mass disappears after aspiration leaving no residual lump and the fluid is not bloodstained.

Management

Cysts are managed conservatively by aspiration (occasionally repeated). Surgery is rarely necessary even if the same cyst fills on several occasions. Suspicion of a coexisting tumour is increased if:

- FNA fails to produce complete resolution of the lump
- the fluid is persistently bloodstained
- there are features on breast imaging that raise the suspicion of malignancy.

Image-guided FNA or WBN biopsy is often diagnostic.

Follow-up is not essential, and common practice is to allow the patient an open-access appointment if the cyst refills or if new cysts appear. Repeated presentation with cysts should not induce complacency. New lesions should be investigated appropriately.

Mastalgia (breast pain)

Mastalgia may be cyclical (related to menstrual cycle) or noncyclical, and unilateral or bilateral. There are no consistent histological changes in the breast. However, because it arises at an age when other changes such as the development of cysts are also common, it has attracted a number of misleading terms implying true pathology, for example mastitis, dysplasia and cystic mastopathy. The symptoms may occur in breasts of all consistencies, from the very soft to the very nodular. As with benign nodularity it should not be regarded as a pathological entity.

Breast pain is very rarely due to carcinoma. It may be severe when caused by a breast abscess, but features of inflammation should then be obvious. Pain referred from musculoskeletal structures in the chest wall can be felt as mastalgia resulting in a referral to a breast clinic (particularly in postmenopausal women who by definition cannot have cyclical mastalgia).

Recognizing the pattern
Mastalgia usually arises in otherwise normal breasts in women of reproductive age. The onset, duration, severity and relief can be very variable. Symptoms usually do improve with time, although this may take weeks or months. The history is very variable in pattern and severity.

Cyclical pain has the following features:
• worse at the time of periods or just before
• awareness of breast swelling
• locally tender to touch.

By contrast non-cyclical pain is:
• Pain throughout or at random intervals during the menstrual cycle. Many women in this age group have undergone hysterectomies with ovarian preservation, and so cannot be precise about their cycle, although they remain susceptible to hormone-associated mastalgia.
• otherwise as for cyclical mastalgia but symptoms more random. Women often describe stress-related symptoms.

Proving the diagnosis
The clinician's role in the management of these women is reassurance often by the exclusion of malignancy. Biopsy is rarely helpful except as a process of exclusion in nodular breasts but imaging by ultrasound or X-ray mammography alone or combined is often very useful in providing the necessary reassurance of the absence of serious pathology.

Management
Most mastalgic pains will settle with time. Sympathetic support and reassurance are essential. A host of medical remedies have been proposed, of which most are ineffective. Evening primrose oil or starflower oil in their various formulations are sometimes of help. Endocrine manipulations such as danazol or bromocryptine are somewhat drastic (and can cause unwanted side-effects) and are rarely indicated, but may be effective in cases of disablingly severe and persistent pain.

Nipple discharge

Nipple discharge takes a variety of forms, and may be either physiological or pathological. Milky or serous discharge can persist for many months after cessation of breast-feeding. Most non-lactational presentations are minor physiological or involutional discharges of clear, milky, greenish or brownish discharge. Most are minor and self-limiting. One form that can be troublesome is mammary duct ectasia, in which ducts fill with degenerate epithelium, often producing a thick green fluid.

Bloody discharge may be suggestive of a duct papilloma (benign), or rarely a carcinoma, particularly of the early intraductal variety which may present in this way long before a lump becomes palpable.

Recognizing the pattern

Nipple discharges may occur at any time in the adult years. Physiological and duct ectasia discharges are frequently minor, intermittent, of low volume and persist for several months. Blood usually brings the patient much more rapidly to the clinic.

Proving the diagnosis

A careful clinical examination is performed to exclude the presence of lumps and confirm the discharge site, type and character. Smear cytology of the discharge may be helpful. The patient may be encouraged to express any fluid herself at the consultation. Mammography is usually necessary in the over 40s to exclude an underlying malignancy but mammography is nearly always normal, particularly when no suspicious features are found on examination.

Persistent non-lactational milk production (galactorrhoea) is rarely associated with the increased production of prolactin from a pituitary adenoma. Routine serum prolactin estimations are, however, not recommended unless there is a concomitant history of headache and/or visual disturbance.

Management

Surgical intervention is not indicated for physiological discharge and only occasionally for duct ectasia. In the case of persistent bleeding from a duct, with or without positive cytology, surgical biopsy by microdochectomy may be indicated.

The site of bleeding is noted and the patient is encouraged not to express fluid preoperatively. A microdochectomy is indicated where the discharge is from a single, defined duct. A subareolar resection of the ducts (Hadfield's operation) is undertaken where a bloodstained discharge issues from several ducts or where the sites of the discharges have not been determined.

OPERATION: MICRODOCHECTOMY

At operation, a fine probe is passed down the involved duct, allowing its accurate excision by either an ellipsoid or a periareolar incision. The tissue is sent for histological examination.

Antibiotic prophylaxis is achieved with a single-dose broad-spectrum antibiotic at induction (e.g. co-amoxiclav).

Procedure profile

Blood requirement	0
Anaesthetic	GA
Operation time	30 minutes
Hospital stay	Day case or planned overnight
Return to normal activity	1–2 weeks

Complicated/symptomatic mammary duct ectasia

In this variety of a normally benign and self-limiting condition the dilated ducts containing inflammatory cells (macrophages) may rupture and cause a foreign body reaction. This reaction is characterized by the presence of plasma cells and is known as 'plasma cell mastitis'. It can be painful due to local inflammation and go on to cause frank infection or abscess formation. Surgery is indicated to prevent further episodes of inflammation or abscess formation and involves total subareolar duct excision. Plasma cell mastitis may occur without evidence of duct ectasia. Sometimes needle-like calcifications are visible on mammography.

OPERATION: SUBAREOLAR TOTAL DUCT EXCISION
(HADFIELD'S OPERATION)

In this case the nipple is again raised off the underlying tissues through a periareolar incision. The main ducts underneath the nipple are then excised as a block and sent for histology. Antibiotic prophylaxis is achieved with a single-dose broad-spectrum antibiotic at induction (e.g. co-amoxiclav).

Procedure profile

Blood requirement	0
Anaesthetic	GA
Operation time	30–60 minutes
Hospital stay	24 hours
Return to normal activity	1–2 weeks

Postoperatively bruising and haematoma may occur. Persistent and recurrent abscess formation may follow incomplete subareolar resection, in particular for symptomatic duct ectasia particularly when previous episodes of inflammation or abscess formation have occurred. Patients should be warned of the risk of altered nipple sensation and cosmetic distortion as well as the risk of infection and recurrent symptoms.

Nipple inversion

Although not a pathology, this is a frequent cause of presentation to a symptomatic breast clinic. It may be unilateral or bilateral.

Many women develop nipple inversion naturally as part of the normal process of involution and postpartum change. The nipple is then often easily everted by gentle manipulation. In benign simple inversion a horizontal slit is often seen across the nipple.

Recent change, or that associated with an underlying mass, may be caused by a tumour and is an indication for further investigation but the experienced clinician will easily recognise the difference between benign inversion and that associated with a breast cancer.

Other causes of benign breast lumps
Post-traumatic haematoma and fat necrosis
Bruising following traumatic injury to the breast may lead to residual organized scar tissue. Even when the history is clear, the examining surgeon cannot be certain whether the lesion is indeed scar tissue or a tumour arising de novo, and the lesion must be fully assessed. Beware the patient with cancer who claims a history of injury.

Recognizing the pattern
The patient will often give a history of trauma, nowadays following a road traffic accident (seat belt injury), although domestic violence may be concealed. On examination there may be bruising associated with an underlying lump.

Management
Usually conservative once a carcinoma has been excluded. Sometimes repeated ultrasound-guided aspiration of liquefying haematomas may relieve discomfort and provide reassurance.

Galactocoele
A galactocoele is a milk-containing cyst which arises during late pregnancy or lactation. Ultrasound is helpful. Milk may be aspirated from the cyst. The cyst may recur, in which case repeated aspirations may be necessary.

Breast abscess
Breast abscesses occur either in the lactating breast, as a result of infection from the baby's mouth entering a cracked nipple, or in non-lactating breasts throughout adult life usually as a complication of the mammary duct ectasia/plasma cell mastitis syndrome.

Recognizing the pattern
The patient complains of a rapid onset of severe localized pain, which may be associated with a lump, skin erythema or discharge of pus. On examination there may be signs of inflammation with a hot, tender swelling of the infected area. This may become indurated or fluctuant.

Proving the diagnosis
Clinical assessment, ultrasound and bacteriology of aspirated pus.

Management
Lactational abscesses are nearly always the result of *Staphylococcus aureus* infection and are best managed by repeated aspirations (preferably under ultrasound control) and antistaphylococcal antibiotics (e.g. flucloxacillin). Surgery is rarely necessary nowadays. The mother can safely continue to breast-feed if she wishes. Non-lactational abscesses are nearly always retroareolar and contain a mixed growth of organisms often with anaerobic bacteria. Repeated aspiration and antibiotics may relieve the acute episode but surgery is often required to treat the underlying condition (duct ectasia/plasma cell mastitis). Where the condition fails to respond to antibiotics alone, incision and drainage may be necessary.

OPERATION: DRAINAGE OF BREAST ABSCESS
The abscess is incised and curetted. Periareolar incisions give excellent long-term cosmesis. The wound is irrigated, and packed or drained. If a periareolar incision is not possible the incision should be carefully chosen to give dependent drainage and the best possible late cosmetic result.

Procedure profile

Blood requirement	0
Anaesthetic	GA (LA with topical cream if abscess very superficial)
Operation time	15 minutes
Hospital stay	1–2 days
Return to normal activity	Variable

Most wounds can be managed on an outpatient basis by district nursing staff.

Mamillary fistula

Occasionally, when an abscess has been incised surgically or has drained spontaneously, a fistula occurs between the skin and the affected duct, and continues to discharge. Treatment is to excise or lay open the fistula using a modified microdochectomy approach. The areola usually heals remarkably well.

Plastic surgery for benign disorders

Procedures undertaken primarily for cosmetic reasons are predominantly not available in the public health service. Breast augmentation and reduction surgery does have a place in the management of women with developmental breast disorders, and in the aftermath of breast cancer surgery as a part of reconstructive surgery.

Disorders of breast development are common and range from minor differences in breast size and shape to gross asymmetries or misshapen breasts which young women in particular find extremely distressing. Often no cause for these abnormalities can be identified and there are no predisposing familial or genetic disorders.

Management

Minor asymmetries are best managed conservatively, with strong reassurance that this is a normal variant. Gross asymmetries can be corrected by either augmentation of the smaller breast or reduction of the larger breasts or combinations of the two. Occasionally complex reshaping procedures are required also (e.g. in tuberous breast abnormality).

In breast augmentation an implant is positioned in a pocket dissected usually between the natural breast tissue and the pectoral muscle often using a small incision placed in the inframammary crease. Patients should be warned of the risk of haemorrhage and infection in the early postoperative period, both of which are rare. The risk of interrupting the sensory nerve supply to the nipple with a permanent loss of (erotic) sensation should be discussed. The risk of capsular contracture and implant failure (and therefore the need for further surgery) should also be discussed in addition to the problems of mammography and FNA biopsy in the presence of a breast implant should the woman develop a breast lump and require investigation later in life.

Breast reduction procedures aim to relieve excessive unilateral or bilateral breast development relative to a woman's size and build, which can be a very disabling problem. Gross hypertrophy can occasionally follow lactation. A variety of breast reduction procedures have been developed. Resected breast tissue should be examined histologically after a reduction mammoplasty. Unexpected tumours and ductal carcinoma in situ (DCIS) are occasionally found. Women over 40 about to undergo breast reduction ideally should have preoperative screening mammography.

5.2 Carcinoma of the breast

Introduction

Carcinoma of the breast is the most common malignant disease in women in the Western world. The incidence is rising but the mortality is gradually falling. There are approximately 35 000 new cases per year in the UK, and approximately 15 000 deaths. Six per cent of women will develop the disease in the UK (50 per 100 000 per annum) but over 80% occur in women over the age of the menopause. Most carcinomas of the breast are invasive ductal carcinomas. Other histological subtypes include lobular, tubular, mucinous and medullary tumours.

The natural history of established breast cancer is variable. Some tumours progress in a logical pattern from primary tumour to regional node metastases to distant metastases while others spread in a less predictable fashion. Axillary node status, however, remains the best indicator of metastatic potential and also for planning adjuvant treatment.

Many biological factors are associated with poorer prognosis, and in particular the tumour grade, which correlates broadly with the degree of tumour differentiation. Unfortunately, there are no absolutely certain predictors of future behaviour which can be gleaned from study of the primary tumour. This unpredictability of behaviour has a major influence on the variety of treatments practised in different specialist breast units and on the many controversies that still surround the disease.

Cancers are identified by presenting:

- through breast screening programmes
- as ductal carcinoma in situ
- as symptomatic breast cancer.

After the general management principles have been described more detailed accounts include:

- surgery for invasive breast cancer
- postoperative adjuvant therapy
- breast reconstruction and plastic surgery
- late problems and metastatic disease.

UK breast screening programme

Two-thirds of women presenting with breast cancer in the UK have symptoms (usually a lump) which will have been investigated in a specialist breast clinic. One-third present in the absence of symptoms, the cancer detected through the National Breast Screening Programme.

Women aged between 50 and 69 (programme extended from 64 to 69 in 2004) are invited for community-based mammographic screening every 3 years. The invitation is by general practice list so unfortunately does not include the adult women (up to 10%) not registered with a GP. Two mammographic views are taken of each breast and read independently by two specialist radiologists. The majority are passed as normal after this initial assessment and simply recalled for a further examination in another 3 years. A small number will have a mammographic abnormality which requires further 'triple assessment' (see pp. 204–211). The abnormality is investigated by clinical examination, further mammographic views, ultrasound and FNA or WBN biopsies (see below). Following this assessment the woman may be passed as normal or benign, indeterminate (requiring further assessment) or malignant (requiring treatment).

A small number with indeterminate radiological abnormalities will require open surgical biopsy to confirm or exclude malignancy. These biopsies often require image guidance by the insertion of a mammographic wire using stereotactic techniques or by surface marking with ultrasound as many of these abnormalities are impalpable to the clinician's finger.

Ductal carcinoma in situ (DCIS)

Up to 20% of malignant lesions detected through the mammographic screening programme are DCIS rather than invasive cancer. DCIS is a malignant proliferation of cells within the microscopic milk ducts (ductules) which has not invaded through the basement membrane. At this stage it is not a true breast cancer since a cancer is an invasive malignancy which can spread by infiltration across basement membranes into blood vessels and lymphatic channels.

DCIS is detected on mammograms because microcalcifications develop which are visible as tiny white dots (which often have a branching pattern) on the X-ray film. Often no lump is palpable at this stage and mammographic (image) guidance is required to mark the position in the breast for the surgeon.

Management
Localized DCIS may be fully excised by local wide excision. Paradoxically, widespread DCIS may mandate a mastectomy to pre-empt the progression to invasive malignancy. In these cases the mastectomy is often followed by an immediate breast reconstruction if the woman wishes.

Following wide excision of localized DCIS some women are referred for adjuvant radiotherapy in the same way as following wide excision of an invasive carcinoma.

Symptomatic breast cancer

Recognizing the pattern
The incidence of cancer increases from the late teens, but is rare under the age of 30 years. Over 30 the incidence begins to rise rapidly and continues to increase into old age. The cancer may present in the following ways.

- As a lump. The patient usually finds this herself but it may be noticed by a partner or during a routine medical examination.
- With indrawing or other deformity of the nipple or skin (occasionally the skin dimple is far more obvious than the lump).
- With erosion/ulceration of the nipple (Paget's disease – see p. 243).
- With pain (uncommonly).
- With bloody nipple discharge (uncommonly).

Women still present de novo (usually delayed through fear rather than ignorance) with grossly advanced disease, including huge masses with ulceration, erosion, oedema ('peau d'orange') and erythema (inflammatory tumours). Involvement of axillary and supraclavicular lymph nodes may be obvious. They may also present as a result of metastatic disease e.g. bone pain or pathological fracture (to orthopaedic surgeons), jaundice from liver metastases or breathlessness from pleural effusions.

On examination the lesion may be firm or soft and of any size. Look for puckering of the skin over the lump. The clinical size should be estimated and the state of regional lymph nodes noted.

Proving the diagnosis

The diagnosis is made by triple assessment as previously described (see pp. 204–11).

The patient should have a chest X-ray and a careful examination carried out to look for axillary or more distant metastases. A full blood count to exclude anaemia (which may indicate bone marrow infiltration) and biochemistry of bone metabolism (calcium, alkaline phosphatase) and liver function is also useful in screening for metastatic disease. The routine addition of more complex investigations in the absence of symptoms or abnormalities of these simple screening tests (e.g. liver scanning by CT or USS, bone scan etc.) is not considered efficient or cost-effective and is no longer recommended.

STAGING OF INVASIVE BREAST CANCER

Following the diagnosis of an invasive breast cancer clinical staging is performed in order to plan initial treatment. Neither cancer staging system currently in use is ideal for the staging of breast cancer but the TNM (tumour, node, metastasis) system based on clinical measurement of tumour size and assessment of

Table 5.2.1 The TNM classification of breast cancer.

Tis	Cancer in situ
T1	< 2 cm (T1a < 0.5 cm, T1b > 0.5–1, T1c > 1–2 cm)
T2	> 2 cm – 5 cm
T3	> 5 cm
T4a	Involvement of chest wall
T4b	Involvement of skin (includes ulceration, direct infiltration, peau d'orange and satellite nodules)
T4c	T4a and T4b together
T4d	Inflammatory cancer
N0	No regional nodal metastases
N1	Palpable mobile involved ipsilateral axillary nodes
N2	Fixed involved ipsilateral axillary nodes
N3	Ipsilateral internal mammary node involvement (rarely clinically detectable)
M0	No evidence of metastases
M1	Distant metastases (includes ipsilateral supraclavicular nodes)

Table 5.2.2 UICC staging of breast carcinoma based on TNM system.

UICC stage	TNM classification of tumours
I	T1, N0, M0
II	T1, N1, M0; T2, N0–1, M0
III	Any T, N2–3, M0; T3, any N, M0; T4, any N, M0
IV	Any T, any N, M1

nodal status (Table 5.2.1) can be combined into the UICC (International Union Against Cancer or Union Internationale Contre Cancer) system to give a guide to best management (Table 5.2.2). A more useful system, however, utilizes pathological assessments of tumour size and nodal status (pTNM) but has the disadvantage that it can only be completed postoperatively.

Another system increasingly used is the Nottingham Prognostic Index (NPI). This system is based on tumour size (measured pathologically), tumour grade and axillary node status. A

Table 5.2.3 Prognostic groups derived by the Nottingham Prognostic Index (NPI).

Prognostic group	NPI	Predicted 10-year survival % without systemic adjuvant treatment
Excellent	< 2.4	94
Good	2.41–3.4	83
Moderate 1	3.41–4.4	70
Moderate 2	4.41–5.3	51
Poor	> 5.4	19

formula is used to give a numerical value which then places the patient into a prognostic group (Table 5.2.3). This can help in subsequent treatment planning, particularly when combined with hormone receptor (ER) status.

The NPI = $0.2 \times$ tumour diameter in centimetres + node status + tumour grade (1–3)

The node status is:
- 1 when nodes are free of disease (N0 – TNM)
- 2 where 1–3 nodes contain metastatic disease
- 3 where 4 or more nodes contain metastatic disease.

Similarly the tumour grade is scored as either:
- 1 for a grade I, less aggressive appearance
- 2 for a grade II, intermediate appearance or
- 3 for a grade III, more aggressive appearance.

Management

Breast cancer is a complex and unpredictable disease. Treatment will be planned on an individual basis, taking into account many factors, including the patient's age and well-being, the size and position of the tumour, and the patient's view of how she wishes to be treated. Age alone is not a contraindication to surgery. Provided the woman is fit for surgery, this probably remains the best option for long-term disease control or 'cure'.

Generally patients judged to have operable tumours and no overt evidence of metastases (including a clear chest X-ray) will be offered surgery. This will either be a wide local excision (WLE) of the primary tumour, or a total (simple) mastectomy.

Most units have a policy of axillary sampling or dissection to obtain sufficient lymph nodes to stage the disease.

It is necessary to use the clinical TNM/UICC systems preoperatively to plan initial treatment with those patients in stages I and II usually undergoing surgical treatment. Patients in stage IV (established distant metastatic disease) will almost certainly not be offered surgery and are treated by combination of endocrine therapy, chemotherapy and radiotherapy. Patients in stage III are increasingly offered neoadjuvant therapy to downstage their clinical disease thus making subsequent surgical management simpler, safer and probably more successful.

BREAST CANCER IN ELDERLY WOMEN
The definition of elderly nowadays is not clear-cut. As with younger women the treatment of an elderly woman with breast cancer should be based on a careful assessment of her fitness, mental and emotional state, the biology of her cancer and her own wishes for treatment.

Generally surgery alone or in combination with systemic therapies and/or radiotherapy offers the best prospect of achieving long-term disease control. Some elderly women, however, are so frail (physically and/or mentally) that surgery would be undesirable or inappropriate. She may also refuse surgical treatment. In these women hormone receptor-positive breast cancers (as confirmed by immunohistochemistry on a WBN biopsy) can be treated by antiestrogens (e.g. tamoxifen) or aromatase inhibitors (e.g. anastrozole, letrozole, exemestane) alone and response measured by regular tumour measures (clinical +/– radiological).

Surgery is then reserved for those tumours that progress despite treatment when followed up for a number of months or years. The specific management will always be guided by an assessment of the woman's 'biological' age, circumstances and coexisting infirmities.

Surgery for invasive breast cancer

The choice of primary surgical procedure is dependent upon many factors. These include the following.

- Tumour size (particularly in comparison with breast size).
- Position of the tumour in the breast (central tumours often require mastectomy irrespective of size).
- Patient choice (some women will choose mastectomy for small tumours for which the surgeon may think breast conservation is appropriate).
- Mammographic features. Large diffuse carcinoma (often lobular) may be unsuitable for breast conservation as are cases where there is evidence of widespread DCIS in association with an invasive carcinoma (as shown by extensive malignant microcalcification on mammogram).
- Patient age is an important factor. Breast cancer in very young women (under 35 years) may be best treated by mastectomy and in very elderly women mastectomy may also be a good option to avoid the need for postoperative radiotherapy which must usually follow breast-conserving surgery.
- The requirement for postoperative radiotherapy may be a factor in a woman's own decision-making when choosing between conservation and mastectomy. With the increasing use of postmastectomy radiotherapy, however, the situation nowadays is less clear cut (see later).

By the time a woman is admitted for breast cancer surgery she should have had extensive information, both verbal and written (and increasingly audiovisual), so that the decision has been made on the choice of surgical procedure to be performed. All these factors need to be discussed between the surgeon, patient (and her family) and the multidisciplinary team responsible for her care, and cross checks made on the confirmed diagnosis, stage and metastatic screen (chest X-ray and bloods).

At the preoperative ward round the surgeon (ideally accompanied by the ward doctor, ward nurse and breast care nurse) will check the results and consent form for surgery and confirm with the patient the side and site to be operated upon, marking with a 'permanent' skin marker.

OPERATION: WIDE LOCAL EXCISION (WLE)
The aim of this procedure is to achieve complete pathological removal of the malignant lesion (minimum of 2 mm clear histological circumferential margin) with minimum distortion of the cosmetic contour of the breast (not always possible). Generally

an incision is placed over the lesion (as this marks the precise site of excision for the radiotherapist) and a cylinder of breast tissue is excised, preserving just the subcutaneous fat and skin over the tumour and the pectoral muscle deep to it. The specimen should be carefully marked by the surgeon (to orientate its position for the pathologist) before it is sent from the operating table to the pathology department. Careful haemostasis is obtained before skin closure, and drains are generally not used. The subcutaneous tissue and skin are closed with absorbable (subcuticular) sutures to leave a fine neat scar.

Procedure profile

Blood requirement	0
Anaesthetic	GA
Operation time	30 minutes
Hospital stay	24–48 hours
Return to normal activity	2–3 weeks but depends on adjuvant therapy.

OPERATION: TOTAL (SIMPLE) MASTECTOMY

Despite modern trends to conservative surgery, the total (simple) mastectomy remains an important operation for central tumours, for those tumours that are large relative to the patient's breast size, and for multifocal or diffuse tumours. Mastectomy also reduces the risk of local recurrence compared to WLE and it remains the preferred operation by and for many women. The breast is excised, usually using a transverse elliptical incision to include the entire breast pad.

Procedure profile

Blood requirement	0/group and save
Anaesthetic	GA
Operation time	45–60 minutes
Hospital stay	3–5 days
Return to normal activity	3–4 weeks but depends on adjuvant therapy.

The operation of radical mastectomy in which the whole breast is removed en bloc with the pectoral muscles and axillary nodes has largely been confined to the history books. It may have a place in the management of locally advanced breast cancer in countries where advanced adjuvant therapy techniques are unavailable (or unaffordable), but in modern UK practice preoperative downstaging (neoadjuvant therapy) can reduce tumour bulk and allow for conventional less radical surgical procedures (total mastectomy or WLE).

OPERATION: AXILLARY DISSECTION

The management of the axilla remains controversial but should not be influenced by the choice between breast conservation or mastectomy. Axillary lymph node staging remains the single most important factor in evaluation of prognosis and in planning adjuvant therapy. The principles of axillary surgery are:

- to obtain information on the metastatic potential of the tumour (prognosis) and for planning of adjuvant therapy
- to remove any malignant disease from the axilla
- to minimize the morbidity of axillary staging.

The anatomy of the axillary nodes is described in terms of levels 1, 2 and 3. In a full axillary clearance all 3 levels are dissected. This yields large numbers of nodes for pathological analysis but women with axillary node-negative disease (60%) have been exposed to significant risk of morbidity without any advantage over a less radical approach. The more extensive the axillary dissection the greater the risk of:

- postoperative seroma (fluid collection)
- sensory changes (numbness, neuralgia)
- reduced shoulder mobility (frozen shoulder in extreme cases)
- lymphoedema (a chronic and disabling swelling of the arm).

For this reason most specialist breast surgeons adopt a less radical approach and dissect just level 1 or sometimes 1 and 2 unless there is evidence of extensive axillary disease macroscopically when a full clearance is appropriate. Some surgeons adopt an even less radical approach and sample nodes in level 1, removing a minimum of four for analysis. Whichever approach is used the surgeon must take care to avoid damage to major motor nerves, especially the long thoracic nerve (to serratus anterior) and the neurovascular bundle to the latissimus dorsi muscle.

SENTINEL LYMPH NODE BIOPSY

A recent development in axillary surgery allows the surgeon to identify and remove the first draining node or 'sentinel' node through which draining lymph from the breast cancer initially passes. As a result a more 'focused' sample (usually of level 1) nodes can be made, ensuring accurate staging. If these nodes are clear of disease it is assumed the remaining axilla is clear and no further axillary treatment is required. If the sentinel lymph nodes are affected (confirmed pathologically) the axilla can be treated at a second operation by further dissection or treated non-surgically by radiotherapy.

The sentinel node is 'marked' preoperatively using a variety of techniques but most commonly by a combination of radiological marking using a radiolabelled colloid solution and a visible (blue) dye which are injected just beneath the skin near the tumour. Both are carried via the breast lymphatics to the sentinel node which is then identified by the surgeon through a small axillary incision using a gamma probe (radiolabelled colloid) and the naked eye (blue dye).

Axillary staging is usually performed through the same incision as used for a mastectomy but requires a separate axillary incision when performed in combination with wide local excision. Most surgeons drain the axillary site using a closed suction drain removed after 2–3 days when the drainage turns serous (not heavily bloodstained) and daily volumes fall to around 50 mL or less.

Whenever drains are removed (early or delayed) postoperative seromas (collections of serous fluid) are common following axillary surgery and may require repeated percutaneous aspirations for 2–3 weeks postoperatively. Postoperatively dressing removal, wound inspection and seroma aspiration is often performed by the breast care nursing component of the modern multidisciplinary team.

The breast care nurse plays an important part in the pre-, peri- and postoperative care, and psychological support. She will ensure that arrangements have been made for fitting an external prosthesis (after mastectomy) when the patient is discharged from hospital. In the early phase after mastectomy, patients may be issued with a lightweight external prosthesis, which may be replaced by a more permanent model after swelling has resolved and wound healing is complete. When the woman is dressed the effect of surgery is disguised. As a result many women do not request reconstructive surgery.

Postoperative adjuvant therapy

Planning of postoperative adjuvant therapy is again a function of the multidisciplinary team comprising surgeon, pathologist, oncologist as well as nurses and radiologists who meet to discuss the results of the pathology analysis following surgery. The final decision rests with the patient and her family. Many factors are taken into account including the pathological staging (pTNM), the hormone receptor status of the primary tumour, and the age and menopausal status of the patient. In addition prognostic scoring systems such as the NPI can be used.

Radiotherapy

The use of high-energy ionizing radiation in the treatment of cancer is planned by clinical (radiation) oncologists and administered in specialist units by therapy radiographers. Radiotherapy finds four general applications in breast cancer care. Details of technique, timing and dosage may vary from one unit to another.

Breast following WLE

Radiotherapy to the remaining breast tissue following breast-conserving surgery (WLE) reduces the risk of local recurrence (within the same breast) by up to 70%. It is therefore the standard of care following WLE in the majority of women. There are selected cases where the omission of radiotherapy following breast-conserving surgery may be safe since the risk of local recurrence is so low. This may mean that older women (over 70) with small (< 2 cm) low-grade (Grade 1) ER-positive carcinomas (see below) which have been completely excised with a satisfactory margin (> 2 mm) can be safely treated with postoperative antiestrogens (tamoxifen) or aromatase inhibitors (e.g. anastrozole) alone (NPI excellent prognostic group). Trials of partial volume radiotherapy are under way in which only the breast tissue immediately adjacent to the excised tumour is treated.

Chest wall after mastectomy

Postmastectomy chest wall radiotherapy is being increasingly used. Indications would include large primary tumours (> 5 cm), pectoral muscle infiltration, extensive nodal involvement (4 or more axillary nodes affected), and extensive lymphatic invasion seen on pathological analysis.

Lymphatic field

Axillary radiotherapy is sometimes used following axillary sampling (or sentinel lymph node biopsy) when positive nodes have been found to avoid the need for further axillary surgery. In women who have extensive axillary nodal disease (4 or more nodes affected) the inclusion of a supraclavicular radiotherapy field is increasingly recommended. Some units also include an internal mammary field, although evidence of long-term benefit is lacking and morbidity is increased.

Palliative

In patients with locally advanced ulcerated or bleeding tumours, radiotherapy may be useful in combination with systemic adjuvant therapies in giving relief of distressing symptoms. It is also useful in the palliation of symptoms of metastatic disease, particularly painful bony metastases.

Systemic adjuvant therapy
Endocrine treatment
HORMONE RECEPTORS, ANTIESTROGENS AND
AROMATASE INHIBITORS

Estrogen receptor (ER) measurements are now used routinely as predictors of response to endocrine therapy. Some units also analyse for progesterone receptors (PgR). Both can be measured by immunohistochemical techniques staining for the receptors on tissue sections similar to those used for routine histopathology. Many primary breast cancers are receptor positive. Fewer metastases are receptor positive. Most well-differentiated and lobular cancers are receptor positive. Premenopausal women have lower rates of ER-positive cancers.

Several drugs are now available which act on the hormone receptor pathways of breast cancer growth. They are only effective in women with ER-positive primary tumours. The use of endocrine therapy in women with ER-negative breast cancer is no longer supported. In units not routinely measuring PgR some women with ER-negative (but PgR-positive) disease may be denied effective endocrine treatment. PgR should therefore be assessed at least in ER-negative tumours.

Menopausal status also needs to be considered, since only antiestrogens (which block the ER pharmacologically) are effective in premenopausal women. The most tried and tested agent is tamoxifen which, when administered for 5 years after surgery, can reduce the risk of relapse by 20–25%.

In postmenopausal women an alternative to antiestrogen (tamoxifen) therapy is the group of newer agents known as selective aromatase inhibitors. These drugs act on the enzymes (aromatase) that convert estrogen precursors into estrogen. These enzymes are found in the liver, adrenal and peripheral fat. Aromatase inhibitors (e.g. anastrozole, exemestane) are not active against ovarian aromatase enzymes and are therefore of no use in premenopausal women unless they are pharmacologically rendered postmenopausal by the use of LH/RH antagonists concurrently.

In deciding on the most appropriate endocrine therapy the side-effects of the agents should be taken into account. Tamoxifen, for example, improves bone density (prevents osteoporosis) in postmenopausal women but carries a small risk of inducing an endometrial (uterine lining) carcinoma in women who have not had a hysterectomy. Aromatase inhibitors do not cause endometrial cancer but do not provide bone protection and at the moment are significantly more expensive (30-fold) than tamoxifen.

OVARIAN ABLATION

For premenopausal women with ER-positive breast cancer, ovarian ablation may be as effective as cytotoxic chemotherapy in preventing relapse. Surgical oophorectomy is, however, rarely performed because 'oophorectomy' can be achieved by radiotherapy or drugs that block the hypothalamopituitary control of ovarian function (e.g. goserelin, an LH/RH antagonist).

The only remaining indication for surgical oophorectomy is in the treatment of a woman with a proven BRCA1 or BRCA2 genetic abnormality since these predispose to the risk of ovarian cancer as well as breast cancer.

Cytotoxic chemotherapy

Drugs may be used singly or in combination, and the treatment may be intermittent or continuous. The agents commonly used are doxorubicin (Adriamycin), epirubicin cyclophosphamide, methotrexate, 5-fluorouracil and vincristine. There is not yet complete agreement about the indications for postoperative chemotherapy. In general 'chemo', usually meaning serial courses of cytotoxic drugs in various combinations, is used in the following circumstances.

- Where one or more axillary nodes are positive at primary surgery in the under 70s, especially if the primary tumour is hormone receptor negative.
- For grade III, histologically aggressive but node-negative primary tumours in the under 50s, particularly if the tumour is hormone receptor negative.
- For very large, advanced or inflammatory tumours at presentation.
- For recurrent disease not responsive to other treatment modalities.

Chemotherapy does not guarantee cure. Meta-analysis of numerous clinical trials suggests that cytotoxic polychemotherapy reduces the overall risk of death by up to 14%. In premenopausal patients the reduction may be 20% or so. It may render an apparently locally inoperable tumour operable (neoadjuvant therapy). Side-effects of these drugs may be severe, including bone marrow suppression, hair loss, nausea, diarrhoea and vomiting.

These treatment options are summarized in Tables 5.2.4 and 5.2.5.

Breast reconstruction and plastic surgery

Following mastectomy many women adapt to wearing an external prosthesis over the mastectomy scar. Provided the scar is neat, smooth and well sited once the prosthesis is positioned in the bra, the mastectomy site is usually well hidden.

Table 5.2.4 Planning systemic adjuvant therapy in postmenopausal women (> 50 years).

	NPI group		
	Excellent and good prognosis	Moderate prognosis	Poor prognosis
Hormone receptor positive	Antiestrogen or aromatase inhibitor	Antiestrogen or aromatase inhibitor	Antiestrogen or aromatase inhibitor + chemotherapy
Hormone receptor negative	None	Chemotherapy considered	Chemotherapy

Table 5.2.5 Planning systemic adjuvant therapy in premenopausal women.

	NPI group		
	Excellent and good prognosis	Moderate prognosis	Poor prognosis
Hormone receptor positive	Antiestrogen +/− LH/RH antagonist	Antiestrogen +/− LH/RH antagonist +/− chemotherapy	Antiestrogen +/− LH/RH antagonist and chemotherapy
Hormone receptor negative	Chemotherapy considered	Chemotherapy	Chemotherapy

For others, however, the prospective and actual loss of a breast can have profound consequences for both themselves and their partners. Depression, altered body image and psychosexual problems are all encountered. Breast reconstruction is beneficial in selected cases but should not be perceived to be, or offered as, a panacea to all psychological problems following the diagnosis and treatment of breast cancer. It does not reduce, for example, the fear associated with the possibility of disease recurrence.

Much debate continues as to the optimum method and the ideal timing of breast reconstruction. As with decisions relating to the cancer treatment a multidisciplinary approach gives the best results, with input from reconstructive surgeons (plastic or specialist breast oncoplastic surgeons), specialist nurses and the patient herself.

Several options for breast reconstruction are available and can either be applied immediately (at the time of the mastectomy) or delayed until the initial phase of cancer treatment is completed. The most frequently used methods are:

- tissue expansion techniques and implants
- tissue transfer techniques based on myocutaneous flaps with or without implants.

The use of permanently implanted prosthetic implants (usually silicone gel filled) offers a relatively straightforward method of reconstruction and is increasing in popularity again as historical fears of silicone leakage have been dispelled and as the quality and choice of implants has increased over the last few years.

In general terms, however, a breast reconstruction based predominantly or totally on the use of the woman's own tissues (autologous) give the best results in terms of cosmetic appearance and feel, and lack of deterioration over time. Reconstruction based on myocutaneous flaps in which soft tissue is brought into the mastectomy area dependent on the blood supply from a major muscle are more complex than tissue expansion techniques but can give very natural looking (and feeling) reconstructions. Morbidity from the donor site (from where the flap is raised) should, however, be carefully considered when selecting patients for these procedures. Options include:

- latissimus dorsi myocutaneous flaps using tissue from the back
- TRAM (transverse rectus abdominis muscle) flaps or variations using tissue from the inferior anterior abdominal wall.

There is no evidence that the inclusion of reconstruction at the same time as the initial mastectomy impedes cancer treatment or compromises results in any way. The increasing use of postmastectomy radiotherapy, however, has a deleterious result on the quality of the reconstruction by causing fibrosis within the soft tissues (particularly around an implant but also with TRAM flaps). Many surgeons no longer offer immediate reconstruction to patients with invasive breast cancer but it remains the best option in the management of the woman with widespread DCIS where much of the skin envelope of the breast can be retained (skin-sparing mastectomy).

Following reconstruction of the breast it is necessary in many women to carry out 'cosmetic' procedures on the opposite breast to restore the best symmetry. This may involve unilateral breast reduction, breast uplift procedures to correct droop (mastopexy) or occasionally breast augmentation. These symmetrizing procedures should be considered an integral part of the 'process' of reconstruction and the woman should be fully aware of what may be needed before embarking on this process.

There is no convincing evidence that a breast reconstruction, if properly and appropriately performed, masks the development of a subsequent recurrence since the tissue most at risk is usually in front of and not behind the reconstruction. With modern breast imaging and image-guided biopsy techniques it is usually possible to assess any area of concern safely without endangering a breast implant.

Late problems and metastatic disease

Lymphoedema

This condition is characterized by a chronic swelling (oedema) of the arm on the side of breast cancer treatment. It most commonly affects the forearm and hand but can affect the upper arm. The oedema is characteristically non-pitting. It is uncomfortable and unsightly and can lead to problems with arm/hand function. Episodes of lymphatic infection (lymphangitis) can follow minor injury (minor cuts, abrasions or even insect bites) leading to a worsening of the condition.

Severe lymphoedema is seen less frequently since the demise of radical mastectomy and radical axillary radiotherapy, but remains a problem in up to one-fifth of patients undergoing axillary surgery for breast cancer.

Management
Once lymphoedema develops there is no cure but it can be effectively controlled using techniques of elevation, lymphatic massage

and wearing elasticated compression sleeves. Most larger centres now have specialist lymphoedema therapists.

The less radical the axillary surgery the lower the risk; hence the drive to develop new techniques such as sentinel lymph node biopsy.

Metastatic disease

Carcinoma of the breast typically metastasizes to the bone marrow, lungs, brain and liver. It may also recur locally, despite seemingly adequate earlier treatment.

Many authorities now recommend that a widespread search for metastases should not be undertaken in the absence of symptoms at the time of presentation. The yield is very low, while the economic and emotional costs are very high. A chest X-ray is sufficient in most primary cases, along with simple blood tests as described earlier.

Metastatic spread and evidence of advanced disease may be revealed from a variety of investigations, which should only be used very selectively in response to specific symptoms. Possible tests include the following.

- Biochemistry. Alterations in the liver function tests – bilirubin, alkaline phosphatase and transaminase enzymes (ALT) – may indicate the presence of liver metastases. An elevated serum calcium and (bony) alkaline phosphatase indicates skeletal (bony) metastases.
- Plain X-rays. Chest X-ray in a breathless patient or one with a cough may reveal pulmonary metastases or pleural effusion. Plain X-rays to investigate localized bony pain may reveal bone destruction from skeletal metastases.
- Specialized radiology.
  - Isotope bone scan indicates skeletal metastases.
  - Ultrasound of liver or CT shows liver metastases.
  - CT chest and abdomen may be more sensitive than chest X-ray and abdominal ultrasound.
  - MRI or CT may be useful in investigating subtle bone scan changes where plain X-rays (skeletal survey) are normal.

Management of advanced or recurrent disease

Many cases of recurrent disease in the breast following previous breast-conserving therapy (WLE and radiotherapy) can be salvaged by mastectomy. Some patients with isolated local (chest wall) recurrence following mastectomy can be treated surgically. If evidence of more distant metastatic disease is confirmed, however, the likelihood of long-term cure is remote and management is aimed at improving and sustaining the quality of life as far as is possible and at preventing undue physical and emotional suffering. The early involvement of doctors and nurses specialising in palliative care may be helpful.

If patients with ER-positive disease relapse while taking anti-estrogen (tamoxifen) changing to an aromatase inhibitor (e.g. anastrozole) may be helpful and vice versa. Patients with ER-negative disease or those with ER-positive disease clearly not responding to endocrine treatment may be offered palliative chemotherapy. Newer agents include the taxanes and immunotherapy with agents such as trastuzumab (in selected patients).

Terminal care

Advanced carcinoma of the breast requires positive management. It can produce profound distress, fear and unpleasant physical symptoms. Analgesia should be given frequently and in sufficient doses to keep the patient out of pain. Hypercalcaemia may be managed by intravenous fluids and by osteoclast inhibitors such as pamidronate and etomidate. Corticosteroids and aspiration of the effusion can help breathlessness from a pleural effusion or lymphangitis carcinomatosa. Symptoms from hepatic metastases (e.g. pain and anorexia) may also respond to corticosteroids. Cerebral metastases may cause severe headache and focal neurological deficits and these may respond to corticosteroids (dexamethasone) and/or radiotherapy.

Multiprofessional, specialist palliative care teams have significantly improved the preservation of a woman's dignity and quality of life in the final days of this disease.

Paget's disease (carcinoma in the nipple)

Paget's disease is an eczematous, scaling plaque which appears in the nipple and spreads out to the areola, caused by malignant cells infiltrating the epithelium of the overlying skin. There is an associated underlying ductal carcinoma in situ or sometimes an invasive carcinoma.

Recognizing the pattern
There is a red, scaly or weeping plaque involving part of the nipple and areola. There may be a lump beneath the areola if an invasive carcinoma has developed. The lesion is never bilateral and always affects the nipple first, spreading out centrifugally to the areola. Eczema (a benign skin condition) often affects the areola first and is often bilateral. It also tends to occur in younger women than those developing Paget's disease.

Proving the diagnosis
The diagnosis of Paget's disease is confirmed on biopsy of the affected skin carried out as an outpatient under local anaesthetic.

Management
The lesion is managed as an early carcinoma of the breast. Because the carcinoma is central, a simple mastectomy will often be necessary although in many cases in the absence of invasive carcinoma excision of the nipple areolar complex alone may suffice.

5.3 Conditions of the male breast

The male breast is susceptible to many of the conditions of the female breast, including benign hypertrophy and less commonly, DCIS and invasive cancer.

Gynaecomastia

This is hypertrophy of the male breast. It may occur on one or both sides. There are many causes, the most important of which are listed in Table 5.3.1.

Recognizing the pattern
The condition is most commonly seen at puberty, in the 20s and 30s (it also affects users and abusers of anabolic steroids), in the

Table 5.3.1 Causes of gynaecomastia.

Physiological	Neonatal
	Pubertal
Idiopathic	Majority of presentations – no obvious cause found
Hormonal	Hypogonadism e.g. Klinefelter's syndrome
	Hormone-secreting tumours, e.g. testis, adrenal, liver
	Estrogen and antiandrogen therapy in advanced prostate cancer
	Deranged estrogen metabolism in chronic liver disease (cirrhosis)
	Hypothyroidism
Drug misuse	Anabolic steroids
	Cannabis
Pharmacological	Recognized side-effects of prescribed drugs in correct doses
	Digoxin
	Spironolactone
	Cimetidine

elderly and obese (idiopathic), and in men undergoing endocrine treatment for prostate cancer. In young men the possibility of a testicular tumour should be considered, although this is a rare presentation.

The presenting complaint is of unilateral or bilateral swelling beneath the nipple. There may be some discomfort. It may be discovered as part of more widespread disease, e.g. cirrhosis. It is important to take a careful drug history.

On examination the breast pad is enlarged. Tenderness is common. Inspect the testes for a tumour and look for evidence of liver failure or hyperthyroidism. Ask about medication and the use of recreational drugs.

Management

Pubertal gynaecomastia usually settles within months. The patient should be reassured. If it causes persisting embarrassment, a subareolar mastectomy may occasionally be carried out. The management of other forms of gynaecomastia depends on the cause. A short (up to 2 months) course of tamoxifen is sometimes helpful in reducing tenderness and swelling.

OPERATION: SUBAREOLAR MASTECTOMY FOR GYNAECOMASTIA

A semicircular incision is made around the edge of the areola and the nipple raised as a skin flap. The enlarged breast tissue is separated from the skin and underlying muscle, and removed through the central incision. The wound is drained using suction. The excised breast pad should be sent for histology. This operation may be indicated where the gynaecomastia consists of firm glandular tissue but gives poor results in cases of a more generalized fatty swelling. For these liposuction may be appropriate in extreme cases.

Procedure profile

Blood requirement	Group and save
Anaesthetic	GA
Operation time	30–60 minutes per side
Hospital stay	1–2 days
Return to normal activity	1–2 weeks

Removal of the breast pad may leave a large subcutaneous space which tends to fill with blood and serum. It is important to maintain suction drainage and external pressure to minimize troublesome haematoma formation. Day-case surgery can be inappropriate.

Carcinoma of the male breast

Approximately 0.6–1% of breast malignancies occur in men. There is an association with Klinefelter's syndrome. Male breast cancer usually affects older men and is rare under the age of 40.

Recognizing the pattern
The patient may notice a lump beneath the areola. Bloody discharge may rarely occur from the nipple.

On examination there is a lump within the breast pad, which is usually painless. There may be palpable, involved, axillary lymph nodes.

Proving the diagnosis
Triple assessment clinics. FNA or WBN biopsy are usually diagnostic. Sometimes imaging with mammography and ultrasound can be useful.

Management
Operable carcinoma is treated as in the female patient by mastectomy, axillary dissection and/or radiotherapy and/or chemotherapy. Many male breast carcinomas are ER positive and in these cases tamoxifen is also used. Postmastectomy radiotherapy is increasingly used in the management of male breast cancers. If a man develops breast cancer below the age of 60 it could indicate a possible genetic abnormality. A detailed family history should be ascertained. If he has a daughter she may be at increased risk and this should be sensitively discussed.

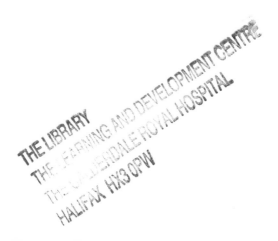

6 Chest surgery

6.1 Chest drainage and thoracotomy

Chest drains

The indications for chest drainage are:
- pneumothorax and tension pneumothorax (see pp. 625–26)
- pleural effusion
- haemothorax
- to prevent the collection of fluid or air after thoracotomy.

  The procedure of insertion is described in some detail as it is something most junior doctors will have to do.

OPERATION: INSERTING A CHEST DRAIN

Make sure that all the equipment you require is ready before you start. This includes the following.
- Local anaesthetic (1 or 2% lidocaine).
- Skin disinfection.
- A suitable tube drain (24–26 Ch) preferably with a radio-opaque line.
- Sutures needed for:
  - holding the drain in
  - closure of the skin.
- The underwater seal bottle containing saline.
- Straight artery forceps and a no. 11 scalpel blade.
- Wall suction and a suitable connection.
- A tube clamp.

  The procedure should be done in a treatment room. The drain is usually inserted in the fourth or fifth intercostal space in the mid-axillary line (practically this is the first rib space palpable below the axillary hair). The patient should be sitting up at 45°,

Surgery: Diagnosis and Management, 4th edition. Edited by N. Rawlinson and D. Alderson. © 2009 Blackwell Publishing, ISBN: 978-1-4051-2921-3

with an assistant holding the patient's arm up behind their head for an anterior approach. Alternatively the patient can lean forward over a suitably placed bed table with arms folded in front of the body (for a posterior or lateral approach). If you are about to drain an effusion check the presence of fluid by inserting a 19-gauge needle on a syringe at your chosen site. This entry site is guided by the size and location of the effusion.

- Clean the skin.
- Inject local anaesthetic, infiltrating the underlying tissues down to the parietal pleura. The presence of fluid or air can also be checked during this manoeuvre.
- Incise the skin with a scalpel and cut down on to the rib below the intercostal space chosen.
- Insert closed artery forceps and open to clean the fascia off the rib.
- Move up to enter just above the rib (Fig. 6.1.1) and enlarge and deepen the hole by opening the closed artery forceps until you penetrate the parietal pleura, thus creating a track for the drain. There may be an egress of air or fluid. Any tension is relieved.
- You may then enter a gloved finger into the pleural space to confirm that you are in the pleural cavity. Your finger will also

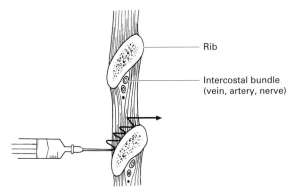

Fig. 6.1.1 Avoid damage to the intercostal bundle when entering the pleural cavity by 'walking up and over the rib'.

ensure that the track is wide enough to accommodate the
drain.

- Put in two sutures:
  - a 0 nylon or silk suture for securing the drain
  - a 2/0 nylon purse string suture left loose to close the wound
    when the drain is removed (optional).
- Mount the tip of the chest drain tube onto the plastic introducer. Alternatively a long curved artery forceps (Roberts)
  may be used. Introduce the chest drain into the track you have
  created and angle its direction into the appropriate position.
  Be sure that you put the chest drain in far enough.
- Connect the drain to the underwater seal as shown in Fig. 6.1.2.

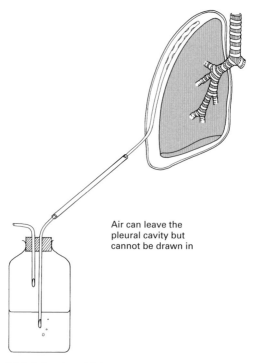

Air can leave the
pleural cavity but
cannot be drawn in

Fig. 6.1.2 Underwater seal drainage.

- Tie it in securely and check that the meniscus is fluctuating. If there is a pneumothorax air will be seen to bubble out on expiration.

USE OF SUCTION

Suction is applied to the chest drain to maintain a negative pressure within the hemithorax. Suction is needed if there is a continuing air leak from the lung into the pleural space as this prevents the lung expanding. Once a lung has collapsed its compliance will increase, often dramatically. This will tend to cause the lung to remain collapsed if suction is not applied.

Suction should be applied to the venting tube of the bottle. For preference use wall suction providing a high volume at low pressure (5–10 kPa).

Postoperatively:

- Check the position of the tube and the expansion of the lung by an early chest X-ray.
- If the tube is in too far it can be withdrawn. This often relieves postoperative discomfort.
- Position the bottle so that the water seal is at all times below the patient, ideally on the floor.
- Tube clamps are not necessary when moving the patient provided that the bottle is kept below the bed. *Never clamp a bubbling drain*.
- The tube can be seen to be patent by observing the meniscus fluctuate on breathing or coughing. The swing reflects changes in pressure in the pleural space.
- Re-expansion of the lung is encouraged by early ambulation and breathing exercises. If there is no 'swing' on the meniscus, the tube is blocked and is performing no useful function. Take a chest X-ray. If the lung is expanded, then the tube may be removed.
- This is done in two ways. After lung puncture or following spontaneous pneumothorax, it is usual to leave the clamped tube in situ for 24 h, then X-ray again. If the lung is still expanded, then the tube is removed.
- In other circumstances this practice is unnecessary provided:
  ◦ there is no air leak present, nor has there been for a minimum of 24 h

    ◦ there is a minimal or non-existent 'swing' of the meniscus within the drain.

Here the tube may simply be removed.
- As you remove the chest drain, ask the patient to breathe in and then hold their breath (i.e. a Valsalva manoeuvre). In this way no air is sucked into the pleural space as the tube is withdrawn. After the tube comes out, tie the skin closure stitch.

Some common problems with chest drainage
Tube bubbling on suction
- There is a continuing air leak from the lung, or a major airway.
- The drain has slipped out and exposed one of the side holes.
- There is a leak somewhere in the circuit.

No bubbling on suction, but the lung is still partially or wholly collapsed
- Tube blocked.
- Tube in wrong place.
- Tube kinked or clamped.

Thoracotomy

A thoracotomy may be performed on a general surgical unit and you should be familiar with the pre- and postoperative care that this entails. This is usually related to oesophageal surgery and this is covered on p. 272. Patients with trauma affecting both the abdominal and thoracic cavities may be under your care. Remember that every effort must be made to achieve full expansion of both lungs. In practice for the patient having chest surgery, this means making sure that no fluid (simple effusion, chyle, pus, blood) is allowed to accumulate in the pleural space.

    Preoperatively explain to the patient that they will have one or two tubes draining the chest postoperatively and tell them why. It will be important that they breathe fully and cough adequately and to do this they must be given adequate analgesia.

    The following approaches may be used.

OPERATION: POSTEROLATERAL THORACOTOMY
This may be used for access to the lung, oesophagus or descending aorta. The patient is placed in a prone or lateral position. The fifth, sixth or seventh intercostal space is opened.

OPERATION: MEDIAN STERNOTOMY
This is the best approach for the heart, pericardium, great vessels and anterior mediastinal structures. The patient lies supine and the sternum is split longitudinally with a reciprocating saw.

OPERATION: ANTEROLATERAL THORACOTOMY
This is the fastest way to gain access to the pleural cavity and (on the left side) the pericardium. It is used in the resuscitation room e.g. for cardiac tamponade after stabbing. The chest is opened through the seventh–eighth space and the costal cartilage divided to help spread the ribs. The access may be extended across the midline by dividing the sternum transversely.

During closure, chest drains are inserted. There are usually two – one at the apex and one at the base. They are brought out through separate stab incisions. The chest drains are attached to underwater seal drainage.

Procedure profile

Blood requirement	Check with operating surgeon
Anaesthetic	GA
Operation time	Depends on indication for operation
Hospital stay	7–10 days depending on procedure
Return to normal activity	2–6 weeks depending on procedure

Postoperatively it is most important that the patient has sufficient analgesia to breathe adequately and cough. This is usually achieved with a thoracic epidural (which requires careful nursing) or parenteral opiate drugs. The management of the chest drain has already been described.

Thoracoscopic surgery

An increasing number of intrathoracic techniques are now being carried out thoracoscopically. The lung on the side of the lesion is collapsed using a double-lumen endotracheal tube. An endoscope attached to a video camera is introduced through a suitable intercostal space, and instruments through other ports.

Lung resections, oesophageal operations and even cardiac procedures are now being done by these techniques. The advantage lies with the more rapid and less painful recovery achieved by avoiding an open thoracotomy.

Surgical airway

A surgical airway is indicated in three situations.
- Upper airways obstruction, e.g.
  - impacted foreign body
  - laryngeal oedema due to epiglottitis, angioneurotic oedema of the tongue or spreading infection of the floor of the mouth (Ludwig's angina)
  - severe facial injury
  - facial burns
  - assault with direct laryngeal injury.
- Conditions requiring prolonged ventilation.
- In severe respiratory disease, to decrease the dead space and allow regular direct suction of the airways.

In an emergency situation the simplest and fastest method of establishing an airway is through the cricothyroid membrane (cricothyroidotomy). Tracheostomy is, however, the method of choice when there is rather less urgency (Fig. 6.1.3). Percutaneous tracheostomy kits are widely available and you should make yourself familiar with the design used in your hospital. The open techniques are described in some detail as, again, the junior doctor may need to do them.

OPERATION: CRICOTHYROIDOTOMY
- Hold the head still.

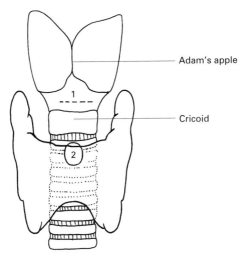

Fig. 6.1.3 Sites for cricothyroidotomy (1) and tracheostomy (2).

- Stand with your dominant (operating) hand nearer the head (so working downwards).
- Make a longitudinal skin incision (minimising the risk of venous bleeding from anterior jugular veins in an emergency) over the cricothyroid membrane (palpable in the space between the thyroid and cricoid cartilage) using any available knife blade.
- Stay in the midline and divide the cricothyroid membrane transversely until air is heard hissing in and out.
- The passage may be enlarged by inserting the handle of the scalpel and rotating it 90°.
- Insert a sterile cricothyroidotomy tube or any tube that will help keep the hole open.

OPERATION: TRACHEOSTOMY
- The patient is positioned supine on the table with the neck extended.
- A 3-cm transverse incision is made two fingerbreadths above the sternal notch.

- The strap muscles are separated in the midline and retracted sideways.
- The thyroid isthmus is either retracted or divided and sutured.
- When all bleeding has been controlled, a 1-cm disc is excised or an n-shaped flap is made in the trachea over the third or fourth ring.
- A tracheostomy tube is inserted and secured.
- The skin is loosely sutured around the tube.

Procedure profile

Blood requirement	0
Anaesthetic	LA/GA
Operation time	30–45 minutes
Hospital stay	Depends on underlying condition
Return to normal activity	Depends on underlying condition

Postoperatively a spare tube, introducer, retractor and sucker should be available by the patient's bed. The airways must be aspirated regularly to remove retained secretions. The inspired air must be humidified to prevent the secretions becoming too viscid.

7 Upper gastrointestinal and small bowel surgery

7.1 Oesophageal problems

Dysphagia

Dysphagia is defined as difficulty in swallowing. When there is a problem with swallowing in the voluntary (oral and pharyngeal) phases, patients do not characteristically describe 'food sticking'. Instead food fails to enter the oesophagus, stays in the mouth or enters the airway, causing coughing, spluttering or recurring chest infections. Virtually all causes of this type of dysphagia are chronic neurological or muscular diseases and it is rare for dysphagia to be the presenting feature of the underlying disorder. These causes are not considered further in this chapter. Oesophageal dysphagia occurs in the involuntary phase and is characterized by a sensation of food sticking.

A list of common causes of dysphagia is shown in Table 7.1.1.

Recognizing the pattern
The characteristic clinical patterns of various conditions are given in the subsequent pages but certain points in the history and examination are helpful in pointing towards a likely diagnosis. However, all patients with dysphagia should be investigated properly as it is not possible to be confident as to the cause from the history alone.
- Onset. Dysphagia due to a foreign body is sudden in onset whereas that due to carcinoma may develop more slowly with a final obstruction. With achalasia and benign stricture, the symptoms develop over several years, and are often accompanied by pain.

Surgery: Diagnosis and Management, 4th edition. Edited by N. Rawlinson and D. Alderson. © 2009 Blackwell Publishing, ISBN: 978-1-4051-2921-3

Table 7.1.1 Causes of dysphagia.

Arising within the oesophagus	Carcinoma of the oesophagus or gastro-oesophageal junction
	Chronic benign stricture
	Achalasia and other dysmotility states
	Foreign body
	CREST syndrome
	Oesophageal perforation
	Acute caustic stricture
	Pharyngeal pouch
	Plummer–Vinson syndrome
	Oesophageal candidiasis
Compressing the oesophagus from outside	Bronchial carcinoma
	Thoracic aneurysm
	Enlarged left atrium
	Enlarged mediastinal lymph nodes
	Large retrosternal goitre
Neuromuscular conditions	Bulbar palsies (related to stroke, motor neurone disease, multiple sclerosis, Parkinsonism)
	Myasthenia and muscular dystrophies
	Hysteria

- Site. Patients often point to the level at which they feel blockage. This is completely unreliable as an indicator of either the nature or site of obstruction.
- Severity. Is the dysphagia for fluids or solids? This gives an indication of how tight the stricture is. If the degree of dysphagia varies from day to day it is often due to dysmotility. In addition, motility problems usually cause dysphagia to both solids and liquids whereas mechanical obstructions cause dysphagia to solids only until they are very severe.
- Pain. Oesophageal pain is usually felt retrosternally and may be referred through into the back and radiate up into the neck and throat. Severe pain may occur from structural or functional oesophageal disease and can be difficult to differentiate from

cardiac pain except in that it is usually precipitated by swallowing. Painful swallowing (odynophagia) is common in infective oesophagitis (candida, herpes, cytomegalovirus). It is wrong to assume that patients with heartburn who develop dysphagia have benign strictures. All patients with dysphagia should be investigated.

- Regurgitation. Patients may begin to regurgitate oesophageal contents from any tight obstructive lesion once oesophageal stasis develops. This symptom is often associated with the onset of paroxysms of coughing at night due to tracheal aspirations.

- Systemic symptoms. Weight loss is a worrying symptom, although it can be due to either benign or malignant oesophageal disease. Patients with a neurological cause may have a past history of stroke or symptoms from other neurological deficits. Patients with the CREST syndrome have Calcinosis, Raynaud's disease, Esophageal dysmotility, the typical pinched facial appearance of Scleroderma and Telangiectasia.

On examination look for cervical or other lymphadenopathy (spreading from a lesion in the chest), and for hepatomegaly or an abdominal mass. A neurological examination may give a clue to the presence of more generalized neurological disease.

Proving the diagnosis

Every patient with dysphagia should have an urgent flexible endoscopy +/– a barium swallow and be referred to an oesophageal specialist.

Oesophageal physiology studies may be used to investigate some patients further.

- 24-h oesophageal pH measurement is the most accurate method of documenting pathological gastro-oesophageal reflux and relating it to the patient's symptoms.

- Oesophageal manometry demonstrates oesophageal peristalsis and the pressures of the oesophageal sphincters. It can be done briefly in the laboratory (station pull-through manometry) or over a longer period (24 h or ambulatory manometry).

- A video swallow records the passage of barium in moving pictures and gives more accurate information on the act of swallowing.

Routine blood tests should look for anaemia, deranged electrolytes, raised inflammatory markers (ESR or CRP) and abnormal liver function tests. A plain chest X-ray may reveal a fluid level behind the heart, evidence of aspiration or a mediastinal mass.

OPERATION: FLEXIBLE UPPER GI ENDOSCOPY
This is usually performed on a day-case basis under either benzodiazepine intravenous sedation or local anaesthetic throat spray. The endoscopist can carefully examine the pharynx, oesophagus, stomach and duodenum, taking biopsies or brushings if necessary. An oesophageal stricture can be dilated if this is appropriate and consent obtained for this procedure as described on p. 266.

Procedure profile

Blood requirement	0
Anaesthetic	LA
Operation time	15 minutes
Hospital stay	Day case
Return to normal activity	1–2 days

If the patient complains of chest or abdominal pain after a therapeutic endoscopy or if surgical emphysema develops in the neck, an urgent barium swallow should be performed to look for perforation. He or she should be kept nil by mouth and given intravenous fluids until the result is known.

Management
The further management of lesions in the oesophagus is discussed below. Lesions causing dysphagia which are outside the oesophagus or which are neurological are not discussed further.

Impacted foreign body
This can occur either in a normal oesophagus or at the site of a carcinoma or a stricture. In a normal oesophagus there are three sites of narrowing:
- at the level of the cricopharyngeus
- where the oesophagus passes behind the left main bronchus with the arch of the aorta crossing its left side

• at the level of the diaphragm.

These three positions are, respectively, at about 15, 25 and 40 cm from the incisor teeth.

Recognizing the pattern

The patient notices that something has stuck in the back of the throat resulting in acute difficulty in swallowing. There is pain which is increased by any attempt to swallow. The patient will notice excessive salivation.

On examination the patient is distressed and retching. Occasionally there may be signs of perforation or mediastinitis (surgical emphysema, tachycardia and fever).

Proving the diagnosis

The foreign body may occasionally be seen on plain chest X-ray if it is radio-opaque.

OPERATION: FLEXIBLE UPPER GI ENDOSCOPY AND REMOVAL FOREIGN BODY

This should always be by an experienced endoscopist. An overtube may be necessary to safely remove sharp objects and occasionally it is necessary for the patient to have a general anaesthetic and be intubated.

Procedure profile

Blood requirement	0
Anaesthetic	LA/GA
Operation time	30 minutes
Hospital stay	Day case
Return to normal activity	1–2 days

After the procedure a careful check is made for signs of perforation.

Although rare, the oesophagus may be injured during endoscopy, particularly if a therapeutic dilatation has been done. Since rigid oesophagoscopy has been abandoned by most clinicians, the incidence of iatrogenic oesophageal injury has fallen dramatically. The decision to manage endoscopic perforations non-operatively depends upon location and size of the tear, the nature of the underlying pathology, the presence of distal obstruction, whether or not there is free communication with the pleural space, and the degree of contamination of the oesophagus at the time that the injury occurred. The mainstay of treatment is to keep the patient nil by mouth, give broad-spectrum antibiotics and initiate either parenteral or distal (jejunostomy) feeding. For elderly and infirm patients who might not be fit for a thoracotomy, early placement of a covered self-expanding stent may be appropriate.

Spontaneous oesophageal perforation

Spontaneous rupture or tearing of the distal oesophagus (Boerhaave's syndrome) usually follows retching and vomiting. It should always be considered as a possible diagnosis in any patient who has collapsed and become rapidly unwell after a vomit. Spreading mediastinitis and septic shock lead to a very high mortality rate, particularly if the diagnosis is delayed and treatment is not instigated in a specialist oesophageal centre immediately.

Recognizing the pattern

A history of violent or prolonged vomiting is followed by severe chest and back pain. There may also be dyspnoea if the pleural space is involved (pneumothorax and/or pleural effusion).

The patient's general condition deteriorates quickly with hypotension, tachycardia, hypoxia, oliguria and a falling Glasgow Coma Score. Surgical emphysema may be felt in the neck and there may be the chest signs of a pleural effusion.

Proving the diagnosis

- A chest X-ray (normal and overpenetrated) may demonstrate surgical emphysema in the mediastinum. It may also show widening of the mediastinum. Look for a pleural effusion or pneumothorax.
- An urgent water-soluble contrast study usually, but not always, demonstrates the perforation.

- An urgent spiral CT scan will accurately detect air in the mediastinum and, if oral contrast is given, show the site and size of the perforation.
- General bloods include full blood count, renal function assessment and arterial blood gases.

Management

All patients require intravenous hydration, a urinary catheter, opiate analgesia, oxygen therapy and intravenous broad-spectrum antibiotics and antifungal agents. They should be kept strictly nil by mouth and transferred to a specialist oesophageal centre as soon as possible.

If the leak is small and contained within the mediastinum and there are no pleural effusions or pneumothorax, the patient may be treated conservatively. Parenteral nutrition is given via a dedicated central line or distal feeding initiated by jejunostomy. Closure of the tear is monitored by serial contrast swallows. Any septic complications must be investigated thoroughly and intrathoracic or mediastinal collections adequately drained by percutaneous CT guided techniques.

If, however, the tear is larger, an urgent operation will be necessary.

OPERATION: REPAIR OF OESOPHAGEAL PERFORATION

The upper oesophagus is approached through the neck. The incision is made anterior to the left sternocleidomastoid and the carotid sheath is retracted laterally. Tears in this region are nearly always iatrogenic and more likely to be amenable to conservative therapy. For perforation of the middle or lower oesophagus a thoracotomy is performed. The side of perforation dictates the surgical approach.

The oesophagus may be repaired primarily if the diagnosis is made early or, if the presentation is late, repaired around a T-tube to create a controlled fistula. Occasionally, severe mediastinitis can mandate emergency oesophagectomy with delayed reconstruction of the GI tract. Enteral nutrition is maintained by a feeding jejunostomy.

Procedure profile

Blood requirement	4
Anaesthetic	GA
Operation time	3–4 hours
Hospital stay	7–10 days
Return to normal activity	6–8 weeks

The postoperative care is as for an oesophagectomy (see p. 276).

Acute caustic injury

Ingestion of strong acid or alkali may be an accident or attempted suicide. They cause chemical burns in the mouth, pharynx, oesophagus and stomach. There is oedema, congestion and ulceration which can lead to acute obstruction at any level. This is followed by fibrosis with potential stricture formation.

Recognizing the pattern

The patient may be of any age or sex, although accidental ingestion of caustic fluids is common in children.

The history is one of severe pain which is continuous and increased by any attempt at swallowing. There may be hypersalivation. Find out the nature of the fluid swallowed and estimate the volume. The need for treatment is urgent, and further enquiry as to motive can be carried out when the patient has recovered.

On examination there may be signs of oropharyngeal inflammation. Look for evidence of circulatory collapse.

Management

Give immediate, strong, intravenous opiate analgesia. As soon as the patient has calmed down, wash away any remaining fluid with mouthwashes. Check for oral and glottic oedema. Consider the need for intubation or tracheostomy.

Do not attempt to wash out the stomach or provoke vomiting because the oesophagus is easily perforated.

Early endoscopy is mandatory to evaluate the extent of mucosal damage so that risks of perforation and stricture development can be estimated. Strong acids cause intense pyloro-spasm leading to pooling in the antrum and considerable later damage. This can be aspirated at endoscopy and diluted by water irrigation. A decision can then be made about the safety of oral feeding or the need for nutritional support via endoscopic gastrostomy, jejunostomy or parenteral route. The patient must then be observed very carefully for evidence of oesophageal per-foration. He or she will already be in pain, but signs of fluid in the chest, developing pyrexia and the development of surgical emphysema may indicate that this complication has occurred. Regular chest X-rays should also be carried out.

Repeat flexible upper GI endoscopy is performed to monitor healing of the oesophagus. Should oesophageal dilatation be required, it is usually started 3–4 weeks after the incident. Long-term management of long strictures that are resistant to dilata-tion may require resection of the oesophagus. Remember to check for and manage any systemic manifestations of poisoning, e.g. renal failure (see relevant medical texts).

Chronic benign stricture

Recurrent gastro-oesophageal reflux can result in a benign inflammatory stricture. However, this is now relatively uncom-mon in Western countries as most patients receive effective acid suppression early on from their primary care physician in the form of proton pump inhibitors (PPIs).

Recognizing the pattern

The patient is most frequently middle aged or elderly but can be any age and either sex. There may be a long history of reflux oeso-phagitis with a more recent onset of dysphagia, the food sticking at the lower sternal level. If the obstruction is severe there is usu-ally regurgitation of food immediately after swallowing and there may be episodes of aspiration of gastric contents into the chest associated with paroxysms of coughing, especially at night.

On examination there is usually very little to find.

Proving the diagnosis

Flexible upper GI endoscopy allows the stricture to be biopsied and this is essential to prove its benign nature. A barium swallow may be requested as an alternative if access to endoscopy is poor or the patient is very frail. The stricture is characteristically short (< 2 cm long) and usually close to the oesophagogastric junction.

Management

Most strictures can be adequately dealt with by endoscopic dilatation in combination with PPIs. This may need to be repeated. Few patients require surgery.

OPERATION: DILATATION OF OESOPHAGEAL STRICTURE

This should be carried out through a flexible endoscope. There is no place nowadays for rigid oesophagoscopy in relation to these strictures. Under direct vision a guide wire is passed through the stricture and bougies are then threaded down over the guide wire and the stricture dilated.

Procedure profile

Blood requirement	0
Anaesthetic	GA
Operation time	30 minutes
Hospital stay	24 hours
Return to normal activity	2–3 days

Postoperatively the main potential complication is perforation (see above).

Longer-term control of gastro-oesophageal reflux disease is achieved by maintenance PPIs or a laparoscopic antireflux operation such as Nissen fundoplication (see p. 281).

Achalasia

Achalasia is a condition in which there is failure of peristalsis and non-relaxation of the lower oesophageal sphincter (LOS) during swallowing. It occurs due to loss of ganglion cells in the myenteric plexus. The cause is unknown in the west.

Recognizing the pattern

The patient is typically aged 30–40 years old and the condition is slightly more common in females.

In the early stages of disease, there are still oesophageal contractions (although uncoordinated) and symptoms can be very intermittent. When these contractions are powerful, patients often complain of chest pain as well as dysphagia. Fluids and food can be equally troublesome. Progression may take years, but gradually the oesophagus dilates and becomes atonic. At this stage, the oesophagus essentially empties only as a result of the hydrostatic pressure of its contents. It hardly ever empties completely. Regurgitation of stagnant, undigested food occurs, together with foul belching. Aspiration can take place at night when the patient lies down, and results in a fit of coughing. This is referred to as nocturnal asthma. Recurrent chest infections due to aspiration pneumonia are common. There may be loss of weight.

On examination there may be signs of chronic chest infection and possibly loss of weight.

Proving the diagnosis

- On a chest X-ray the mediastinum may be widened with a fluid level behind the heart. This represents the dilated oesophagus. There may also be evidence of pneumonitis. None of these signs may be present, however, particularly in the early stages.
- Barium swallow shows dilatation and tortuosity of the oesophagus, which tapers down to a narrow lower segment of achalasia.
- Flexible upper GI endoscopy may reveal a grossly dilated oesophagus containing a pool of stagnant undigested food.

Management

There are three treatment options.

- Endoscopic injection of the LOS with botulinum toxin (Botox). This is an effective short-term treatment but has to be repeated every 3 months. It is best used for elderly patients who are unfit for other interventions.
- Forceful dilatation using a 3-cm diameter balloon disrupts the LOS without damaging the mucosa and is an effective treatment in the majority of patients but does have a small risk of perforation and does not always work.

- Surgical division of the LOS can be achieved laparoscopically (Heller's myotomy).

LAPAROSCOPIC HELLER'S MYOTOMY

Using a 4–5 port upper abdominal approach, the gastro-oesophageal junction and distal oesophagus are exposed and the LOS musculature divided, great care being taken not to damage the underlying mucosa. Confirmation of complete LOS division is provided by an on-table endoscopy and an anterior hemifundoplication (Dor) is fashioned as an antireflux procedure to prevent gastrooesophageal reflux disease (GORD). Surgery is more difficult if there have been previous failed attempts at balloon dilatation.

Procedure profile

Blood requirement	Group and save
Anaesthetic	GA
Operation time	60–90 minutes
Hospital stay	2–3 days
Return to normal activity	2 weeks

Postoperatively no nasogastric tube is used and oral fluids are allowed immediately. Once free fluids are established, a light diet is allowed, usually on the second postoperative day, and mobilization is encouraged with appropriate analgesia. If there is any concern about the patient's early recovery a water-soluble contrast study should be done immediately to exclude a leak.

Pharyngeal pouch

This is a rare cause of dysphagia due to a pulsion diverticulum occurring as a result of cricopharyngeal muscle spasm. It is described on p. 140.

Plummer–Vinson syndrome

This rare syndrome consists of:
- iron deficiency anaemia

- dysphagia due to a postcricoid web in the oesophagus.

It was described by Plummer and Vinson in 1921, and by Paterson and Kelly 2 years earlier.

There is hyperplasia of the squamous epithelium with hyperkeratosis in the mucosa of the upper oesophagus associated with patches of desquamation. This can lead to the formation of a web, which usually lies anteriorly.

Recognizing the pattern

The patient is typically a woman aged between 40 and 50 years. The history is one of high dysphagia, the patient complaining that food appears to stick in the back of the throat. This may be associated with retching and a choking sensation. There may be symptoms of anaemia.

On examination the patient is usually anaemic with spoon-shaped nails (koilonychia), smooth tongue and angular stomatitis. She may also occasionally have a palpable spleen.

Proving the diagnosis

- A barium meal shows a narrowing of the upper oesophagus due to a web-like fold in the anterior wall.
- A full blood count shows anaemia with a hypochromic, microcytic picture.
- Upper GI endoscopy shows a friable web across the lumen of the oesophagus.
- Biopsy of the bone marrow shows absent iron stores.

Management

The web is dilated at the time of endoscopy. The condition is said to be premalignant leading to the development of postcricoid carcinoma. Although the number of documented cases is miniscule, biopsies of this region are advisable to exclude any dysplasia.

Postoperatively the patient is treated with iron therapy and vitamin supplements. Provided the anaemia is corrected, the condition does not usually recur. Occasionally a blood transfusion is required.

If the biopsy shows malignant cells, then the lesion is treated as a postcricoid carcinoma (see p. 274).

Barrett's oesophagus

This is a term that describes the replacement of normal squamous oesophageal epithelium by specialized intestinal metaplasia and it appears to be an adaptive response to chronic GORD. Endoscopically, the squamocolumnar junction is moved proximally up the oesophagus to varying degrees. It is a risk factor for the development of oesophageal adenocarcinoma, a condition which has increased by more than 300% in males in the UK in the last 30 years. The reasons for this are unclear. Many patients with Barrett's will develop dysplasia prior to invasive cancer, the so-called 'dysplasia–carcinoma sequence', providing a window of opportunity for intervention to prevent progression. Multiple biopsies must be taken to detect dysplasia and patients are usually offered endoscopic surveillance, although there is currently limited evidence that it saves many lives. About 1% of Barrett's patients in surveillance will develop malignant change each year.

High-grade dysplasia should be diagnosed by two separate histopathologists from biopsies taken on two separate occasions. Treatment of high-grade dysplasia may be endoscopic using photodynamic therapy or by a transhiatal oesophagectomy.

Carcinoma of the oesophagus

Most carcinomas of the cervical and proximal third oesophagus are squamous. Below this level, the proportion of squamous to adenocarcinomas varies depending upon where the patient lives in the world. Internationally, squamous tumours still make up 90% of all oesophageal malignancies but in North America, UK and Northern Europe, adenocarcinoma is now the predominant disease.

The Siewert classification of adenocarcinomas of the gastro-oesophageal junction (GOJ) describes:

- type I tumours as those in the tubular oesophagus within 5 cm of the GOJ
- type II as those straddling the GOJ, and
- type III as those arising in the cardia of the stomach growing up into the GOJ.

Predisposing factors for squamous cancers include cigarette smoking, high alcohol intake, poor diet, achalasia, and Plummer–Vinson syndrome. Adenocarcinomas appear to be related to GORD and obesity but the relationship is poorly understood at present.

Oesophageal tumours have a poor prognosis. They meta-stasise early along nerves, via lymphatics, through venous blood vessels to the liver and lungs, directly into adjacent tissues such as the diaphragm or airways, and via the peritoneal cavity. Patients generally present with dysphagia, by which time 60% have blood-borne metastases and are incurable. Of the remaining 40% who receive aggressive treatment, only about a third of them will be cured. The most important prognostic factor for this group is nodal spread.

Recognizing the pattern

The patient is usually a male over the age of 50 years but the inci-dence in younger people and women is showing a disturbing increase. Adenocarcinomas are seven times more common in men than in women.

The patient typically presents with a short history of progres-sive dysphagia which may have been preceded by long-term GORD. This initially affects solids only, but gradually increases until even swallowing liquids becomes a problem. Retrosternal pain may occur but is usually a late symptom. There may be regurgitation of food or fluids, or bloodstained vomiting. There is frequently a history of significant weight loss.

On examination there is often nothing to find except evidence of some recent weight loss. The finding of an abdominal mass, hepatomegaly or lymphadenopathy are very bad signs and usu-ally means that the patient is incurable.

Proving the diagnosis

- Urgent flexible upper GI endoscopy and biopsy.
- Barium swallow may be appropriate if the patient is very frail, or as a first-line investigation when availability of endoscopy is limited.

Management

The patient and relatives should be brought to an appropriate clinic for the diagnosis to be explained, preferably in the presence of a specialist upper GI nurse who can help provide information, support and practical advice.

Investigations to stage the tumour include the following.

- Full blood count to exclude anaemia.
- Urea and electrolytes to exclude renal disease.

- Liver function tests. These may suggest the presence of metastases (elevated bilirubin and alkaline phosphatase) or show evidence of malnutrition (hypoproteinaemia).
- A multislice CT scan of chest and abdomen to look for distant metastases.
- An endoluminal ultrasound scan (EUS) to provide local staging information about the primary tumour (only if a CT scan has excluded distant disease first). This test uses a high-frequency ultrasound probe mounted on a flexible endoscope to provide accurate local staging of the tumour.
- Laparoscopy to rule out peritoneal spread.
- Special tests such as bronchoscopy may be needed in selected patients and an increasing number of centres use positron emission tomography in combination with CT (PET-CT). This relies on the increased uptake of glucose by tumour cells (given as fluorodeoxyglucose) and may disclose metastatic disease not identified by other techniques.

All patients should be discussed by a multidisciplinary team (MDT) before a decision is made about treatment. The conclusions of the MDT and the treatment options are as follows.

- Metastatic disease (haematogenous or peritoneal) – palliate patient's symptoms. This may take the following forms:
  ◦ best supportive care
  ◦ endoscopic stenting for dysphagia
  ◦ endoscopic thermal ablation of tumour using lasers or argon plasma coagulation (APC). This is particularly useful for proximal tumours that cannot be stented
  ◦ radiotherapy alone or in combination with chemotherapy for squamous tumours
  ◦ chemotherapy.
- Localized but advanced disease in a fit patient – preoperative chemotherapy (neoadjuvant) followed by surgery.
- Localized but advanced disease in an unfit patient – palliate symptoms or, if appropriate, treat with definitive chemo/radiation.
- Localized early disease – surgery alone.

OPERATIONS FOR OESOPHAGEAL CARCINOMA
Surgery has little, if any, role in planned palliation of a patient's symptoms although it is an unfortunate fact that many attempts

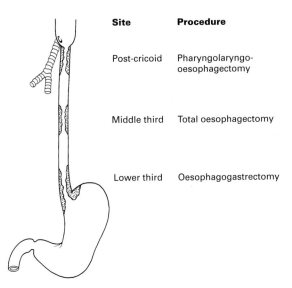

Site	Procedure
Post-cricoid	Pharyngolaryngo-oesophagectomy
Middle third	Total oesophagectomy
Lower third	Oesophagogastrectomy

Fig. 7.1.1 Carcinoma of the oesophagus: the sites of origin and the relevant surgical procedures.

at cure with surgery will turn out to be palliative as the tumour recurs after resection. The type of operation performed depends on the site of the growth (Fig. 7.1.1). The goals of surgery should be as follows.

- To obtain a complete macroscopic and microscopic resection of the primary tumour (described as R0 resection). For this to be achieved, the tumour must be at least 1 mm from all resection margins when analysed by the histopathologist. It may sometimes be necessary to resect structures adjacent to the oesophagus such as the diaphragmatic crura.
- To perform safe reconstruction of the gastrointestinal tract by using anastomotic techniques that have low leak rates.
- To resect an adequate number of lymph nodes to ensure accurate tumour staging (by assessing nodal positivity) and increase the chance of cure in those patients with few involved nodes.
- To operate with an acceptable in-hospital mortality rate. This should be under 10%.

- To give patients an acceptable quality of life after surgery. Overall 5-year survival rates after oesophagectomy are in the region of 25–30%, although 'node-negative' tumours have much better survival rates at about 40–50% compared to 'node-positive' ones at 10–15%.

OPERATION: PHARYNGOLARYNGO-OESOPHAGECTOMY
In this operation for tumours of the cervical oesophagus, it is necessary to resect the larynx as well as the oesophagus and a permanent tracheostomy is fashioned. Abdominal and neck incisions are made, the stomach mobilized, and the mediastinal oesophagus delivered transhiatally. Gut continuity is restored by bringing a gastric tube (conduit) via the posterior mediastinum and suturing it to the lower pharynx in the neck.

Procedure profile

Blood requirement	4
Anaesthetic	GA
Operation time	5 hours
Hospital stay	10–14 days
Return to normal activity	2–3 months

TOTAL OESOPHAGECTOMY
Procedures include the following.

IVOR–LEWIS RESECTION (TWO-PHASE)
This operation is performed for carcinoma of the mid and distal third oesophagus and for type I and type II tumours of the gastro-oesophageal junction. Through an abdominal incision the stomach is mobilized, preserving its blood supply via the gastro-epiploic arcade. The abdomen is then closed, the patient turned onto their left side and the right chest opened. The tumour is removed with a wide margin of normal oesophagus and the stomach is brought up into the chest for anastomosis with the native oesophagus at the apex of the chest.

McKEOWN RESECTION (THREE-PHASE)

This is similar to the Ivor–Lewis procedure, except it begins with a right thoracotomy to mobilize the mediastinal oesophagus. The patient is then turned onto their back and abdominal and left neck incisions are made to mobilize the stomach and cervical oesophagus simultaneously by two surgical teams. After resection, a gastric conduit is brought via the posterior mediastinum and is anastomosed to the native cervical oesophagus.

LEFT THORACOABDOMINAL RESECTION

This operation involves an oblique incision from the left chest, across the costal margin and into the abdomen. It gives simultaneous access to both sides of the diaphragm and is favoured by some surgeons for tumours of the GOJ. Gut continuity is again re-established with a gastric conduit anastomosed to the oesophagus as high as possible in the chest.

TRANSHIATAL RESECTION

This operation is mainly used for early tumours or high grade dysplasia in Barrett's oesophagus, although some surgeons use it for more advanced tumours of the gastro-oesophageal junction as well. Via an abdominal incision the diaphragmatic hiatus is opened widely and the oesophagus mobilized under direct vision up to the level of the carina. The left neck is then opened, the cervical oesophagus mobilized and divided, and the proximal third of the oesophagus mobilized by blunt dissection or using a vein stripper. The mobilized oesophagus is then removed via the abdomen and a gastric conduit brought via the posterior mediastinum to the neck and anastomosed to the cervical oesophagus.

Procedure profile

Blood requirement	2
Anaesthetic	GA
Operation time	4–5 hours
Hospital stay	10–14 days
Return to normal activity	3 months

EXTENDED TOTAL GASTRECTOMY

For Siewert type III tumours and some smaller type II lesions, it may be possible to avoid a thoracotomy by using a transhiatal approach to resecting a short segment of distal oesophagus in continuity with the GOJ. This is particularly appropriate if the lesion is clearly gastric and a total gastrectomy is needed to confidently resect all involved lymph nodes. In this case, reconstruction is by a long Roux-en-Y jejunal limb. For early lesions of the GOJ it may be possible to preserve some of the distal stomach and restore continuity either by anastomosing the stomach directly to the distal oesophagus or with a jejunal interposition segment (Merendino procedure).

Procedure profile

Blood requirement	6
Anaesthetic	GA
Operation time	3–4 hours
Hospital stay	10–14 days
Return to normal activity	2–3 months

Postoperatively a thoracic epidural is used for pain control. Patients who have had a thoracotomy and resection are usually nursed in intensive care or a high-dependency unit. Daily chest physiotherapy is important as is the early detection and aggressive treatment of any complications.

Complications include atelectasis, hypoxia and pneumonia. Anastomotic leakage occurs in 5–7% of cases and has a high mortality if not identified and dealt with promptly. Other problems include cardiac dysrythmias, myocardial infarct, conduit necrosis, wound infection, deep vein thrombosis and pulmonary embolism, infected collections and bowel obstruction.

Many surgeons feed patients via feeding jejunostomies for the first 5–7 postoperative days. Nasogastric tubes are left in situ for 5–7 days and oral fluids started when nasogastric decompression is discontinued. Parenteral feeding is still used by some but there is evidence that it is less effective than enteral feeding and septic complications from the central line are common.

A contrast swallow or endoscopy is essential if the patient becomes unwell and no other clear cause is evident. Routine swallows in all patients have been shown to be of no value. Small leaks are usually managed conservatively but major disruptions or conduit necrosis require urgent surgical revision.

Some patients will experience dysphagia weeks or months after their surgery due to an anastomotic stricture. Endoscopic dilatation is the treatment of choice and many surgeons have an 'open access' policy for their patients so that dilatation can happen without delay.

Radiotherapy can be combined with chemotherapy as definitive treatment or as a neoadjuvant therapy prior to surgery. However, this increases postoperative mortality considerably and remains experimental at present.

7.2 Stomach and duodenum

Abdominal pain

When a patient presents with abdominal pain the site of pain gives a primary clue as to the organ involved (Fig. 7.2.1). In this book abdominal conditions are grouped according to the site where the pain typically presents. Disease states may of course present in other ways apart from pain (e.g. haematemesis, jaundice, change in bowel habit, etc.) and the more important of these are included as seems appropriate in relation to other conditions discussed.

Acute and chronic presentations of abdominal pain are discussed under appropriate disease headings, but it is worth remembering that upper abdominal pain can arise from chest pathology and a variety of systemic disorders.

Important conditions presenting with upper abdominal pain, together with their complications and management, are dealt with on the following pages.
- Hiatus hernia/GORD (p. 278).
- Gastric ulcer (p. 284).
- Duodenal ulcer, including perforation, pyloric stenosis, haematemesis and melaena (p. 284).

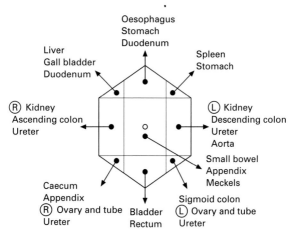

Fig. 7.2.1 Typical sites of presentation of visceral pain from different organs.

- Gallstones, including obstructive jaundice (p. 318).
- Carcinoma of the stomach (p. 294).
- Carcinoma of the pancreas (p. 342).
- Pancreatitis (p. 347).

  Less commonly, upper abdominal pain may arise from disease in the liver, spleen or diaphragm. Examples are as follows.
- Hepatic abscess (p. 72).
- Hepatic metastases, secondary to malignant disease from many sites.
- Subphrenic abscess (p. 70).
- Ruptured spleen (p. 636).
- Liver injury (p. 334).

Gastroduodenal disease

Hiatus hernia/GORD

Many clinicians use the term hiatus hernia as a diagnosis or a specific disease entity. It is rarely appropriate to do this. Hiatus hernia is really only an anatomical description of a hernia where some part or all of the stomach lies in the posterior mediastinum above the diaphragm. There are two main types of hiatus hernia (Fig. 7.2.2). In the sliding variety, the gastro-oesophageal angle is straightened out and the junction between the oesophageal mucosa and gastric mucosa slides up into the chest. This is associated with the presence of reflux disease, but is not an essential prerequisite for its development. Symptoms are due to reflux of gastric contents into the oesophagus (hence GORD – gastro-oesophageal reflux disease). In the rolling variety of hiatus hernia, there is a large hiatal defect and the fundus of the stomach tends to roll up next to the oesophagus, forming a paraoesophageal hernia. In this type of hernia, symptoms, when present, are often due to partial obstruction of the herniated stomach so that the patients suffer epigastric pain and early satiety when they eat. In addition, they may vomit after eating to obtain relief. Large hernias can twist around on the long axis of the stomach within the chest and cause a gastric volvulus. This is a life-threatening condition. The two main types of hiatus hernia may be combined but not necessarily symptomatic. Patients with a paraoesophageal hernia can have GORD.

Recognizing the pattern

Reflux symptoms may occur in any age group in either sex.

In GORD, the patient complains of heartburn (related to reflux of acid), regurgitation and epigastric pain. Heartburn is an epigastric or low retrosternal burning pain, which may radiate to the back, neck or even down the arms. The symptoms are worse on stooping or lying flat at night. Symptoms often come on when the patient has recently gained weight and are common in the last trimester of pregnancy.

With a gastric volvulus the patient complains of a sudden onset of very severe constricting lower chest and upper abdominal pain. The symptoms may mimic those of a myocardial infarction and lead onto circulatory collapse and septic shock.

Proving the diagnosis

The diagnosis of GORD with or without hiatus hernia is usually made at endoscopy although a third of patients have no visible

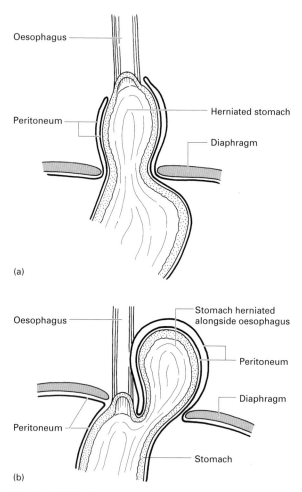

Fig. 7.2.2 (a) Sliding hiatus hernia. (b) Rolling hiatus hernia.

endoscopic damage. A paraoesophageal hernia may be suspected when endoscopy seems difficult, and this diagnosis is best established by performing a barium meal. A chest X-ray may reveal a fluid-filled viscus behind the heart.

Management

The initial management of GORD is acid suppression using a proton pump inhibitor (PPI). Lifestyle changes are helpful; for many patients weight loss, cessation of smoking and avoidance of irritating foodstuffs such as coffee, spices, acids etc. may allow them to stop taking PPIs. However, the reality is that many will not make any major changes and become dependent upon medication to control their symptoms.

Laparoscopic antireflux surgery is very effective at controlling reflux symptoms but has some common consequences. These are dysphagia to solids during the first few months of recovery, early satiety, bloating and increased flatus. Surgery can cure up to 90% of patients but great care is needed in patient selection and the technical aspects of the surgery. Surgery should be considered for young patients who are PPI dependent, for those who cannot tolerate PPIs and for those whose symptoms are poorly controlled despite adequate dosage. Patients with a rolling hernia who have had a possible episode of strangulation should always be considered for an operation, although many are elderly and frail and careful judgement is required. Laparoscopic techniques have made this type of surgery safer.

LAPAROSCOPIC NISSEN FUNDOPLICATION (Fig. 7.2.3)

Patients should be carefully counselled prior to surgery and have quantifiable GORD (best done by 24 h pH measurement) or mechanical symptoms related to a large hiatus hernia.

The hiatus is approached laparoscopically using a 4–5 port upper GI approach. Conversion rates to open surgery should be no more than 5% but may rise to 20% for large hiatus hernias. Any hiatus hernia is reduced into the abdomen, the peritoneal sac excised and the diaphragmatic hiatus narrowed with sutures into the crura posterior to the oesophagus. Occasionally it may be necessary to repair the diaphragm using a non-absorbable mesh. A 360° fundoplication is then performed. Alternative

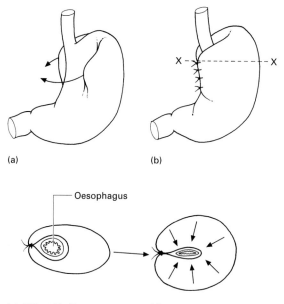

(a)

(b)

Oesophagus

(c) T.S. at X---X

(d)

Fig. 7.2.3 Nissen fundoplication. (a) The gastric fundus is mobilized by division of the short gastric vessels. (b) This is then brought behind and in front of the intra-abdominal oesophagus and sutured. (c) This makes a 360° wrap of fundus around the distal oesophagus. (d) As the wrap is made of the hollow stomach, raised intragastric pressure distends it and occludes the enclosed portion of the oesophagus preventing reflux.

laparoscopic antireflux operations involve incomplete wraps of between 180 and 270°, brought either anteriorly or posteriorly around the oesophagus. The results of all of these variants are similar. They may have a slightly lower side-effect profile in the first few months compared to the Nissen operation. The drawback is slightly more reflux in the long term.

Procedure profile

Blood requirement	Group and save
Anaesthetic	GA
Operation time	60–90 minutes
Hospital stay	1–3 days
Return to normal activity	2 weeks

Postoperatively no nasogastric tube is necessary and the patient is allowed oral fluids immediately. Regular antiemetics are given to prevent retching and vomiting as this can disrupt the crural repair and force the wrap up into the chest. A light soft diet is introduced 24–36 h after surgery and the patient discharged for convalescence at home. Inability to swallow liquids is an indication for an early return to theatre as the crural repair or the wrap have been made too tight and will require release. This is easily done laparoscopically before the 10th postoperative day. If there are any concerns about the patient, an urgent contrast swallow should be done to exclude perforation or wrap migration.

Patients should be warned to expect dysphagia to solids during the first few weeks after the operation and should stay on a soft diet until this resolves. Patients may also suffer from the 'gas bloat syndrome'. In this, swallowed air becomes trapped in the stomach because the patient is unable to belch and as intragastric pressure increases, the wrap tightens making the problem worse. Patients should use a straw to take liquids and avoid hot drinks for the first few weeks after surgery as this reduces the degree of swallowed air. All patients should be able to belch after a variable period following surgery but this may take some time to return.

Peptic ulcers

Peptic ulcers are becoming rarer but are of two types – those in the stomach and those in the duodenum. Although there are classical symptom patterns for each type, in clinical practice the distinction is often not straightforward and flexible endoscopy is needed to differentiate between them. Most patients have chronic symptoms, but do not forget that both gastric and duodenal ulcers can present for the first time with either perforation or bleeding.

Gastric ulcer
Recognizing the pattern
The patient is typically middle aged or elderly, debilitated and thin, and complains of poor appetite, loss of weight and pain that comes on immediately after eating. The pain may be relieved by lying flat (when the gastric contents fall back into the fundus of the stomach and away from the ulcer on the lesser curve) and also by antacids. The patient may also present with melaena or symptoms related to anaemia.

On examination there may be tenderness in the epigastrium or left hypochondrium.

Proving the diagnosis
The diagnosis is confirmed by a flexible upper GI endoscopy. All gastric ulcers should be biopsied as a proportion will be ulcerating gastric cancers.

Management
Tests for *Helicobacter pylori* should be performed as this is a common cause of gastric ulcers. If detected, it should be eradicated using a combination of a PPI and two antibiotics (see the *British National Formulary*). Non-steroidal anti-inflammatory drugs (NSAIDs) should be stopped and the patient started immediately on a healing dose of a PPI.

It is essential to monitor healing by repeated endoscopy. If the ulcer fails to heal completely then further biopsies are indicated to exclude a missed neoplasm.

Elective surgery for benign gastric ulcer is now very rarely indicated and is usually done for pyloric stenosis causing gastric outlet obstruction. A limited resection to encompass the ulcer with Roux-en-Y reconstruction is the treatment of choice.

Duodenal ulcer
The condition is usually due to *Helicobacter pylori* infection but is also associated with NSAIDs and smoking.

Recognizing the pattern

The patient may be young or elderly and the condition is more common in males than in females. Eating will often ease the pain and the patient may be overweight as a consequence. Elderly patients who are in hospital with other illnesses may develop duodenal stress ulcers which are a frequent cause of upper GI bleeding.

The pain is situated in the epigastrium and may radiate through to the small of the back. It comes on 1–2 h after meals and also when the patient is hungry. It has a tendency to wake the patient up in the early hours of the morning when acidity is high and the stomach is empty. There may also be 'periodicity' with periods (often weeks) when the ulcer is active and painful, followed by periods (often months) of inactivity and absent symptoms.

If the ulcer is chronic, the patient may develop scarring and stenosis of the duodenum or pylorus which can result in gastric outlet obstruction.

On examination there is tenderness to the right of and above the umbilicus, deep in the abdomen.

Proving the diagnosis

The diagnosis is proved by a flexible upper GI endoscopy and all patients with a history of haematemesis or melaena should undergo this test within 24 h of such an event.

Management

This is conservative. There is little if any role for performing definitive 'anti-ulcer surgery' as PPIs are so effective at reducing gastric acid production. A patient with recurrent peptic ulceration who cannot tolerate or is poorly compliant with medical therapy should be considered for a definitive ulcer surgery only after all possible contributing causes have been eliminated (e.g. hypercalcaemia, gastrinoma).

Perforated peptic ulcer

Gastric and duodenal ulcers may perforate, although perforation of the latter is more common. As gastric ulcers are frequently posterior, they may perforate into the lesser sac. Anterior duodenal ulcers perforate direct into the main peritoneal cavity.

Recognizing the pattern

The typical pattern of symptoms suggesting gastric or duodenal ulcer has already been described. Not infrequently, however, patients present with a perforation without much in the way of a past history of indigestion. There is a sudden, defined onset of severe epigastric pain. The patient frequently remembers the precise time it started. The pain rapidly spreads first to the right iliac fossa and later all over the abdomen. When a gastric ulcer perforates into the lesser sac, the symptoms are much more localized until gastric contents leak out of the foramen of Winslow, giving rise to a right-sided peritonitis. On examination there is typically marked tenderness over the whole of the abdomen with 'board-like rigidity'. Percussion of the liver may reveal absent liver dullness. This sign is due to gas lying between the liver and the anterior abdominal wall. The patient may be tachycardic, hypotensive, hypoxic and pyrexial.

Proving the diagnosis

The diagnosis is proved by doing an erect chest X-ray. Gas may be seen under the diaphragm. This is not foolproof though, and if negative in the face of a strong clinical suspicion of a perforation, an urgent CT scan should be requested.

Management

The management of an acute perforation is usually surgical. It is, however, possible on occasion to manage these lesions conservatively if the patient does not have signs of generalized peritonitis. This usually occurs when the presentation is 'late' and the perforation has become sealed off from the rest of the peritoneal cavity by the omentum. The protocol for conservative management involves the following.

- A nasogastric tube is positioned in the stomach and regularly aspirated. It is essential that the stomach is kept empty.
- Adequate intravenous fluid replacement is given. These patients have usually lost a lot of fluid into the peritoneal cavity and are markedly dehydrated. A urinary catheter is essential for adequate resuscitation. A central venous pressure (CVP) line may also be needed when large amounts of fluid have to be given, especially in the elderly patient with cardiac disease.

- The patient is given broad-spectrum antibiotic cover.
- Intravenous PPIs are started to suppress gastric acid production.
- Four-hourly review is necessary to ensure that the patient's condition has not deteriorated. If at any time there is a worsening of the patient's symptoms or signs they should have urgent surgery to close the perforation.

Approximately 50% of patients presenting with localized signs from a perforated ulcer will avoid an operation with this regimen. For all other patients, rapid resuscitation should be followed by a prompt operation to minimize the consequences of peritonitis.

OPERATION: FOR PERFORATED PEPTIC ULCER
This may be performed laparoscopically if the surgeon has the appropriate skills. Otherwise the abdomen is opened through an upper midline vertical incision. Deep sutures are placed through the oedematous tissue around the perforation and a patch of omentum sewn over to close the defect (Fig. 7.2.4). Sometimes it is better to use the omentum to plug the hole and sew this to the duodenal wall when the tissues are particularly friable. In the worst circumstance, closure of the duodenum may be impossible and a Foley catheter is then placed in the duodenum, using the inflated balloon to keep it in place. This results in a controlled duodenal fistula. The peritoneum is carefully washed out and all food residue removed. Drains are placed at the site of the perforation.

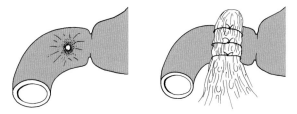

Fig. 7.2.4 Oversewing a perforated duodenal ulcer.

Procedure profile

Blood requirement	Group and save
Anaesthetic	GA
Operation time	60–90 minutes
Hospital stay	5–7 days
Return to normal activity	2–4 weeks

Postoperatively oral intake is limited to 30 mL per hour for at least 48 h. If well, the patient can then resume oral intake but it may be 3–5 days before solids are tolerated. The main complication is recurrent leakage from the ulcer and intra-abdominal sepsis, either in the subphrenic regions or in the pelvis. An oral contrast study will diagnose the former and CT scanning the latter. Infected collections should be drained percutaneously under radiological guidance.

Pyloric stenosis

The condition known as 'pyloric stenosis' in adults is usually, in fact, a duodenal stenosis secondary to scarring from a chronic duodenal ulcer.

Recognizing the pattern

Pyloric stenosis can arise in any patient with a duodenal ulcer and the developing obstruction is usually heralded by the onset of vomiting. Characteristically this is copious and contains food ingested a day or two previously. In long-standing pyloric stenosis the patient may become very ill with lassitude and loss of weight. In some elderly patients there is very little history of previous indigestion until the stenosis develops.

If the vomiting has been prolonged the patient is dehydrated and weak. There may be tenderness over the duodenal region. The characteristic sign is a 'succussion splash'. A stethoscope is placed over the stomach and the patient gently shaken from side to side. Food can be heard splashing in the stomach several hours after the previous meal.

Proving the diagnosis

The diagnosis is proved either radiologically or by upper GI endoscopy. The grossly distended stomach may be visible on a plain abdominal X-ray. Endoscopy can be difficult due to food debris but biopsies should be taken to exclude malignancy if a view of the stenosis can be obtained. There is a characteristic biochemical picture of a hypochloraemic alkalosis due to loss of hydrochloric acid. Inability to exchange potassium ions for hydrogen in the kidneys means that hypokalaemia occurs.

Management

Pyloric stenosis secondary to duodenal ulceration is usually an indication for surgery although some strictures can be successfully dilated with a balloon. Before surgery is undertaken, electrolyte and nutritional disturbances must be corrected. Several days of conservative management may be needed to achieve this. Adequate intravenous therapy including potassium and chloride ions must therefore be given. A nasogastric tube is passed and the stomach kept empty. A PPI is prescribed. Not infrequently the stomach begins to empty again with this management. Nevertheless, once obstruction has developed it is likely to recur and surgical treatment should be undertaken.

OPERATION: FOR PYLORIC STENOSIS

The most common procedure performed is a truncal vagotomy and pyloroplasty or gastroenterostomy. Some surgeons prefer to perform a highly selective vagotomy and in this case the stenosis is dealt with either by a duodenoplasty or by dilatation. In a duodenoplasty the stenosis in the duodenum is incised longitudinally and sewn up vertically, thus widening the area. These manoeuvres allow the pylorus to be retained and thus obviate the development of problems related to abnormal gastric emptying after a drainage procedure. An alternative strategy in an elderly frail patient might be a laparoscopic gastroenterostomy and long-term acid suppression with a PPI.

Procedure profile

Blood requirement	2
Anaesthetic	GA
Operation time	1–2 hours
Hospital stay	7–10 days
Return to normal activity	3–6 weeks

Bleeding peptic ulcer

Haematemesis (vomiting blood) and melaena (tarry black motions) are due to bleeding from the upper gastrointestinal tract. Bleeding from the lower gastrointestinal tract is discussed on p. 368.

Upper gastrointestinal haemorrhage may be from the following sites.

- The pharynx:
  - usually swallowed blood from a nasal haemorrhage.
- The oesophagus:
  - oesophagitis with ulceration secondary to GORD
  - oesophageal varices secondary to portal hypertension.
- The stomach:
  - gastritis, nearly always due to NSAIDs
  - gastric ulcer
  - benign tumours, especially GIST
  - carcinoma
  - Mallory–Weiss tear – a mucosal injury to the gastro-oesophageal junction secondary to repeated vomiting
  - vascular anomalies, especially Dieulafoy malformation.
- The duodenum:
  - duodenal ulcer.

The shocked patient vomiting blood is a common and dramatic surgical emergency. A junior surgical trainee can be severely tested in these circumstances and the condition will be dealt with in some detail here.

Management

A suggested scheme of management is as follows:

- initial assessment with simultaneous resuscitation

- secondary assessment
- special tests and definitive treatment.

*INITIAL ASSESSMENT AND SIMULTANEOUS
RESUSCITATION*

An assessment must be made of the following.

- The ABC scheme of assessment to evaluate the patient's *a*irway, *b*reathing and *c*irculation.
- 100% oxygen is administered via a rebreathing mask. Oxygen saturations are measured with a pulse oximeter.
- Estimate the amount of blood lost by the patient. After a sudden bleed a patient who is unconscious with a minimal blood pressure, a rapid, thin pulse and cold clammy extremities has probably lost 1.5–2 L of blood. A patient who is conscious but mildly shocked, with a low blood pressure and a tachycardia, may have lost about 1 L. Signs of shock are not usually present when the patient has lost less than 500 mL.
- Two wide-bore intravenous catheters are placed, one in each antecubital fossa, and blood samples taken for haemoglobin level, clotting studies and cross-matching of 8 units of blood. With ongoing bleeding it is wise to warn the laboratory that more may be needed.
- Intravenous fluid is given, starting with a litre of saline given immediately.
- Blood pressure is monitored every 15 min.

SECONDARY ASSESSMENT

A thorough history and examination is now taken and a urinary catheter inserted to measure hourly urine output. Patients who are haemodynamically unstable should be nursed in an appropriate area of the hospital such as an HDU or in a designated facility for patients with acute GI bleeding (usually on the gastroenterology ward). Results from the blood tests are collated and used to guide management. Significant anaemia in a shocked bleeding patient (suggesting an acute-on-chronic bleed) warrants urgent blood transfusion.

SPECIAL TESTS AND DEFINITIVE TREATMENT

Patients with upper GI bleeding should have an endoscopy within

24 h of admission. Unstable patients will need this immediately and most hospitals now have arrangements for emergency endoscopy 24 h a day. Endoscopy should locate the bleeding source and provide haemostasis by injections of adrenaline, application of a heater probe or endoscopic clips. Oesophageal varices can be banded or injected with sclerosant.

These endoscopic techniques have greatly reduced the need for emergency surgery to control haemorrhage. However, a shocked patient who continues to bleed or who rebleeds despite endoscopic therapy should have urgent open surgery to stop bleeding. Close liaison between the endoscopist and surgeon (if they are different people) is needed to ensure appropriate surgical intervention when it is needed. Local protocols should exist to facilitate this.

The risk of further bleeding after admission can be predicted using scoring systems such as the Rockall score (Fig. 7.2.5).

OPERATION: FOR BLEEDING PEPTIC ULCER
Surgery for bleeding ulcers has changed in the last 20 years. The focus is now exclusively upon saving the patient's life by stopping the bleeding. This needs to be done quickly and with minimal trauma to the patient using an adequate incision, good retraction and good lighting. Usually this can be achieved by performing an anterior gastrotomy or duodenotomy (depending on where the ulcer is) and inserting a figure of eight prolene suture into the base of the ulcer and around the bleeding vessels to control it. The enterostomy is simply closed with a running absorbable suture and the patient recovered in ICU or HDU, depending upon their comorbidities and degree of blood loss. Gastric ulcers should always be biopsied to exclude malignancy.

Procedure profile

Blood requirement	8
Anaesthetic	GA
Operation time	1–2 hours
Hospital stay	5–7 days
Return to normal activity	4 weeks

Assessment of patients with haematemesis or melaena

The 'Rockall Score' is an externally validated mortality risk assessment score for patients admitted with upper gastrointestinal bleeding. It is simple and practical to use, helping identify those at highest risk of dying and needing active intervention. It also identifies those for safe, early discharge (initial score 0, final <2).

Initial Rockall score

AGE
<60 years	0
60–79 years	1
>80 years	2

SHOCK
None	0
Pulse >100 and syst BP >100	1
syst BP <100	2

COMORBIDITY
None	0
Cardiac failure, IHD, or any major comorbidity	2
Renal/liver failure or disseminated malignancy	3

Total initial Rockall score (max score 7) ☐

Predicted mortality		
	Initial risk score	Initial risk score
	Pre-endoscopy	Post-endoscopy
0	0.2%	0.0%
1	2.4%	0.0%
2	5.6%	0.2%
3	11.0%	2.9%
4	24.6%	5.3%
5	39.6%	10.8%
6	48.9%	17.3%
7	50.0%	27.0%
8+	–	41.1%

Full Rockall score after endoscopy

ENDOSCOPIC DIAGNOSIS
M-W tear or no lesion and no sign of bleeding	0
All other diagnoses	1
Malignancy of upper GI tract	2

MAJOR STIGMATA OF RECENT HAEMORRHAGE
None or dark spot only	0
Blood in upper GI tract, adherent clot, visible or spurting vessel	2

Final Rockall score (Max score 11) ☐

Fig 7.2.5 The Rockall score.

Proton pump inhibitors are started immediately after surgery and continued until ulcer healing is confirmed on follow-up endoscopy. Definitive 'anti-ulcer surgery' has been abandoned by most surgeons in the emergency setting as it increases mortality and is usually unnecessary due to effective medical healing of ulcers.

Acute gastritis

This is a frequent source of gastric haemorrhage. There may be a history of drug ingestion, particularly of drugs used in the management of arthritis, such as phenylbutazone, indomethacin, NSAIDs, steroids and aspirin compounds. Acute gastritis can also occur in septicaemia.

Management

In most cases the condition settles with adequate acid suppression using PPIs and withdrawal of the offending drug. Rarely bleeding continues unabated and, if diffuse bleeding from the stomach is confirmed at urgent endoscopy, an emergency total gastrectomy may be necessary. Luckily this is very uncommon as surgery in this scenario has a high mortality.

Oesophagitis

Bleeding from oesophagitis will usually stop spontaneously. If discrete areas of bleeding are seen at endoscopy, adrenaline injections can be used. A PPI should be given.

Rarities

A variety of unusual lesions can present with acute upper GI bleeding. The Mallory–Weiss lesion is a tear at the oesophago-gastric junction that usually follows prolonged retching. It is seen mainly in young men who are inebriated and who notice blood in their vomit. Bleeding is rarely dramatic and in the absence of any haemodynamic instability, when the history is clear, this is probably the only upper GI bleed that does not need endoscopy. Conversely, GI stromal tumours (GISTs) arising from the stomach and Dieulafoy malformation (an unusual vascular anomaly where an ectatic artery erodes the gastric mucosa), can produce catastrophic haemorrhage.

It is for this reason that resuscitation of the patient with an upper GI bleed should be prompt and aggressive. The recognition of unusual lesions by the endoscopist is important. Always try and attend when acute endoscopy is being performed. You will have a much clearer idea of the likelihood that further bleeding might occur.

Carcinoma of the stomach

Any gastric lesion is potentially malignant until it has been biopsied and proved to be benign. If suspicions continue of possible malignancy in a non-healing ulcer, repeated biopsies must be taken.

Adenocarcinoma of the stomach is one of the commonest malignancies worldwide but it ranks about seventh in the UK, with incidence rates of between 15 and 22 cases per 100 000 population, depending upon geographical area. Higher rates are seen in the 'postindustrial' urban areas such as the Midlands and South Wales. *Helicobacter pylori* infection is thought to be the major cause of gastric cancer worldwide and as socioeconomic factors improve in a developing country, so the helicobacter rates fall and the incidence of gastric cancer falls as well. This association is mainly true for distal gastric cancer. Proximal tumours are now commoner in many areas of the UK and may be associated with gastro-oesophageal reflux disease although this is still uncertain.

Tumours that are detected early have an excellent prognosis. However, over 80% of tumours in the UK are detected late and the survival rate for these patients is poor.

Early detection is therefore essential for successful treatment. By the time patients have 'alarm symptoms' such as weight loss, anaemia, a mass or dysphagia, two-thirds will have incurable disease. Tumours spread via lymphatics, venous blood vessels, directly into adjacent organs such as the pancreas and via the peritoneal cavity.

Recognizing the pattern

The patient is typically over 45 years of age and the condition is more common in males. Patients may complain of dyspepsia, epigastric pain, nausea, early satiety and loss of appetite. Fatigue may indicate anaemia; an iron-deficient picture should always trigger investigation of the GI tract unless menorrhagia is clearly the cause. The symptoms will often improve or even disappear with adequate acid suppression from a PPI and this is a common 'catch' for the unwary.

On examination there may be signs of anaemia, tenderness in the epigastrium or even a mass palpable in the left hypochondrium. The later is a bad prognostic sign as is any evidence of nodal enlargement in the supraclavicular fossa (Virchow's node or Troisier's sign) and hepatomegaly. Cachexia, ascites and jaundice are also signs that the disease is unlikely to be curable.

Proving the diagnosis

It is not possible to distinguish between the symptoms of benign gastric pathology and cancers. This is very important and means that all patients with unexplained symptoms must have an endoscopy regardless of age or sex.

Management

The surgical management is to excise the tumour and the local lymph nodes if a cure is to be attempted. Either a subtotal or total gastrectomy may be required in order to achieve adequate clearance of the tumour. The latter may be carried out through the abdomen alone, or through a thoracoabdominal incision. The extent of the resection is based on the stage, site of tumour and the lymph nodes involved.

Early small (< 2 cm diameter) tumours which are confined to the mucosa (T1) have a low risk of having spread to adjacent lymph nodes and local resection is safe and has high cure rates. This can be achieved endoscopically (endoscopic mucosal resection, EMR) or surgically using laparoscopic techniques.

More advanced tumours that have invaded the submucosal layer or the muscularis propria have a high chance of having metastasized to regional lymph nodes. In addition, they may have spread further to the liver, lungs or peritoneum. Consequently, patients with tumours which are deemed to be 'endoscopically advanced' must have a CT scan of their chest and abdomen and a staging laparoscopy before their management is discussed in a multidisciplinary meeting. If no evidence of distant spread is found then the patient should be considered for surgery. There is now strong evidence for the use of neoadjuvant chemotherapy in gastric cancer. Surgery for gastric cancer should occur in high volume cancer centres as there is a strong correlation between number of operations done and outcome.

Preoperatively both the patient and their relatives will need careful counselling. A specialist nurse should ideally be involved in this process. Assessment of the patient's fitness for major surgery is essential and may require lung function tests, blood gases, ECG, and echocardiography depending upon the degree of comorbidity. Nutritional needs must be met.

Gastrectomies for cancer are classified according to the degree of radicality.
- D1: Resection of the perigastric nodes lymph nodes along the greater and lesser curve of the stomach. The majority of

resections undertaken in the UK are D1 gastrectomies although this is changing.

- D2: Resection of lymph nodes along the main arteries of the stomach (left and right gastric, coeliac, left and right gastro-epiploic and splenic). This is usually achieved without resection of the spleen or tail of the pancreas and is called a 'modified D2 resection'. This is safer than the original D2 operation.
- D3: This is similar to a D2 resection but includes all the lymph nodes around the porta hepatis and behind the head of the pancreas. It is selectively used by some surgeons for distal gastric tumours.
- D4: This is as for a D3 resection but also involves an extensive retroperitoneal dissection to remove para-aortic nodes up to the level of the diaphragm. It is experimental.

OPERATION: TOTAL GASTRECTOMY, EXTENDED TOTAL GASTRECTOMY AND DISTAL GASTRECTOMY

In this operation the whole of the stomach is removed with varying amounts of the distal oesophagus depending on how proximal the tumour is. The oesophagus is anastomosed to a mobilized limb of jejunum (Roux-en Y), end to side. A feeding jejunostomy may be sited to feed the patient until oral intake is permitted. In a distal gastrectomy a small proximal gastric remnant is left and the jejunum is anastomosed to this rather than the oesophagus. It has lower complication rates than total gastrectomy and generally a better functional result for the patient.

Procedure profile

Blood requirement	2
Anaesthetic	GA
Operation time	3–4 hours
Hospital stay	2 weeks
Return to normal activity	10–12 weeks

OPERATION: THORACOABDOMINAL GASTRECTOMY

This operation may be used where the carcinoma of the stomach involves the lower oesophagus or gastro-oesophageal junction. In this case an oblique incision is extended up along the bed of the eighth rib and the chest opened. The anastomosis to the oesophagus is then carried out inside the chest. This is an alternative to the extended gastrectomy when safe proximal clearance cannot be achieved through the hiatus and more oesophagus must be resected above the tumour to ensure clear margins (R0 resection).

Procedure profile

Blood requirement	2
Anaesthetic	GA
Operation time	3–5 hours
Hospital stay	2 weeks
Return to normal activity	10–12 weeks

Postoperatively the patient is allowed 30 mL of water only per hour by mouth for the first 3–5 days. Care of the patient is essentially the same as for a patient who has undergone oesophagectomy. Respiratory complications are common, and effective analgesia is essential to ensure adequate coughing post surgery. Early mobilization is important.

Postgastrectomy syndromes

These are becoming less common as the number of gastric resections for benign disease diminishes. They include the following:
- bilious vomiting
- dumping
- diarrhoea
- long-term nutritional problems.

Bilious vomiting

This is vomiting of pure bile and occurs in up to 10% of patients following a gastrectomy. It is more common after simple gastroenterostomy when a loop of proximal jejunum is anastomosed to the gastric remnant and bile is inevitably diverted into the stomach. The Roux-en-Y reconstruction avoids this.

Management

Bilious vomiting is more common immediately after a gastric operation and tends to settle as time passes. Medical management includes substances which help to bind bile salts such aluminium hydroxide (Aludrox and Maalox). Metoclopramide may also be of value as a prokinetic agent.

The patient should be reassured that the symptoms usually settle. Avoidance is better still by using the Roux-en-Y reconstruction in the primary procedure.

If the symptoms persist, bile diversion by conversion to a Roux-en-Y reconstruction should be considered.

OPERATION: GASTRIC RECONSTRUCTION FOR BILIOUS VOMITING

Bile diversion is best achieved by converting the standard enterostomy loop to a Roux-en-Y procedure (see Fig. 7.2.6). This results in the bile entering the intestine well away from the stomach.

Procedure profile

Blood requirement	2
Anaesthetic	GA
Operation time	2 hours
Hospital stay	7 days
Return to normal activity	4–6 weeks

Postoperatively there are no special problems after this procedure. Oral fluids can be reintroduced as soon as the stomach is seen to be emptying (as evidenced by diminished gastric aspirate and passage of flatus).

Dumping

This is a complex mixture of symptoms and may consist of abdominal pain, distension and colic, and vasomotor disturbance occurring after meals. It is rare after highly selective vagotomy alone. Dumping gradually becomes more common with operations that involve division of the vagal trunks and a

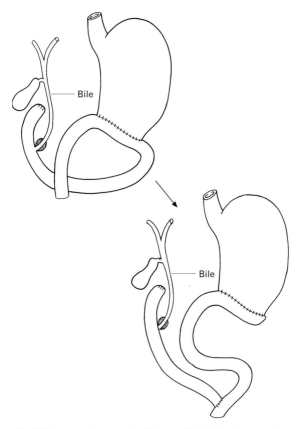

Fig. 7.2.6 Roux-en-Y conversion for biliary gastritis. The bile and pancreatic juice can no longer reach the stomach.

drainage procedure and rises again if part of the stomach is resected. Curiously, with near-total and total gastrectomy, it seems less of a problem, probably because many of these patients have little or no reservoir for food resulting in small calorie intakes at each occasion when they eat.

There are two types.

- Early dumping. This is due to rapid emptying of the stomach, a high osmotic load in the small bowel and an increased splanchnic blood flow resulting in a fluid shift from the vascular compartment to the bowel lumen. This is precipitated particularly by hot, sweet or bulky meals taken with fluid.
- Late dumping. This is due to a reactive hypoglycaemia caused by increased insulin output in response to the earlier hyperglycaemia. The hyperglycaemia itself follows rapid gastric emptying.

Recognizing the pattern

Early dumping starts immediately after a meal and consists of attacks of sweating, flushing, tachycardia, palpitations, epigastric fullness, nausea and occasionally colicky abdominal pain, vomiting and diarrhoea.

Late dumping starts 1–2 h after meals and consists of faintness accompanied by sweating, tremor and nausea.

Proving the diagnosis

The diagnosis of dumping is made on the history. Hypoglycaemia may be confirmed by measuring the blood sugar during an attack. However, many patients get abdominal symptoms after gastrectomy which are not easily classified as early or late dumping. It may therefore be more useful to use the term 'postgastrectomy syndrome' to include all the problems that patients encounter. Many symptoms will improve with time.

Management

The symptoms are difficult to treat and are best managed by persuading the patient to modify their intake of food so as to minimize the rapid gastric emptying of foodstuffs. Patients with dumping must have the causes explained to them and should be reassured that the condition usually settles with time. After a year, less than 5% of patients are significantly bothered by dumping.

Early dumping can be prevented by small, dry meals, with a diet consisting of fat and protein and restricted carbohydrate. Drinks should be taken between and not during meals. Late dumping is made worse by exercise after a meal so susceptible patients should rest for an hour after eating.

Severe persistent dumping is sometimes amenable to surgical correction, depending on the initial operation, but this is usually not feasible after a resection for cancer.

Diarrhoea

Truncal vagotomy not only decreases gastric secretion and delays emptying, but also affects the rest of the bowel to a variable extent. Up to 50% of patients after a truncal vagotomy suffer some increase in bowel habit and 5% need treatment for this. The diarrhoea is typically 'episodic'. The patient has normal bowel actions most of the time but is then struck with episodes of urgency and looseness. The mechanism is uncertain and several factors may be responsible. The rapid emptying of the stomach that follows the accompanying gastric drainage procedure results in hyperosmolar contents arriving in the small bowel lumen. As the bowel rapidly dilutes this, vigorous peristalsis ensues, producing some of the symptoms of early dumping and also diarrhoea. There may also be a direct effect of loss of vagal influence on the small bowel and on the biliary tract. Diarrhoea is also very rare following highly selective vagotomy.

Diarrhoea that comes on for the first time some months after gastrectomy might be due to bacterial overgrowth in the small bowel, potentially as a result of loss of gastric acid. This is an occasional yet treatable cause of diarrhoea. The diagnosis can be proved by a ^{14}C breath test.

Recognizing the pattern

The patient complains of an increase in bowel habit, which in severe cases may consist of attacks of uncontrollable watery diarrhoea. These attacks are episodic and unpredictable.

Management

The diarrhoea sometimes responds to codeine phosphate (45–120 mg daily in three to six divided doses), diphenoxylate (Lomotil) or loperamide (Imodium). Bacterial overgrowth is treated with a short course of antibiotics.

Nutritional problems

Most patients struggle to regain weight after a major gastric resection. Vitamin B12 deficiency is inevitable and for this reason, all patients having a substantial gastric resection should receive B12 injections every 3 months for the rest of their life to prevent pernicious anaemia. Loss of acid may affect iron absorption in the upper small bowel, resulting in an iron-deficient anaemia. Poor dietary calcium intake coupled to poor absorption as a result of inefficient mixing between food and digestive juice, means that there is an insidious loss of bone density. Careful assessment of bone chemistry, iron and iron stores is essential in the late follow-up of these patients.

7.3 Central abdominal pain

Acute appendicitis

This is the commonest surgical emergency in most western European countries. The appendix has a narrow lumen and there is a rich collection of lymphatic tissue in the submucosa. Obstruction of the lumen can follow impaction of a faecolith or swelling of the submucosal lymphatic tissue. Once this occurs, a vicious circle ensues with further swelling and obstruction, blockage of blood supply, infection and ischaemia of the distal appendix.

Recognizing the pattern
Acute appendicitis can occur at any age, although it is particularly common between the ages of 10 and 30 years.

The typical history is of central abdominal colic associated with nausea and vomiting. After a few hours the colic subsides and the pain settles in the right iliac fossa. At this stage the pain is worse on movement (walking, coughing).

The patient looks unwell and is flushed. There is often a foetor. The tongue is furred and the patient has a low-grade pyrexia, typically of 37.5°C. The fever is very rarely above 38.0°C in the early stages of the disease. There is also a tachycardia. Examination of the abdomen discloses marked tenderness in the right iliac fossa with guarding and rebound. By careful palpation it is usually possible to delineate a constant line of tenderness over the site of the appendix.

This localized tenderness is the single most important factor in making the diagnosis. Rectal examination may also disclose tenderness high up on the right side, especially if the appendix is in a pelvic position.

The clinical picture of appendicitis does, of course, vary widely and the presentation may be particularly confusing in the very young and the very old.

Proving the diagnosis

There are no absolute tests to prove or disprove the diagnosis of acute appendicitis. If the suspicion is strong enough, a laparoscopy or laparotomy must be performed in order to exclude the disease.

Management

A localized line of tenderness, together with signs of peritonitis, will indicate the need for operative exploration.

Preoperatively the patient must be adequately rehydrated and the value of giving preoperative antibiotics with the premedication has been demonstrated. A metronidazole suppository is effective.

If the history is very long (e.g. 7 days) and if the pain is settling it may be justified to treat the condition conservatively. In these cases an appendix mass may be palpable in the right iliac fossa. The patient is observed to be sure the mass settles. An 'interval appendicectomy' may be required some months later, as some of these patients do develop chronic pain. The adoption of this as a standard procedure, however, is without proven benefit.

OPERATION: OPEN APPENDICECTOMY

The abdomen is opened through a skin-crease or grid-iron incision situated in the right iliac fossa. The appendix lies under McBurney's point, which is on a line between the anterior superior iliac spine and the umbilicus, two-thirds of the way from the umbilicus. The incision is best made almost horizontally in Langer's lines (see Fig. 7.3.1). The muscles of the abdominal wall are split in the line of their fibres (grid-iron incision) and the peritoneum opened. The presence or absence of purulent peritoneal fluid is noted and a swab taken.

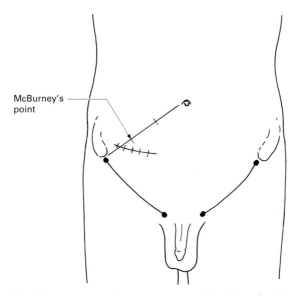

Fig. 7.3.1 Appendicectomy. The incision is made just below McBurney's point, horizontally, parallel to Langer's skin lines.

The upper part of the caecum is grasped and pulled out of the wound towards the patient's feet. After completing this manoeuvre, the caecum is then pulled upward towards the patient's head and the appendix is thus delivered. It may be necessary to free adhesions in order to achieve this. With a retrocaecal appendix it is necessary to mobilize the lower pole of the caecum by dividing the peritoneum laterally. The appendix stump is crushed and tied with a dissolvable suture. The appendicular vessels are ligated and the appendix is removed. Many surgeons invert the appendix stump into the caecal wall using a purse-string or 'Z' sutures. The terminal 100 cm of small bowel is gently examined to see if there is a coincident Meckel's diverticulum. A drain is inserted into the peritoneum only if there was an abscess. The wound is closed in layers with dissolvable sutures and infiltrated with local anaesthetic.

OPERATION: LAPAROSCOPIC APPENDICECTOMY
Young women with an uncertain diagnosis of appendicitis should be laparoscoped, as up to 30% will have other pathologies. If appendicitis is confirmed, the surgeon can proceed to laparoscopic appendicectomy if he or she is suitably experienced. Otherwise they should convert to an open operation. There are different port sites depending upon the surgeon's preferences (see Fig. 7.3.2). The principle of the laparoscopic operation is the same as for open appendicectomy.

Procedure profile

Blood requirement	0
Anaesthetic	GA
Operation time	30–40 minutes
Hospital stay	2–3 days in the absence of residual sepsis
Return to normal activity	10–14 days

The postoperative ileus after open operation is usually short-lived and oral fluids can be reintroduced immediately unless extensive peritoneal contamination was found. If this is the case, antibiotics should be given for 5–7 days or longer if necessary. The patient's temperature is monitored closely for the first 36–48 h after surgery and if it is normal the patient can be discharged home. Oral analgesia is given regularly for the first 3–5 days.

The wound must be inspected before the patient leaves hospital. A water-resistant dressing allows the patient to shower immediately.

Mesenteric adenitis

The mesenteric lymph nodes may become inflamed as part of a general infection or gastroenteritis. The importance of the condition lies in differentiating it from acute appendicitis.

Recognizing the pattern
The patient is commonly under 10 years of age.

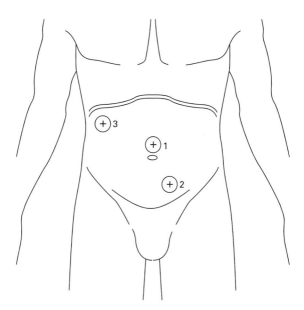

Fig. 7.3.2 Possible port sites for laparoscopic appendicectomy.

The complaint is of abdominal pain. This may be gener-alized or localized, possibly in the right iliac fossa. There may be symptoms of diarrhoea and/or vomiting, or of a recent upper respiratory tract infection.

On examination the tenderness tends to be moderate with lit-tle guarding or rebound, and poorly localized. The patient may be pyrexial, often with a fever above 37.5°C. There may be signs of pharyngeal inflammation and 'shotty' nodes palpable in the neck. The C-reactive protein (CRP) estimation is usually normal as is the white blood count.

Proving the diagnosis
Careful re-examination is important to exclude appendicitis. A CT scan may be helpful and diagnostic laparoscopy may be needed.

Management

If appendicitis can be excluded, the management is conservative with paracetamol +/– ibuprofen and the patient can be allowed home.

Intestinal obstruction

This section should be read in conjunction with large bowel obstruction on p. 370.

The bowel may become obstructed from a variety of causes anywhere along its length. The obstruction may be mechanical or functional (localized or generalized paralytic ileus).

Mechanical causes are usefully divided into those that compress the bowel from the outside, those that arise within the wall of the bowel and obstruct the lumen, and those that arise within the lumen (Table 7.3.1). Paralytic ileus is described on p. 41.

Recognizing the pattern

The patient can be of any age from a newborn baby onwards. Age is sometimes a clue to likely aetiology.

Mechanical intestinal obstruction has three classical features: vomiting, colicky abdominal pain and distension. The level of obstruction and its duration dictate the extent to which these are present. Vomiting occurs early with proximal obstructions, there is little colic and virtually no discernable distension. Think of pyloric stenosis as a good example. Obstruction in the small bowel produces intense colic, followed by vomiting. As the level of obstruction becomes more distal in the small bowel, vomiting occurs later and distension becomes increasingly apparent. In the large bowel, distension predominates, and the competence of the ileocaecal valve influences the extent to which decompression into the small bowel can occur. Vomiting is a late feature.

Irrespective of cause, the patient may be dehydrated due to fluid losses into the intestine and vomiting. A change in the pain from the intermittency of colic to the persistent pain of ischaemia is a strong indicator there is a cause that has imperilled the blood supply. This is often accompanied by tachycardia and the onset of fever. Look carefully for visible peristalsis under the

Table 7.3.1 Mechanical causes of intestinal obstruction.

Outside the bowel	
Adhesions or bands	p. 311
Volvulus	p. 373
Invasion by neighbouring malignant growths	
Strangulated hernia, etc.	p. 424
In the bowel wall	
Tumours	pp. 315, 373
Infarction	p. 313
Congenital atresia	pp. 579–81
Hirschsprung's disease	p. 586
Inflammatory bowel disease	pp. 359
Diverticulitis	p. 385
In the lumen	
Impacted faeces	p. 36
Bolus obstruction	
Gallstone ileus	p. 318
Intussusception	pp. 315, 590
Large polyps	p. 373

abdominal wall. Distended loops of obstructed small bowel are often tender on palpation, but focal tenderness may indicate perforation. On auscultation there may be hyperactive high-pitched bowel sounds. Never forget to look carefully for old abdominal scars and be absolutely sure that there are no abdominal wall hernias.

Proving the diagnosis

The diagnosis is proved by performing a supine and erect abdominal X-ray, which shows the presence of distended loops of small bowel together with fluid levels (see Fig. 7.3.3). Small bowel loops have transverse lines like a 'coiled spring' – the valvulae conniventes. Distended large bowel has haustra – transverse lines interrupted by the taeniae coli. If the colon is obstructed the caecum will also be distended. CT scanning is becoming increasingly important in making accurate diagnoses in patients with suspected gut obstruction. Closed loop obstruction can occur in

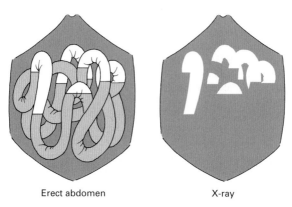

Erect abdomen   X-ray

Fig. 7.3.3 Fluid levels in obstructed small bowel.

both the small and large bowel and because of the high risk of strangulation and perforation, demands urgent action. All patients must have urgent blood tests (urea, electrolytes and full blood count). These provide useful information about the degree of dehydration. The white cell count is often elevated with strangulation.

Management

The first step is to decide on whether obstruction is simple or potentially strangulated, based on the clinical features, test results and likely cause. This determines the need for urgent action. The next step is to replenish the fluid loss and keep the bowel empty by nasogastric suction. A urinary catheter should be inserted to assess the response to fluid replacement. Conservative therapy is often successful in the management of small bowel obstruction that is secondary to adhesions from previous surgery. Sigmoid volvulus can often be decompressed by sigmoidoscopy and obstruction due to faecal impaction by enemas, but failure of any conservative approach to achieve resolution after 48 h should lead to re-evaluation and consideration of surgery. General deterioration in the patient's condition, increasing abdominal tenderness and tachycardia are all indications for operation. These latter signs may indicate that part of the bowel is becoming ischaemic.

OPERATION: FOR INTESTINAL OBSTRUCTION
The procedure undertaken depends on the underlying cause.

- Intestinal adhesions are divided and loops of bowel mobilized so as to free the obstruction. Occasionally it is necessary to resect a damaged segment of small bowel.
- A volvulus is untwisted and the viability of the bowel checked. The surgeon may wait to see whether a dubious segment of bowel regains its colour satisfactorily after a period.
- A strangulated hernia is repaired and the bowel dealt with as above.

Procedure profile

Blood requirement	0
Anaesthetic	GA
Operation time	Variable – depends on the cause
Hospital stay	1–2 weeks
Return to normal activity	Variable

Other causes of intestinal obstruction are dealt with in other sections (see Table 7.3.1).

Meckel's diverticulum

This lesion is a remnant of the attachment of the small bowel to the embryological yolk sac. It arises from the antemesenteric border somewhere along the distal 100 cm of small bowel. The diverticulum may contain remnants of all types of intestinal mucosa (including acid-secreting gastric mucosa).

Recognizing the pattern
The patient may be of any age, although problems from a Meckel's diverticulum are more common in children.

The lesion may remain asymptomatic for the whole of the patient's life. If it does cause trouble, however, the presentation is in one of three ways.

- The picture of acute appendicitis. This is due to obstruction of the lumen of the diverticulum in exactly the same way as the appendix becomes obstructed. This presentation is not common, as the diverticulum usually has a wide neck.
- The picture of intestinal obstruction. This is often due to the fact that the Meckel's diverticulum is associated with a band running up to the umbilicus and this may obstruct other loops of bowel.
- Intestinal bleeding. If the diverticulum contains gastric mucosa a peptic ulcer may arise in the adjacent ileum. This bleeds and the patient passes fresh blood per rectum. This is perhaps the most common presentation of a Meckel's diverticulum in children.

Proving the diagnosis

This is difficult and frequently a laparotomy is necessary. An attempt should be made to define the diverticulum using radioactive technetium scanning, but this is not always reliable. The lesion may be demonstrated on a barium meal and 'follow through', or even a barium enema, but again the investigation is unreliable.

Management

If there is a strong suspicion that a Meckel's diverticulum might be present, a laparotomy is undertaken.

OPERATION: FOR MECKEL'S DIVERTICULUM

The diverticulum is resected and the small bowel closed. If there is an ulcer in the ileum, this segment of ileum is resected together with the diverticulum. The appendix may be taken out in the same operation to avoid diagnostic confusion later. This operation can also be performed laparoscopically and is very similar to laparoscopic appendicectomy (see p. 306).

Procedure profile

Blood requirement	0 (babies may require 1)
Anaesthetic	GA
Operation time	1 hour
Hospital stay	4–7 days
Return to normal activity	3–4 weeks

Ischaemic bowel

Ischaemic bowel may arise either secondary to some of the causes of intestinal obstruction, or as a primary condition from interruption of the arterial or venous blood supply. Arterial blockage is usually due to an embolus from the heart or great vessels, usually when there is already a degree of atherosclerosis at or close to the origin of the superior mesenteric artery. Mesenteric venous thrombosis is seen in patients with acquired (e.g. neoplasia) or inherited (e.g. protein C, protein S deficiencies). Bowel infarction is a life-threatening condition and early laparotomy is mandatory. In this section primary ischaemia of the bowel will be considered.

Recognizing the pattern

The patient is usually elderly and may have other signs of cardiac or vascular disease.

The patient complains of a sudden onset of severe colicky abdominal pain which rapidly becomes constant. The patient becomes very distressed and shocked. There may be a history of recent myocardial infarction or dysrhythmia.

On examination the signs may not seem to coincide with the severity of the patient's pain. There is usually some localized tenderness but not a lot in the way of guarding or rebound tenderness in the early stages. Rectal examination may reveal blood. The patient may be in atrial fibrillation. There is often profound metabolic derangement. The patient may be shocked, hypoxic, tachycardic, tachyopneic, oliguric and acidotic.

Proving the diagnosis

Urgent blood tests (urea, electrolytes, full blood count, arterial blood gases, amylase) will usually confirm the above features and exclude acute pancreatitis. Resuscitation and a laparotomy may be the next step. If there is doubt about the diagnosis an urgent abdominal CT scan should be arranged. If an inherited coagulopathy seems possible, ensure blood is taken preoperatively as the patient may need anticoagulation after surgery.

Management

Before laparotomy, resuscitation may be required to treat shock. Broad-spectrum parenteral antibiotics, intravenous fluids, analgesia and oxygen must be given.

OPERATION: LAPAROTOMY FOR ISCHAEMIC BOWEL

At operation the ischaemic loop of bowel is identified. Various causes may be found. The ischaemia may be secondary to a volvulus or band causing obstruction of the mesenteric vessels. In this case treatment of the cause may result in adequate perfusion of the ischaemic segment.

Another possible cause is embolism or thrombosis of one of the major arteries supplying the bowel. If the bowel is still potentially viable, an embolectomy or bypass operation may be performed to restore the blood supply. Any bowel that fails to recover must be resected. Occasionally where there is a long loop of ischaemic bowel and viability is dubious, it may be permissible to close the abdomen and take a second look after 24 h to determine the viability of the bowel.

Procedure profile

Blood requirement	0
Anaesthetic	GA
Operation time	1–2 hours
Hospital stay	7–10 days
Return to normal activity	4 weeks, depending on patient's condition

Postoperatively the patient is given intravenous fluids and nasogastric suction until flatus is passed, and bowel function restored. Good analgesia, probably via an epidural, is essential. Early mobilization with chest physiotherapy is also important.

Massive small bowel resections may result in a need for parenteral nutrition on either a temporary or permanent basis. There is considerable adaptation over about a 3-month period, and during this time deliberate restriction of oral intake may be necessary, so that the patient does not have metabolic and nutritional problems related to secretory diarrhoea that overwhelms the colon's capacity for water reabsorption. Early input from a nutritional care team is important. Adult patients left with less than a metre of small bowel may need permanent intravenous feeding, or at least electrolyte supplementation.

Intussusception in adults

Intussusceptions are much commoner in children and are dealt with on p. 590. The management in the adult is very similar, although open operation through a vertical incision, and not reduction by barium enema, is the method of choice. This is because there is almost always a causative lesion in an adult, such as a polyp, which forms the head of the intussusception. This will need to be resected.

Small bowel tumours

Small bowel tumours are rare. Benign tumours include adenomas, lipomas and GISTs (gastrointestinal stromal tumours – a type of soft tissue sarcoma). They may bleed, causing melaena and anaemia, and they can cause intussusception. Multiple hamartomatous polyps of the small bowel occur in association with melanin pigmentation of the lips and oral mucosa as part of the Peutz–Jeghers syndrome. Malignant change is rare.

Primary malignant tumours include lymphosarcoma, spindle cell sarcoma and carcinoma. Small bowel secondaries can occur with most epithelial tumours but it is an unusual site.

Carcinoid tumour is a potentially malignant growth of the Kulchitsky cells (argentaffin cells, amine precursor uptake and decarboxylation system); 65% arise in the appendix and 25% in the ileum. Other primary sites include the rest of the gut and, very rarely, the bronchus, testis and ovary. They spread to local nodes and via the bloodstream to the liver. They are often found as a coincidental finding after an appendicectomy. Size and completeness of excision will often dictate the need for further surgery. Some tumours produce serotonin and kinins (and possibly prostaglandins and histamine), but the carcinoid syndrome (flushing, abdominal cramps, diarrhoea) only occurs when the tumour has metastasized to the liver and these substances are able to escape hepatic metabolism.

Recognizing the pattern

They present with symptoms of bleeding (melaena and anaemia), intestinal obstruction or general carcinomatosis. The bowel wall may perforate, causing acute peritonitis.

The main features of carcinoid are flushing attacks (sometimes precipitated by alcohol), colic and diarrhoea. Episodic bronchospasm and pulmonary stenosis are features of pulmonary carcinoids because vasoactive amines enter the pulmonary circulation.

Proving the diagnosis

Small bowel tumours are often only found at laparotomy (e.g. for intussusception or bleeding). Occasionally, a barium meal may reveal a lesion in the duodenum or upper jejunum. Carcinoid syndrome is proved by demonstrating elevated levels of 5-hydroxyindole-acetic acid (5-HIAA, the breakdown product of serotonin) in the urine (normal range is 2–20 mg in 24 h). In this case a CT scan will show evidence of secondaries in the liver.

Management

Benign tumours are resected if they are causing symptoms of bleeding or obstruction. Malignant tumours are treated by wide excision including the local mesenteric nodes.

Metastases in the liver are often found at operation for carcinoid. Partial hepatectomy may be considered for metastases although the distribution of metastases does not often make this feasible. In addition, the tumour can be very slow growing with the disease running a relatively indolent course so that the patient may be managed conservatively for many years. Octreotide and its long-acting derivatives will often provide good symptomatic control. Transarterial catheter embolization via the hepatic artery can help some patients.

OPERATIONS
See right hemicolectomy on p. 378.

8 Hepatobiliary, pancreatic and splenic surgery

8.1 Hepatobiliary disease

Gallstones

Gallstones precipitate from bile concentrated in the gall bladder. They may be formed purely from cholesterol or bile pigment though most stones are mixed. Ten per cent of gallstones are radio-opaque due to the presence of calcium salts. Stones tend to cause symptoms when they obstruct the neck of the gall bladder or bile duct. Rarely a large gallstone may ulcerate through the gall bladder wall and enter the gut. The stone may then cause intestinal obstruction (gallstone ileus).

Recognizing the pattern

Gallstones are classically said to occur in the 'fat, fertile female in her 40s', but nowadays many age groups are affected and the condition is not uncommon in men. Typical symptoms are of two types.

- 'Flatulent dyspepsia' consists of discomfort and fullness in the epigastric region coming on an hour or two after meals and particularly after fatty food. Often the patient has subconsciously decided to keep off fats and therefore does not give a positive history of fat intolerance. The dyspepsia commonly occurs in the evenings. Both the intensity and frequency of pain are highly variable. These symptoms are certainly not specific to gallstones and functional dyspepsia can occur in the same pattern. Caution is advised before recommending cholecystectomy in such patients, even when gallstones have been unequivocally demonstrated.

Surgery: Diagnosis and Management, 4th edition. Edited by N. Rawlinson and D. Alderson. © 2009 Blackwell Publishing, ISBN: 978-1-4051-2921-3

- Acute gall bladder pain (often referred to as 'biliary colic') is probably due to obstruction of the outlet of the gall bladder. It is a much more severe pain, also coming on after food. The pain usually begins in the epigastrium or right hypochondrium and radiates around the costal margin to the right shoulder blade. The pain is not truly colicky (it does not come in waves) in that it often comes on suddenly, remains intense and then abates over a relatively long period. It frequently lasts a few hours and often results in the patient seeking medical advice. It settles with an injection of pethidine but there may be soreness under the right hypochondrium for several days. The pain is made worse by deep inspiration, coughing or movement.

If the contents of the gall bladder become secondarily infected (acute cholecystitis), the patient becomes systemically unwell with pyrexia often accompanied by anorexia, nausea and vomiting. With repeated attacks of pain and inflammation the gall bladder tends to become thick-walled and incapable of contraction. A stone passing into the common bile duct (CBD) can cause obstructive jaundice or acute pancreatitis. In the case of the former, secondary infection in the entire biliary tree can occur (acute cholangitis) and this is a severe illness demanding urgent action. Gallstone pancreatitis is discussed later in this chapter.

Patients with intermittent dyspeptic symptoms usually have no abnormal findings in the abdomen except during an episode of pain. In an acute attack of biliary pain, there is tenderness maximal beneath the right 9th costal cartilage over the gall bladder. If the examining hand is placed 2–3 finger-breadths below the costal margin and the patient asked to inspire deeply, a sharp pain is typically felt that stops further inspiration, as the gall bladder descends (Murphy's sign). In acute cholecystitis the patient may have a fever or be slightly jaundiced due to oedema around the gall bladder neck that presses on the bile duct (Mirizzi syndrome). If a stone blocks the outlet of the gall bladder without causing infection and the wall is thickened from previous attacks, it will distend and be palpable as a smooth swelling (mucocoele) in the right upper quadrant contiguous with the liver dullness. When infected, this is an empyema and the gall bladder usually becomes walled off by the omentum so that it can no longer easily be felt. In acute cholangitis, there is often a high fever, jaundice and diffuse hepatic tenderness, as infection spreads through the biliary tree.

Proving the diagnosis

During an acute attack there may be mild derangement of liver function tests. The presence of gallstones is confirmed by an ultrasound scan that will also demonstrate wall thickness, bile duct diameter and wall oedema in an acute attack. Occasionally, body habitus or overlying bowel gas can make ultrasound inconclusive. Alternative tests to detect gall bladder disease include magnetic resonance cholangiography (MRC) or HIDA (an iminodiacetic acid derivative, excreted by the hepatocytes into the bile) scanning.

Management

Cholesterol stones can sometimes be dissolved by medical treatment using bile acid derivatives (urso- or chenodeoxycholic acid). These agents have side-effects and are often poorly tolerated. Stone recurrence is common as soon as the treatment is stopped and dissolution therapy is therefore rarely used nowadays. Shattering stones by extracorporeal shock-wave lithotripsy has also been tried, but the fragments have to pass through the sphincter of Oddi and can cause jaundice or pancreatitis. With the advent of laparoscopic cholecystectomy in the early 1990s, these alternatives have become virtually obsolete.

The definitive management of gallstones for most patients is removal of the gall bladder. In elderly or frail patients, complications of gallstones such as pancreatitis can occur, where removal of stones from the bile duct alone may be adequate treatment.

Acute cholecystitis can be managed conservatively with bed rest and antibiotics (e.g. a cephalosporin or a quinolone derivative), but most surgeons perform urgent cholecystectomy during the acute attack. The gall bladder is usually easy to remove in the early stages (48 h) as it is surrounded by oedema.

Jaundice related to gallstones is a complex topic and a number of management strategies can be adopted that often reflect the resources available in a particular hospital. All patients should be given an antibiotic which is effective in bile (as above) to treat or minimize risks from cholangitis. Patients with transient abnormalities and a normal-calibre (usually 7 mm or less on ultrasound) bile duct or those with mild gallstone pancreatitis can undergo cholecystectomy with or without bile duct exploration as appropriate. The management of severe gallstone pancreatitis is discussed later. Acute cholangitis is a serious condition with high risks of end-organ damage secondary to sepsis. It is important to maintain adequate hydration to minimise the risk of renal failure and failure of the patient to respond promptly to antibiotics is an indication for urgent drainage of the biliary system either by endoscopic sphincterotomy (ES) or at operation.

OPERATION: LAPAROSCOPIC CHOLECYSTECTOMY
The gall bladder area is visualized on a video screen connected to a camera on a laparoscope. Operative manoeuvres are carried out through secondary laparoscopic ports (Fig. 8.1.1). The cystic duct and artery are clipped and divided and the gall bladder

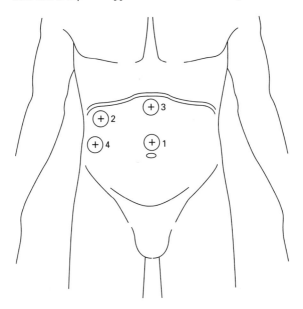

Fig. 8.1.1 Port sites for laparoscopic cholecystectomy.

removed. A cholangiogram can also be performed. A major abdominal incision is therefore avoided in favour of three or more stab wounds for the laparoscopic cannulae. Postoperative pain is less and recovery faster than after open surgery.

Procedure profile

Blood requirement	Group and save
Anaesthetic	GA
Operation time	1–2 hours
Hospital stay	Day case–48 hours
Return to normal activity	1–2 weeks

OPERATION: LAPAROSCOPIC CHOLECYSTECTOMY AND EXPLORATION OF THE COMMON BILE DUCT

Some surgeons still resort to open operation or endoscopic sphincterotomy when stones are found in the bile duct, but the majority will deal with these laparoscopically. A wire (Dormia) basket or a balloon is introduced into the bile duct percutaneously usually via the cystic duct. Stones can be grasped under X-ray control and extracted. If the stone is too large to retrieve through the cystic duct the bile duct can be opened and later closed with sutures directly or over a latex T-tube (make sure that the patient does not have latex allergy). The duct can also be inspected and stones retrieved under vision using a choledochoscope passed through a port. If stones are removed through the cystic duct, the recovery is the same as for a simple cholecystectomy.

Procedure profile

Blood requirement	Group and save
Anaesthetic	GA
Operation time	1–2 hours (with CBD exploration 2–3 hours)
Hospital stay	Day case–48 hours
Return to normal activity	1–2 weeks (3–4 if preoperative jaundice)

Postoperatively the patient suffers very little pain and can usually resume drinking and eating within a few hours after operation. Recovery is remarkably rapid and the patient can return to full activity 1–2 weeks after surgery.

If the CBD has been explored and a T-tube used, a cholangiogram is performed after a week to exclude the presence of further retained stones before the T-tube is removed. If the X-ray is clear, the T-tube can be taken out after 10–14 days when the latex rubber will have caused a track to form that prevents biliary peritonitis.

The development of jaundice or the presence of significant abdominal pain 24 h after laparoscopic cholecystectomy are ominous signs that merit prompt attention to exclude damage to the bile duct and/or biliary peritonitis. An urgent ultrasound scan to look for biliary dilatation or free fluid in the peritoneal cavity is needed. The patient may require repeat laparoscopy or further detailed imaging (MR cholangiogram, ERCP) if biliary injury seems likely. Some bile leaks and minor injuries are amenable to endoscopic stenting, but major injuries require revisional surgery that should only be carried out at specialist centres.

After a cholecystectomy patients can return to a normal diet with no dietary restrictions. They can be reassured that removal of the diseased gall bladder usually has no effect on bowel function.

Surgical jaundice

Patients are referred to surgeons when their jaundice is thought to be due to obstruction. The first task is to establish that the jaundice is indeed obstructive and then to determine the cause of the obstruction. An understanding of the physiology of bile metabolism is necessary.

Jaundice is due to excessive accumulation of bile pigment (bilirubin and its derivatives). The normal metabolism of bile is shown in Fig. 8.1.2. An excess of bilirubin may be due to any of the following.

- Excessive production – prehepatic jaundice, e.g. haemolytic anaemia.
- Defective processing of bilirubin in the liver – hepatic jaundice, e.g. hepatitis.

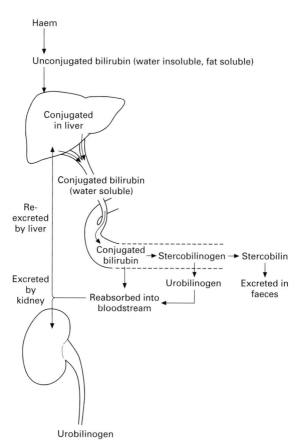

Fig. 8.1.2 Normal bilirubin metabolism: bilirubin is conjugated in the liver and excreted into the gut.

- Blocked excretion of bile from the liver – posthepatic or obstructive jaundice, e.g. stone in the CBD or carcinoma of the pancreas.

The main features of these three types of jaundice are given below.

Prehepatic jaundice
Recognizing the pattern
This occurs in a younger age group and is common in children. There is an excessive production of bilirubin due to an increased red cell turnover. This may be due to a haemolytic disorder such as spherocytosis, drug-induced haemolysis or an incompatible blood transfusion. There is an increased unconjugated bilirubin in the peripheral blood and low haemoglobin. The serum alkaline phosphatase, alanine transaminase (ALT) and the serum albumin are all normal. Blood clotting studies are also normal. The absence of liver damage makes this type of jaundice easy to separate from the other two. Because of the satisfactory liver function the jaundice is always mild and the patient is usually not deeply jaundiced.

Hepatic jaundice
Recognizing the pattern
In this condition there is liver damage from one of a variety of causes including infectious (usually viral) hepatitis, cirrhosis (often due to alcohol) and drug- or chemical-induced liver damage. The patient is usually markedly jaundiced and ill from the effects of the underlying liver disease. Laboratory tests show marked elevations in transaminases and a less marked rise in alkaline phosphatase. Blood clotting is abnormally prolonged and often refractory to vitamin K injection. Some bile is often still being processed in the liver and the stools may remain a normal colour.

On examination the liver is enlarged and tender.

Posthepatic obstructive jaundice (Fig. 8.1.3)
Recognizing the pattern
In this condition the liver function is initially normal but may become secondarily damaged due to back pressure or ascending infection. Characteristically the alkaline phosphatase is very high and the ALT less elevated. The serum albumin should be normal. The jaundice is usually deep but it may be intermittent if the obstruction is intermittent (e.g. gallstones). Abnormal coagulation studies are usually promptly corrected by vitamin K.

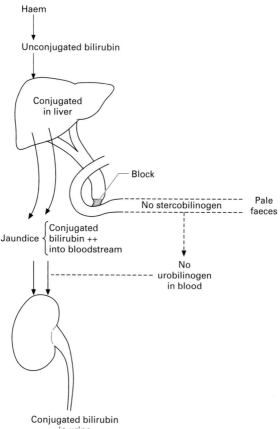

Fig. 8.1.3 Obstructive jaundice. When conjugated bilirubin cannot get into the gut it appears in the bloodstream and is excreted in the urine.

Proving the diagnosis

These three types of jaundice have characteristic laboratory findings.

- Test the urine for urobilinogen and urobilin. Urobilinogen is raised in prehepatic jaundice and bilirubin is present in

Table 8.1.1 Laboratory results in jaundice.

	Prehepatic (haemolytic)	Hepatic (hepatitis)*	Posthepatic (obstructive)
Bilirubin			
Unconjugated	Raised	Raised	May be raised
Conjugated	Normal	Raised	Raised
Alanine transaminase (ALT)	Normal	Raised	May be raised
Alkaline phosphatase	Normal	Slightly raised	Raised
Plasma proteins	Normal	May be low	Normal

*There is often an element of obstruction in hepatic jaundice due to intrahepatic cholestasis.

posthepatic jaundice. Urobilinogen is absent from the urine if the obstruction is complete.
- Liver function tests. The pattern of results in various types of jaundice is shown in Table 8.1.1. In addition, the prothrombin time gives a useful indicator of liver function and may be important in the future management of the patient.
- Ultrasound. If the intrahepatic bile ducts are dilated, the cause is obstructive. The level of obstruction (intra- or extrahepatic) may point to the cause. Ultrasound may also detect the presence of gallstones in the gall bladder or masses within the liver or pancreas.
- Magnetic resonance cholangiogram. An excellent picture of the biliary tree can be obtained without the need for injections or endoscopy. This has largely eliminated the need for diagnostic ERCP.
- ERCP. The ampulla of Vater is inspected using a side-viewing endoscope. The lower end of the CBD is cannulated to show the level of the obstruction and probable cause. Endoscopic sphincterotomy (ES) can be performed to facilitate stone extraction. Tissue can be obtained by biopsy or brush cytology and biliary stents can be placed to overcome obstruction on a temporary or permanent basis.
- CT scanning. CT and MR provide high-quality images of this region. While CT is rarely used to prove that obstructive

jaundice is present, it is widely used to identify and characterize mass lesions causing obstruction.

- EUS (endoscopic ultrasound). Probably the most sensitive method for identifying small lesions not seen by other imaging. It has the advantage that targeted biopsies can be obtained without a percutaneous approach.
- If the ducts in the liver are not dilated, a liver biopsy may be appropriate to identify the cause of hepatic damage.

Management
Before any intervention, patients with obstructive jaundice should be given vitamin K. Adequate hydration is essential to prevent renal failure (hepatorenal syndrome). This is best achieved with intra-venous crystalloid, started at least 12 h prior to intervention. A urinary catheter should always be present to monitor urine output and gauge fluid requirements.

OPERATION: ERCP AND ENDOSCOPIC SPHINCTEROTOMY
The patient is sedated and a side-viewing endoscope passed through the mouth into the duodenum. The ampulla is inspected and cannulated. The biliary and pancreatic ducts are visualized on an X-ray image intensifier. If a stone is seen, a sphincterotomy can be performed using a diathermy wire stretched across an insulated cannula inserted into the ampulla. Stones can be pulled into the duodenum using a balloon or wire basket. They can also be crushed with a lithotrite, or a stent can be inserted. Suspicious lesions can be biopsied.

Procedure profile

Blood requirement	Group and save
Anaesthetic	Sedation
Operation time	30 minutes – 2 hours
Hospital stay	Up to 24 hours
Return to normal activity	Depends on diagnosis

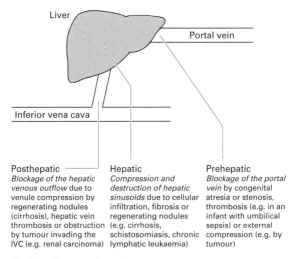

Liver

Portal vein

Inferior vena cava

Posthepatic
Blockage of the hepatic venous outflow due to venule compression by regenerating nodules (cirrhosis), hepatic vein thrombosis or obstruction by tumour invading the IVC (e.g. renal carcinoma)

Hepatic
Compression and destruction of hepatic sinusoids due to cellular infiltration, fibrosis or regenerating nodules (e.g. cirrhosis, schistosomiasis, chronic lymphatic leukaemia)

Prehepatic
Blockage of the portal vein by congenital atresia or stenosis, thrombosis (e.g. in an infant with umbilical sepsis) or external compression (e.g. by tumour)

Fig. 8.1.4 The causes of portal hypertension.

Portal hypertension

The portal venous pressure is raised when there is an obstruction in the portal system. This can be situated before, in or after the liver. Common causes of such an obstruction are shown in Fig. 8.1.4. The commonest aetiology in Western countries is cirrhosis. Schistosomiasis is the main cause worldwide. The normal portal venous pressure is 5–10 mmHg and the pressure may reach 30–40 mmHg in portal hypertension. Elevated portal pressure leads to the development of venous collaterals between the portal and systemic venous circulation. The most important of these are in the oesophagus, where varices may develop. Collaterals also develop at the umbilicus and in the rectum and anal canal (Fig. 8.1.5). The patient also develops ascites if there is coexistent liver failure with hypoproteinaemia and hyperaldosteronism. Splenomegaly is common and there may be a degree of

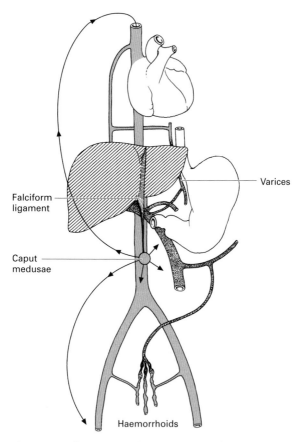

Varices

Falciform
ligament

Caput
medusae

Haemorrhoids

Fig. 8.1.5 Portal hypertension results in the enlargement of veins at the sites of portasystemic venous anastomoses.

hypersplenism with leucopenia and thrombocytopenia. Porto-systemic encephalopathy may occur due to the fact that blood from the gut bypasses the liver and its filtering and detoxifying mechanisms.

This section focuses on those complications of portal hypertension that involve the surgeon. Details of the management of patients with acute and chronic liver disease are covered in many large medical textbooks.

Recognizing the pattern

The usual presentation of portal hypertension is haematemesis and melaena. This is described later. There may also be symptoms of anaemia. There is usually a history of liver disease or alcoholism. The patient may have noticed easy bruising or a purpuric rash.

On examination the signs of portal hypertension include splenomegaly (80–90%), ascites and occasionally dilated veins around the umbilicus (caput medusae) over which there may be a venous hum on auscultation. Look for purpura and stigmata of chronic liver disease. These include jaundice, skin pigmentation, clubbing, spider naevi, palmar erythema, gynaecomastia, testicular atrophy and, in men, a female distribution of pubic hair.

The liver is a variable size in cirrhosis. Hepatosplenomegaly and ascites with no history of alcohol abuse suggest hepatic vein obstruction.

Signs of encephalopathy include confusion, drowsiness and tremor, increased tendon reflexes, upgoing plantar responses and constructional apraxia (e.g. inability to copy a star).

Proving the diagnosis

The presence of oesophageal varices is usually made by endoscopy, confirming the diagnosis together with the source of bleeding. Ultrasound with Doppler study of the vessels allows visualization of the hepatic and portal veins and depicts directional flow. CT and MRI can all provide additional information about liver architecture and a vascular map.

Evidence of liver disease may be found by measuring the serum bilirubin, serum albumin, hepatic enzymes and a coagulation screen. A liver biopsy may help to diagnose the nature of the disease. The hepatitis status of all jaundiced patients should be known. Many patients require specific tests to identify individual causes of chronic liver disease (e.g. haemochromatosis) or to indicate other problems associated with chronic liver disease (e.g. α-fetoprotein to look for hepatoma). A full blood count, urea and electrolytes, and calcium should be measured.

Management

The long-term management of portal hypertension includes the elective management of ascites and the underlying liver disease associated with portal hypertension and these topics are not discussed here.

Surgical management includes a variety of procedures.

- Endoscopic treatment for bleeding (either variceal banding or injection sclerotherapy – this decreases recurrent bleeding, but does not change survival).
- Portosystemic shunt – this is now performed almost exclusively by the transjugular intrahepatic portosystemic shunt (TIPSS) procedure, by specialist radiologists. There is a very small role for surgical shunts in patients with extrahepatic portal hypertension (see below). Other operations (such as oesophageal transection and gastric devascularization) are very rare.
- Liver transplantation is the definitive treatment of portal hypertension and also deals with the underlying disease process and improves survival. Liver transplantation is also used as the treatment of some acute and chronic forms of liver disease without portal hypertension. While waiting for transplantation, endoscopic treatments and/or TIPSS may be needed to control bleeding varices.
- The emergency management of bleeding oesophageal varices is described below.

OPERATION: TRANSJUGULAR INTRAHEPATIC PORTOSYSTEMIC SHUNT (TIPSS)

TIPSS involves the passage of a biopsy needle or stylet through the right internal jugular vein in order to create an intrahepatic track between the hepatic and portal vein under radiological guidance. This track is dilated with an angioplasty balloon catheter and a metallic stent inserted.

The main indication for TIPSS is to control and prevent variceal bleeding after failure of endoscopic methods.

Procedure profile

Blood requirement	2
Anaesthetic	LA
Operation time	2–3 hours
Hospital stay	48 hours
Return to normal activity	Variable

Postoperatively there are usually no problems apart from those associated with the original disease process.

Early complications are rare. Check for a haematoma at the entry site. There is a possibility of the patient developing hepatic encephalopathy if liver function is marginal.

Open operations when the above methods have failed should be restricted to major centres dealing with liver disease including transplantation.

Bleeding oesophageal varices

These occur as part of the syndrome of portal hypertension and can bleed massively. Hospital mortality is high and 60% of those who recover rebleed within 1 year. Blood in the bowel may precipitate encephalopathy. Patients with portal hypertension may bleed from other sites, usually a gastric or duodenal ulcer or haemorrhagic gastritis.

Recognizing the pattern
The haematemesis is usually profuse though often preceded by a small haematemesis ('herald bleed'). There may be a history of similar episodes and also of previous liver disease. The patient may be an alcoholic.

Signs of hypovolaemic shock (tachycardia, hypotension and cold extremities) are common. Stigmata of portal hypertension, liver disease and alcoholism are usually present to a varying degree. Look for the signs of encephalopathy (p. 331).

Proving the diagnosis

The bleeding site must be confirmed by endoscopy as soon as the patient is stabilized. Other emergency investigations include the following.

- Haemoglobin, haematocrit and cross-match.
- Clotting screen.
- Platelet count.
- Urea, electrolytes and calcium.
- Liver function tests and serological assessment of hepatitis A, B and C.

Management

Resuscitation is carried out as on p. 291. A central venous pressure (CVP) line is usually needed. Use fresh blood if possible as this contains more clotting factors and platelets than stored blood. Fresh frozen plasma (FFP) and platelet transfusion may be required. Vitamin K (10 mg i.v) is given. Neomycin (1 g 6-hourly) and lactulose (30–50 mL 8-hourly) are given to decrease the urea-splitting organisms in the bowel and to clear the bowel of blood. This is done to prevent encephalopathy.

Medical treatments to reduce splanchnic blood flow (vaso-pressin analogues or the somatostatin analogue, octreotide) are useful in temporarily arresting haemorrhage so that haemo-dynamic stability can be achieved before endoscopy.

Variceal band ligation or injection sclerotherapy is used to control the bleeding and is effective in the majority of patients. In encephalopathic or unstable patients, this is often safer under general anaesthesia to reduce risks of aspiration. If endoscopic haemostasis is not possible, then oesophageal tamponade using a modified (four-lumen) Sengstaken tube is an effective method of achieving temporary control. This may allow a further attempt at sclerotherapy or banding within the next 12 h.

When sclerotherapy fails (less then 10% of patients) TIPSS should be considered. Heroic operations undertaken by the surgeon unfamiliar with portal hypertension are doomed to failure. Patients should be transferred or assistance obtained from an experienced liver surgeon.

FOUR-LUMEN SENGSTAKEN TUBE (Fig. 8.1.6)

Placement and maintenance of the tube is unpleasant for the

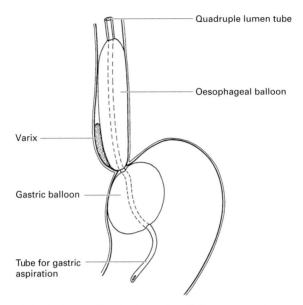

Fig. 8.1.6 The Sengstaken tube: the oesophageal balloon compresses the varices.

patient. The tube is usually inserted at the end of unsuccessful attempts at endoscopic haemostasis. General anaesthesia is again safer in these circumstances. It compresses the varices and fundal veins. The tube is passed into the stomach and the gastric balloon inflated. This balloon is impacted on the lower end of the gastro-oesophageal junction by traction on the tube. The upper oesophageal balloon is then inflated. Regular aspiration of the stomach is carried out through the tube to ensure that bleeding is not continuing. The oesophagus is aspirated to prevent inhalation of nasopharyngeal secretions.

If bleeding is controlled, balloon deflation and the timing of tube removal should be determined by the need for repeat endoscopic therapy.

A Sengstaken tube should not remain in place for more than 24 h. Complications of its use include aspiration, pressure necrosis of the oesophageal and gastric mucosa, rupture of the oesophagus and respiratory obstruction.

Hepatic tumours

These may be benign or malignant.

Benign hepatic tumours
Benign hepatic tumours include the following:
- haemangioma
- focal nodular hyperplasia
- liver cell adenoma.

Benign tumours of the liver are uncommon and frequently asymptomatic, being found incidentally at laparotomy or laparoscopy. The cavernous haemangioma is the most common. It presents in adults most commonly between 30 and 70 years of age and may grow to a very large size. Focal nodular hyperplasia and liver cell adenoma are most commonly found in women of child-bearing age and are associated with the use of the oral contraceptive pill.

Recognizing the pattern and proving the diagnosis
A cavernous haemangioma is usually asymptomatic. Vague abdominal symptoms (pain, nausea, a perception of abdominal swelling) are no more common in these patients than in the general population. The diagnosis is proven by ultrasound, CT scan or MRI. These tumours rarely bleed. Focal nodular hyperplasia tumours are usually small and found incidentally, often during an ultrasound examination for suspected gallstones. The tumours usually have a central scar that is detected by the above imaging. Distinguishing these tumours from malignant hepatoma can, however, be difficult and this may justify excision. Liver cell adenomas are often larger and more likely to present with symptoms. They grow rapidly due to haemorrhage and necrosis within the tumour and first presentation with bleeding into the peritoneal cavity is not rare. The diagnosis is proven as above. Urgent hepatic resection may be required.

Management
The risk of spontaneous haemorrhage from a haemangioma is insignificant. Resection is only required when there is doubt about the nature of the tumour. Patients with focal nodular hyperplasia or liver cell adenoma should be advised to stop the

oral contraceptive pill. Having made the diagnosis, large tumours may require resection and small tumours may be managed conservatively. There is no evidence that these lesions carry any malignant potential.

Malignant hepatic tumours

Malignant hepatic tumours are of the following kinds.

- Primary:
  - primary hepatocellular carcinoma (hepatoma)
  - cholangiocarcinoma
  - fibrolamellar carcinoma
  - epithelioid haemangioendothelioma
  - angiosarcoma.
- Secondary.

The incidence of primary hepatocellular carcinoma shows considerable geographical variation, being common in the Far East and Africa and relatively uncommon in Europe and North America. Its incidence is strongly associated both with chronic hepatitis B infection and with cirrhosis of other aetiologies. It is commoner in males (3 : 1). Other, less significant, aetiological agents include the groundnut fungal toxin (aflatoxin) and the oral contraceptive pill.

Cholangiocarcinoma (primary carcinoma of bile duct) occurs both within the intra- and extrahepatic parts of the biliary system, most commonly occurs after 60 years of age and more frequently in males (2 : 1). It is discussed here and with cancer of the pancreatic head (see p. 342). Within the liver, the most common location is at or close to the main bifurcation into the right and left hepatic ducts (Klatskin tumour). It may develop at an earlier age, particularly in association with sclerosing cholangitis (10%) or as a complication of chronic biliary stasis as a result of choledochal cyst.

The other three primary tumours are all rare but are noteworthy because of the good prognosis in fibrolamellar carcinoma and the associations with anabolic steroids and various organic chemicals leading to the development of angiosarcoma.

The majority of malignant tumours of the liver are secondary to primary tumours in the gastrointestinal tract (stomach, pancreas, colon) or elsewhere.

Proving the diagnosis

The diagnosis of a malignant neoplasm of the liver is usually established by a combination of clinical features (e.g. previous resection for colorectal cancer) and careful imaging. Ultrasound, CT and MRI are complementary. High levels of α-fetoprotein (hepatoma) or carcinoembryonic antigen (follow-up of colorectal cancer patients) may lead to the detection of malignancy in otherwise asymptomatic individuals. Histological confirmation can be obtained by percutaneous CT-guided biopsy but this should never be carried out until it is certain that the patient is not suitable for any type of liver resection.

Management

The aim of hepatic surgery is to achieve a resection with clear pathological margins (R0). Resection may be undertaken in an anatomical fashion according to the segments of the liver, or in a non-anatomical fashion. In hepatoma surgery, the problem is often the size and quality of the liver remnant after resection, bearing in mind that most of these patients have chronic liver disease. For secondary tumours, resection is largely confined to colorectal tumours although highly selected patients with other secondary tumours (kidney, breast) can benefit from hepatic surgery. Hepatic surgery for colorectal secondaries involves a variety of patient groups. Some have synchronous tumours (found at the same time as the primary), some are metachronous (found at follow-up) and some occur after adjuvant therapies. Some cases with unresectable tumours can be rendered resectable by chemotherapy. The precise indications for surgery in these various subgroups is beyond the scope of this book, but the principle that surgery should result in an R0 resection is common to all.

In some cases where a primary liver tumour is small, patients should be considered for hepatic transplantation. Local tumour ablation using radiofrequency current administered percutaneously under ultrasound or CT guidance has also been used as a curative treatment for very small hepatomas, although the technique is usually regarded as a palliative treatment. Relief of pruritus due to obstructive jaundice can be achieved by transhepatic or endoscopic stenting of the biliary system or surgical bypass.

OPERATION: HEPATIC RESECTION
- Left hepatectomy (removal of the anatomical left lobe, Coinaud segments I–IV).
- Right hepatectomy (removal of the anatomical right lobe, Coinaud segments V–VIII).
- Extended right hepatetectomy (removal of the right lobe and medial two segments of the left lobe, Coinaud segments I, II, V–VIII).

The porta hepatis is explored and the appropriate branches of the portal vein, hepatic artery and hepatic duct ligated and divided. The liver parenchyma is then divided, carefully ligating or clipping all vessels that cross the line of section. The appropriate hepatic vein is identified, clamped and oversewn or closed with a stapler. A sealant (derived from thrombin or fibrin) is usually applied to the raw surface to produce perfect haemostasis and minimize bile leaks.

Procedure profile

Blood requirement	2–8
Anaesthetic	GA
Operation time	2–6 hours
Hospital stay	7–14 days
Return to normal activity	2–3 months

Postoperatively the patient requires monitoring in an intensive care or high-dependency setting. The patient should be observed for postoperative haemorrhage, hepatocellular insufficiency, coagulopathy, hypoglycaemia, hypoalbuminaemia and later for signs of bile leak. (Full blood count, coagulation studies and liver function tests should be performed daily until stable.)

Hepatic transplantation

Indications for liver transplantation include the following:
- chronic liver disease

- acute liver failure
- metabolic defects
- liver tumours.

Chronic liver disease

The common causes of chronic liver disease leading to transplantation are:

- primary biliary cirrhosis
- posthepatic cirrhosis (chronic active) hepatitis
- autoimmune chronic active hepatitis
- sclerosing cholangitis
- cryptogenic cirrhosis
- alcoholic cirrhosis (carefully selected cases).

Liver transplantation should be considered in patients who develop life-threatening complications, particularly gastro-oesophageal variceal haemorrhage, encephalopathy, spontaneous bacterial peritonitis or intractable ascites and malnutrition. In some patients without such complications, symptoms of fatigue and itching may be sufficiently severe to warrant transplantation.

Acute liver failure

Patients suffering from fulminant hepatic failure (liver failure within 8 weeks of the onset of symptoms) or subacute hepatic failure (liver failure between 8 and 26 weeks of the onset of symptoms) may require urgent liver transplantation. The most common aetiological agents are viral hepatitis (hepatitis B, non-A, non-B), drug reactions and toxins.

Metabolic diseases

A number of life-threatening metabolic diseases are characterized by the deficiency of a hepatic enzyme. Examples of this include α_1-antitrypsin deficiency, primary hyperoxaluria and Wilson's disease. Successful replacement of the diseased liver results in permanent cure of the condition.

Liver tumours

Patients with primary liver tumours may be suitable candidates for liver transplantation.

Management

Preoperatively the extent of liver disease is assessed by liver function tests, coagulation screen, and the presence or absence of complications of liver disease. The size of the portal vein can be assessed by Doppler ultrasound. The patients undergo a microbiological screen, including looking for cytomegalovirus. Blood grouping and antibody studies are undertaken. A full general medical and anaesthetic assessment is also carried out.

OPERATION: HEPATIC TRANSPLANTATION

The majority of liver transplants involve brain-dead, heart-beating donors. The excised liver must be matched to the size of the recipient. An adult liver can be split for two recipients (e.g. a child and an adult smaller than the donor). Recently, living related transplantation has been undertaken that involves transplantation of the left hemiliver into an adult or segments II and III into a child. In these circumstances, management of the donor is as described above for liver resections. In cadaveric transplantation, the liver is fully mobilized until it is attached only by its vascular connections (inferior vena cava (IVC), portal vein and hepatic artery). Cannulae are placed in the aorta and portal vein and, when the circulation stops (when the heart is excised for transplantation), in situ cooling is carried out. The liver, perfused and stored in suitable preservation solution, can remain ischaemic, at ice temperature, for up to 24 h.

The recipient often has the following complications:
- portal hypertension
- coagulopathy
- adhesions due to previous upper abdominal surgery.

The liver is mobilized with careful attention to haemostasis. The bile duct is divided, the blood vessels clamped and the liver excised. The donor liver is then transplanted, anastomosing the suprahepatic IVC, infrahepatic IVC, portal vein, hepatic artery and bile duct. Some patients tolerate clamping of the IVC and portal vein poorly and require bypass from the infrahepatic IVC and portal vein, back to the right side of the heart.

Procedure profile

Blood requirement	12
Anaesthetic	GA
Operation time	5–6 hours
Hospital stay	2–3 weeks
Return to normal activity	3 months

Postoperatively most liver transplant recipients require a period of ventilation and intensive monitoring of cardiopulmonary, renal and liver function. Immunosuppressive medication is started at the time of operation. Particular problems include bleeding, graft infarction, infection, rejection and biliary complications.

8.2 Pancreas and spleen

For benign tumours of the pancreas, see section 4.3.

Carcinoma of the pancreas

Carcinoma of the pancreas is an adenocarcinoma arising from the ductal epithelium. For the majority of patients, it carries a dismal prognosis with less than 5% of patients alive after 5 years. Histologically it is usually solid and fibrous (scirrhous) or rarely a cystadenocarcinoma. The incidence is increasing in the UK and the USA. Two-thirds of pancreatic carcinomas occur in the head of the gland and these tend to compress the CBD, causing jaundice. A subset of tumours (often referred to as 'peri-ampullary') cluster at or close to the ampulla of Vater. Those arising from the ampulla itself tend to present with jaundice at an earlier stage than those arising from pancreatic ductal epithelium which subsequently invade the ampulla. In addition, there are carcinomas arising from the duodenal wall or terminal bile duct. Ampullary cancers have the best prognosis and ductal adenocarcinomas of the pancreas the worst. A carcinoma in the body and tail may remain undetected until it is quite large. Ductal adenocarcinomas invade locally (frequently involving the superior mesenteric vein and artery) and exhibit perineural spread that is difficult to identify beyond the pancreas. Lymph node involvement is common and further spread occurs to liver, lungs and the peritoneal cavity.

Recognizing the pattern

The patient with this disease is typically middle aged or elderly (aged 50–70 years).

The presentation is often non-specific with a gradual onset of ill health and weight loss. If pain is present, it is usually dull and situated deep in the epigastrium. It radiates through to the back. The pain is characteristically relieved by sitting forwards. The disease is sometimes associated with episodes of spontaneous venous thrombosis, 'thrombophlebitis migrans'.

The patient with a carcinoma of the head of the pancreas may be jaundiced and show signs of weight loss. In the presence of jaundice the gall bladder may be palpable as a smooth, rounded mass below the liver. Courvoisier's dictum states that if the gall bladder is palpable in a case of obstructive jaundice then the cause is unlikely to be stones in the bile duct. (A gall bladder containing stones is usually fibrotic and shrunken.)

Carcinomas of the body or tail of the pancreas present late and by then a mass is often palpable in the epigastrium or left upper quadrant.

Proving the diagnosis

This may be difficult in those patients harbouring small tumours (< 2 cm in diameter). Ultrasound or CT will usually show a mass in the pancreas, the extent of biliary dilatation and whether there is any evidence of liver metastases. Multislice CT provides detailed imaging of the primary tumour and likely extent of spread and a tissue diagnosis is not considered necessary in most patients prior to undertaking resection. As with liver tumours, percutaneous biopsy should only be performed when the patient is not suitable for resection. Cytology of pancreatic secretions, brushings or biopsy during ERCP may confirm the diagnosis.

An ampullary carcinoma can be visualized directly and a biopsy taken. Endoscopic and laparoscopic ultrasound are useful in assessing resectability and the former can also be used to obtain a tissue diagnosis if required. Liver function tests may confirm the obstructive nature of the jaundice (see Table 8.1.1). Faecal occult blood tests may be positive if the duodenum is involved.

Management

Patients with unresectable or metastatic tumours and satisfactory performance status should be offered palliative chemotherapy (a combination of gemcitabine and capecitabine is currently considered the most effective treatment). In this incurable group, those with symptomatic jaundice should be considered for endoscopic biliary stenting or bypass surgery. Palliative gastric and biliary bypasses are also treatment options in young patients with unresectable tumours.

Periampullary tumours that are thought to be localized or resectable on diagnostic imaging in fit patients should be managed by a laparotomy and a traditional Kausch–Whipple resection or its modification, pylorus-preserving pancreatico-duodenectomy. Temporary relief of jaundice prior to planned resection might improve the patient's sense of well-being, but there is no evidence that it is beneficial in reducing complications or enhancing prospects of survival. At operation a bypass procedure can be performed if the tumour is not resectable. There is evidence that adjuvant chemotherapy using 5-FU and gemcitabine improves survival after resection.

Endocrine tumours of the pancreas (especially insulinoma) may be amenable to enucleation. Very few ductal adenocarcinomas arising from the body or tail of the gland are amenable to surgery, but patients with cystic tumours may benefit from distal pancreatic resection even when the tumour is large.

Prophylactic antibiotics are used with all pancreatic operations. The patient's clotting factors should be checked and vitamin K1 given if the patient is jaundiced. Adequate hydration of the patient is vital prior to any intervention. If concomitant splenectomy is a possibility, the instructions given below in relation to splenic surgery should be followed.

OPERATION: DISTAL PANCREATECTOMY (Fig. 8.2.1)
This can be performed with or without spleen preservation. The cut end of the pancreas is closed including careful ligation of the pancreatic duct. This operation can be performed laparoscopically.

Procedure profile

Blood requirement	4
Anaesthetic	GA
Operation time	2–3 hours
Hospital stay	5 days (laparoscopic)–2 weeks (open)
Return to normal activity	1–2 months

OPERATION: KAUSCH–WHIPPLE OPERATION
(Fig. 8.2.1)
In this operation the neck of the pancreas is transected as it runs over the portal vein. The head of the pancreas is removed together with the distal part of the stomach, pylorus and complete duodenal loop along with a short section of jejunum. The CBD is also divided. The gall bladder is removed. A modern variation is to retain the antrum and the first few centimetres of duodenum.

There are many ways of reconstructing the gastrointestinal tract. Some surgeons routinely include a feeding jejunostomy. There are wide variations in the use of transanastomotic stents and intra-abdominal drains.

Procedure profile

Blood requirement	4–6
Anaesthetic	GA
Operation time	3–5 hours
Hospital stay	2–3 weeks
Return to normal activity	3 months

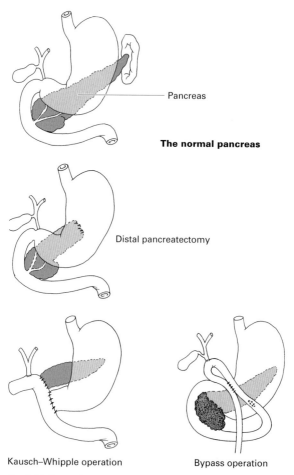

The normal pancreas

Distal pancreatectomy

Kausch–Whipple operation

Bypass operation

Fig. 8.2.1 Pancreatic operations.

Individual surgeons vary widely in their postoperative management of this complex procedure. The most feared complication of this type of surgery is leakage from the anastomosis between the pancreas and the GI tract. Subclinical leaks manifest by high levels of amylase in an intra-abdominal drain are common. Conversely, the absence of drainage is no indicator that a leak has not occurred. A high index of clinical suspicion in patients with unexplained deterioration in their clinical condition should prompt further investigation (CT scan) and possibly revisional surgery.

OPERATION: BYPASS OPERATION FOR CARCINOMA OF PANCREAS (Fig. 8.2.1)

This can be done in two ways, both of which involve three anastomoses. In the first a loop of jejunum is anastomosed to the bile duct to relieve biliary obstruction. The stomach is anastomosed to the side of this loop forming a gastrojejunostomy relieving potential duodenal obstruction. Finally, an anastomosis is made between the two sides of the jejunal loop in order that food may bypass the loop going to the CBD. The alternative is to use the Roux-en-Y technique where the jejunum is divided and the distal end joined to the bile duct. A second anastomosis between the stomach and this loop is created followed by a downstream enteroenterostomy.

Procedure profile

Blood requirement	2
Anaesthetic	GA
Operation time	90 minutes
Hospital stay	7–10 days
Return to normal activity	May be indefinite

Pancreatitis

Pancreatitis is inflammation of the pancreas and may be acute, relapsing or chronic.

Acute pancreatitis

Acute pancreatitis reflects acute inflammation of the pancreas from a variety of causes. It carries a mortality of around 5% in the

UK. Irrespective of aetiology, pancreatic enzyme precursors are prematurely activated within the gland rather than in the lumen of the GI tract. The activated enzymes damage the pancreas, setting up a local inflammatory cascade. In the mildest cases this process is largely contained in and around the gland, but the inflammatory process may progress from oedematous through haemorrhagic to necrotizing pancreatitis with an associated increasingly severe systemic response.

Resolution may occur at any stage without progression to the next. The development of multisystem organ failure consequent upon a systemic inflammatory response syndrome (SIRS) accounts for about half of all deaths from acute pancreatitis. Pseudocyst formation and the development of infection in relation to necrosis usually occur in the second to third week. Pseudocyst formation probably occurs as the residual pancreas recovers. Secretions and transudate accumulate in a damaged pancreatic bed and in the lesser sac creating an amylase-rich encysted collection. Necrosis of the pancreas may lead to secondary infection of the pancreatic bed (infected pancreatic necrosis) and this condition accounts for most of the late fatalities.

Recognized causes of pancreatic damage include:
- biliary disease (55–60% of cases in England)
- idiopathic (35–40%)
- alcoholic (1–5%)
- trauma
- crush injury
- abdominal surgery
- carcinoma of the pancreas
- mumps
- hypothermia
- drugs, e.g. steroids/thiazides
- polyarteritis nodosa
- hyperparathyroidism
- hyperlipidaemia.

Recognizing the pattern

The disease is more common in the middle aged and elderly. In the UK it is usually seen in the type of patient who suffers from gallstones (see p. 318).

The patient presents with a sudden onset of upper abdominal pain, which gradually becomes very severe. It tends to radiate through to the back and is usually associated with vomiting. In patients with a severe attack, there may be signs of organ failure over the next 24 h.

On examination there is generalized abdominal tenderness, maximal in the upper abdomen. The patient also shows signs of dehydration and shock and is generally toxic with a low-grade fever reflecting systemic inflammation. They may also be slightly jaundiced due to obstruction of the CBD by oedema or by the stone causing the pancreatitis. Late examination may disclose bruising in the subcutaneous tissue of the flanks (Grey Turner's sign) or even around the umbilicus (Cullen's sign). These signs are due to bleeding from a severe haemorrhagic pancreatitis.

Both the history and signs are rather non-specific and the differential diagnosis includes perforated peptic ulcer (although these patients rarely vomit), mesenteric infarction, intestinal obstruction and myocardial infarction.

Proving the diagnosis

The diagnosis is proved by measuring the serum amylase (normal range 80–150 international units). If this is above 1000 units in the context of an appropriate clinical picture, acute pancreatitis is extremely likely. Other causes for a moderately raised amylase include a perforated duodenal ulcer, myocardial infarction and acute cholecystitis. The severity of the condition is not related to the amylase level. Prediction of the severity of an attack is important as this will identify those patients who require potential intensive care support.

A number of scoring systems have been used to predict severity (Imrie, Ransom, APACHE II).

Apart from the amylase, other baseline investigations should include the following.

- Urea and electrolytes.
- Haemoglobin and white cell count.
- Liver function tests, calcium, and glucose.
- A chest X-ray and an abdominal X-ray. These help to exclude a perforated ulcer or intestinal obstruction.
- Abdominal ultrasound scan to look for gallstones.

- Electrocardiogram (ECG).
- Blood gases.

  After admission the daily progress of the disease is assessed by daily measurement of the following:
- urea and electrolytes
- white cell count
- calcium
- C-reactive protein (high levels after 48 h indicate a high likelihood of necrosis).

  These detect any developing renal failure, hyperglycaemia (transient diabetes) or hypocalcaemia, which can then be treated accordingly.

  An abdominal CT scan should be performed in patients with a severe biochemical attack within the first week. This is the most accurate way to delineate necrosis and correctly identify the patients at risk of developing later infection.

Management

This condition is usually managed conservatively, though patients with a severe biochemical or clinical attack may need high-dependency or intensive care. There are specific indications for intervention.

MEDICAL TREATMENT

- Analgesia. The pain is often severe. The patient should be written up for pethidine (50–100 mg i.m. 4-hourly). Pain compromises respiratory performance, but so do narcotic analgesics. Epidural anaesthesia should be considered to overcome this.
- Blood and fluid replacement. The oedematous process is associated with a huge loss of fluid into the retroperitoneal tissues, accompanied by a loss of protein and blood if the pancreatitis is severe. This results in oligaemia, which aggravates the tendency to renal failure. It is essential therefore to give the patient adequate fluid replacement early on. This should be sufficient to maintain a good urinary output. In the first 24 h this is mainly fluid and electrolyte replacement. In a severe case of pancreatitis, a CVP line should be set up and a urinary catheter inserted to monitor the adequacy of fluid replacement.

- Nutritional support. Former views about 'resting the pancreas' have proved to be incorrect. Most patients do have a degree of ileus or delayed gastric emptying due to swelling around the duodenum. Fine-bore feeding (nasojejunal) can nearly always be accomplished and it is surprising how many patients still tolerate this when the distal end of the tube is still in the stomach.
- Antibiotics. The use of antibiotics in acute pancreatitis is controversial. Some physicians believe it may delay or prevent the onset of late pancreatic sepsis but a systematic review of the evidence indicated that this strategy does not work.
- In severe gallstone pancreatitis, early ERCP and sphincterotomy and removal of CBD stones should be undertaken.

SURGICAL TREATMENT
- In patients with gallstone pancreatitis, consideration should be given to removing the gall bladder to prevent further attacks. Laparoscopic cholecystectomy during the index admission when the patient has recovered from the initial attack of pancreatitis is recommended.
- Late in the disease there may be a need to operate and remove necrotic and infected pancreatic tissue, or to drain a pancreatic pseudocyst or abscess.

Management of complications
- Renal failure occurs as a complication of the early stage of acute pancreatitis. Treatment is by peritoneal dialysis or in severe cases by haemodialysis.
- Diabetes. A transient episode of hyperglycaemia is not uncommon in severe pancreatitis and insulin therapy may be needed. However, the diabetes usually recovers later.
- Hypocalcaemia. 10% calcium gluconate (10 mL) may be required once or twice a day.
- Pseudocyst formation – see below.
- Duodenal ileus. This is a rare complication. Although the patient's general health improves, they continue to show signs of duodenal obstruction with vomiting. The condition is due to persistent inflammation on the inner aspect of the duodenal loop.
- Haematemesis and melaena. This is usually due to concurrent peptic ulceration.

After recovery from the acute attack, identification and treatment of any other underlying cause must be carried out so as to prevent recurrence (e.g. parathyroidectomy for hypercalcaemia or treatment of alcoholism).

Pancreatic pseudocyst
Recognizing the pattern
The patient continues to have a persistent fever and the white count either remains elevated or begins to climb again. The abdomen should be examined regularly and a mass may become palpable in the epigastrium.

Proving the diagnosis
An ultrasound or CT scan proves the diagnosis. The latter gives more precise information about the anatomical relationships of the cyst and may be used to guide intervention.

Management
Many radiological 'pseudocysts' are confused with acute fluid collections around the pancreas that settle spontaneously and so a policy of patient observation should be adopted. Indications for operation are failure to resolve after 2–3 weeks, the presence of unremitting pain or obstructive symptoms due to compression of adjacent structures by the pseudocyst. Symptomatic fluid collections less than 6 cm in diameter can be aspirated with a reasonable chance that it will not recur, but repeated aspiration should be avoided as this increases the risk of introducing infection into the pseudocyst. Large symptomatic pseudocysts require drainage and this can nearly always be accomplished endoscopically through the back wall of the stomach. Preparation of the patient is the same as for an ERCP and one or more stents are placed between the stomach and the pseudocyst cavity to create an internal fistula.

OPERATION: LAPAROSCOPIC DRAINAGE OF A PSEUDOCYST
The pseudocyst is drained either by a transgastric approach or into a loop of small bowel depending on the anatomical location

of the pseudocyst. The anterior wall of the stomach is opened.
The posterior wall of the stomach is then incised and the pseudocyst, which is adherent to it, is drained into the stomach. A tube
drain is then placed in the pseudocyst and brought out across the
lumen of the stomach through the anterior abdominal wall and
skin to the exterior.

Procedure profile

Blood requirement	Group and save
Anaesthetic	GA
Operation time	1–2 hours
Hospital stay	2–7 days
Return to normal activity	Variable

Postoperatively oral fluids can be introduced once any ileus
recovers. The transgastric tube is left in place until there is evidence that the cavity has shrunk down (usually about 2 weeks).
The size of the cavity can be seen by injecting contrast down the
drain and taking X-rays. Once the tube has been removed, the
exit site at the abdominal wall heals rapidly.

OPERATION: PANCREATIC NECROSECTOMY

The removal of infected pancreatic necrosis is best undertaken
when there is evidence of positive microbiology in the tissues in
and around the area of necrosis (done by image-guided aspiration), but before the patient has signs of generalized sepsis. This
is usually not before the second week after the onset of an attack
of pancreatitis. This infected necrotic slough can be removed
endoscopically by passing a dilating cannula over a radiologically
inserted drain in the left flank. A laparoscope is inserted together
with secondary instruments through other ports. The necrotic
tissue can then be aspirated under vision avoiding damage to the
splenic vessels. This approach usually requires multiple repeat
procedures to remove all contaminated material, but it may still
be less morbid than an open transperitoneal operation.

Procedure profile

Blood requirement	2–4
Anaesthetic	GA
Operation time	2–4 hours
Hospital stay	10 days (can be months)
Return to normal activity	Variable

Chronic pancreatitis

In chronic pancreatitis there is gradual destruction and fibrosis of the gland. The pancreatic duct is distorted with strictures and dilated segments. Calculi or diffuse pancreatic calcification may occur. This condition is associated with diabetes and malabsorption due to the failure of endocrine and exocrine function.

Recognizing the pattern

The patient is in poor health and may have chronic pain. Relapsing chronic pancreatitis is characterized by episodes of epigastric pain and vomiting with associated weakness. Obstructive jaundice may develop. Steatorrhoea, weight loss and diabetes indicate severe disease with failure of pancreatic function. A history of chronic alcohol abuse is nearly always present.

Proving the diagnosis

A plain abdominal X-ray may show calcification. Stool analysis may show frank steatorrhoea (more than 6 g of fat lost per day). There is an elevated level of faecal elastase. Pancreatic function can be measured by performing a glucose tolerance test and analysing pancreatic secretions (including bicarbonate and enzymes) but these tests are only rarely used. Excellent images of the pancreatic and biliary ductal systems can be obtained by magnetic resonance scans (MRCP).

Management

Functional failure is treated medically with a high-protein, high-calorie diet, exogenous enzyme preparations and vitamin replacement. Insulin may be needed.

A variety of interventions have been used in the treatment of chronic pancreatitis. The two main indications for intervention are pain (poor control even with opiates) or jaundice. Bleeding related to the formation of small inflammatory aneurysms on the splenic artery is a rare but nevertheless dramatic reason for intervention. Both endoscopic and surgical procedures are designed to overcome ductal obstruction. As chronic pancreatitis seems to be most severe in the head of the gland, endoscopic stenting of the pancreatic and/or bile ducts is increasingly being used as definitive therapy or as a way of identifying the group of patients that might respond best to surgery.

Operations tend to be of two sorts. A drainage procedure (longitudinal panreaticojejunostomy) is favoured when preservation of functional pancreatic tissue is worthwhile. Resections involving the head of the gland can be undertaken with or without duodenal resection. In some cases of unremitting pain, thoracoscopic splanchnic nerve resection may be performed.

Surgical conditions of the spleen

The spleen is situated in the left upper quadrant of the abdomen protected by the rib cage. It receives blood from the splenic artery, which is a branch of the coeliac plexus. It also receives some blood from the short gastric and left gastroepiploic arteries. Blood returns to the portal system via the splenic vein. The spleen has important immunological functions, clearing antigens from the circulation and producing immunoglobulin M (IgM) and various factors that are important in the phagocytosis of encapsulated bacteria. It is the major site for red cell and platelet destruction. It also produces lymphocytes and plays a role in red cell maturation.

The spleen can become enlarged as a result of a response to infection, connective tissue disorders, myelo- or lymphoproliferative disorders, infiltration by neoplastic cells from other sites and in various types of anaemia.

The indications for splenectomy include the following.
- Hypersplenism.
- Myeloproliferative disorders, e.g. myelofibrosis, chronic myeloid leukaemia.

- Haemolytic anaemia: spherocytosis, elliptocytosis, pyruvate kinase deficiency, thalassaemia, immune haemolytic anaemia.
- Platelet disorders: thrombocytopenic purpura.
- Trauma (see p. 636).
- Neoplasia involving the spleen, e.g. primary splenic lymphoma.

Management

Splenectomy for normal-sized or moderately enlarged spleens is usually undertaken laparoscopically. Spleens weighing over 1 kg are best dealt with by open surgery.

Preoperatively the patient should be vaccinated against pneumococci, haemophilus, influenza B, and meningococcal group C 2 weeks before an elective splenectomy. He or she should also be given pre- and postoperative penicillin (or erythromycin if allergic to penicillin).

OPERATION: OPEN SPLENECTOMY

A left subcostal or paramedian incision is performed. The short gastric vessels are divided. The peritoneum lateral to and above the spleen is opened and the spleen and tail of pancreas mobilized to the midline. The splenic flexure of the colon is freed, the splenic vessels divided between the pancreas and the spleen, and the spleen removed. Any splenunculi should also be removed.

Procedure profile

Blood requirement	2
Anaesthetic	GA
Operation time	60–90 minutes
Hospital stay	7–10 days
Return to normal activity	4 weeks

OPERATION: LAPAROSCOPIC SPLENECTOMY
(Fig. 8.2.2)

The splenic vessels are usually approached through the lesser sac after dissecting the short gastric vessels. The artery and vein are

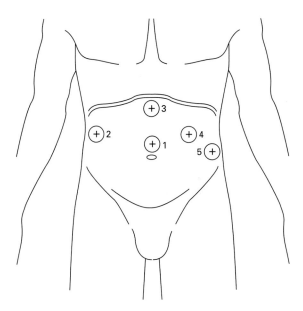

Fig. 8.2.2 Possible port sites for laparoscopic splenectomy.

ligated and the rest of the splenic pedicle divided with a linear stapler. The spleen is placed in a bag. It can either be broken up or removed intact through a short incision anywhere in the abdominal wall (e.g. suprapubically for good cosmesis).

Procedure profile

Blood requirement	Group and save
Anaesthetic	GA
Operation time	2–3 hours
Hospital stay	3–5 days
Return to normal activity	2–3 weeks

Following splenectomy a number of complications can arise.

- Acute dilatation of the stomach (see p. 42). The risk can be minimized by adequate aspiration of the stomach until the gastric ileus has fully recovered.
- Left basal pulmonary collapse and pneumonia. Movements of the left base are diminished and it is important to give adequate analgesia and physiotherapy to protect against this complication.
- Subphrenic abscess. This may follow infection of a haematoma or damage to one of the organs in the neighbourhood of the spleen (see above).
- Thrombotic complications. When the spleen is removed the platelet level rises and if the platelet count goes over 1000×10^9/L there is a risk of thrombotic complications. Aspirin should be given (75 mg daily or 150 mg on alternate days) to decrease platelet stickiness until the platelet count falls to less than 1000×10^9/L.

9 Colorectal surgery and perianal pain

9.1 Colorectal surgery

Inflammatory bowel disease

Crohn's disease (CD) and ulcerative colitis (UC) are the major inflammatory bowel diseases. They are chronic inflammatory disorders of the GI tract of uncertain aetiology. Crohn's can affect any part of the gut from mouth to anus with relative rectal sparing. UC is limited to the large bowel starting in the rectum and extending proximally to a variable degree. Other differences are highlighted in Table 9.1.1.

Both conditions normally have a relapsing and remitting character. UC has an association with a wide variety of extra-GI manifestations. There is also a risk of malignant transformation in patients with long-standing colitis of either aetiology – about 20% after 30 years from diagnosis in UC.

Table 9.1.1 Crohn's disease and ulcerative colitis compared.

	Ulcerative colitis	Crohn's disease
Incidence (UK)	5 per 100 000	5 per 100 000
Peak age of onset	20–39	18–22
Sex distribution	Male = female	1 male : 1.5 female
Geographical distribution	Mostly Anglo-Saxon and European	Mostly Anglo-Saxon and European
Associated factors	HLA-B27	Smoking
Pattern of bowel involvement	Contiguous from rectum proximally	Skip lesions, rectal sparing

Surgery: Diagnosis and Management, 4th edition. Edited by N. Rawlinson and D. Alderson. © 2009 Blackwell Publishing, ISBN: 978-1-4051-2921-3

Recognizing the pattern

COLITIS

Colitis of either aetiology presents as bloody stool of increased frequency. The consistency of stool often depends on the extent of the disease with more extensive involvement often leading to an increased looseness of stool. Exclusively colonic Crohn's occurs in about 25% of CD patients.

During acute attacks the patient may become dehydrated, hypokalaemic (from diarrhoea) and anaemic (from GI blood loss). They may also complain of abdominal pain. Abdominal examination is often unremarkable apart from mild tenderness. Significant tympanitic distension or any evidence of peritonism are of great concern and need urgent attention.

SMALL BOWEL CROHN'S

This is the most common site of CD, affecting more than 80% of sufferers. It is often characterized by acute exacerbations on a chronic background. There tend to be two pathologically distinct patterns of disease which occasionally occur together in the same patient.

- Fibrostenosing disease presents with increasingly frequent attacks of intermittent small bowel obstruction sometimes presenting as an emergency. Always consider CD in young patients with small bowel obstruction and a virgin abdomen.
- Inflammatory/fistulating disease is more likely to be associated with constitutional symptoms such as fever and weight loss during attacks. These attacks can mimic acute appendicitis as the commonest site of disease is ileal or ileocaecal (80%). It may also present with fistulae to the skin, bladder or vagina or to another part of gut causing profuse diarrhoea.

PERIANAL DISEASE

This occurs at some stage in about one-third of patients with CD. Consider CD in patients with multiple or atypical abscesses or fissures. These abscesses are often associated with underlying fistulae which are often complex. If present it is usually associated with CD elsewhere in the GI tract, especially ileocaecal disease.

Proving the diagnosis
- Blood tests often show a chronic or acute-on-chronic inflammatory response. Look for:
  - raised CRP, ESR, WCC
  - low Hb, albumin.
- Radiology/imaging.
  - Colitis: barium enema may show 'drainpipe' colon in chronic cases with loss of haustrations and normal mucosal features.
  - Small bowel CD: small bowel enema is the investigation of choice for ileal disease. Look for strictures ('string sign'), fistulae or ulceration which can lead to the 'cobblestone' effect.
  - Perianal CD: MRI helps define the fistulae that accompany Crohn's perianal abscesses.
- Gentle flexible sigmoidoscopy will also show acute inflammation and allows biopsies to be taken for histology but care is required as the risk of perforation is high in acute disease. Look for demarcation between normal and inflamed bowel to determine the extent of disease in UC. The rectum can often look relatively normal in Crohn's colitis – known as rectal sparing.
- Histology.
  - UC: contiguous disease limited to the colon. Biopsies show an acute-on-chronic inflammatory reaction mostly confined to the mucosa. Always look for reports of dysplasia as these will require closer surveillance or colectomy even in quiescent disease.
  - CD: unlike UC the inflammation is not contiguous but can involve 'skip lesions' where areas of inflammation are separated by uninvolved bowel. Macroscopically at operation fat-wrapping and oedematous thickened mesentery and bowel are characteristic of CD. Microscopically the diagnosis depends on a combination of features. Non-caseating granulomas are found in about 60% of patients and although suggestive of CD when found they are not pathognomonic. Focality of chronic transmural inflammation is the key to diagnosis. Differentiating Crohn's and ulcerative colitis can be difficult.
- Microbiology. Exclude infective causes of diarrhoea by taking stool samples for microscopy, culture and sensitivity (MC&S).

Management

Both conditions are managed jointly by physicians and surgeons. The major difference is that in UC surgery is curative, whereas in CD it should be used to treat symptomatic complications and as such a minimalist approach should be adopted.

ACUTE COLITIS

- Acute colitis should be treated by high-dose i.v. and topical steroids (administered per rectum). Failure to improve within 5 days of treatment (see Table 9.1.2) or deterioration within that period indicates that surgery is required. Frequent clinical evaluation including stool charts as well as daily blood and radiological assessment are vital to prevent progression to toxic megacolon which is liable to perforate. Remember that significant pain may indicate perforation.
- Intravenous cyclosporin has been shown to reduce the colectomy rate in patients not responding to steroids although there is a high relapse rate once the cyclosporin is stopped.
- Oral 5-ASA compounds provide no advantage in acute colitis.
- Broad-spectrum antibiotics can be used in those showing signs of septic complications.
- Anticoagulation is essential in UC given the increased risk of DVT in these patients. Avoid anti-diarrhoeal drugs (e.g. loperamide, codeine), opioids and if possible NSAIDs, all of which increase the risk of perforation.

In quiescent and chronic active colitis oral and rectal 5-ASA compounds are the mainstay of maintaining remission. Azathioprine is helpful in those with frequent relapses and in steroid-dependent patients. Those with distal colitis also benefit from budesonide or beclomethasone enemas as a form of 'weak' steroid.

Table 9.1.2 Features of severe acute colitis.

Stool frequency > 6 per day
Temperature > 38°C
Pulse > 90
Abdominal tenderness +/– distension

Remember to ensure patients that who have had colitis for more than 8 years have annual colonoscopic surveillance booked.

SMALL BOWEL CD

Oral steroids (including budesonide), 5-ASA compounds and immunosuppressants are all used to control symptoms but their role in preventing recurrence following surgical resection is questionable. 50% of patients have a clinical relapse within 5 years of their first resection and 50% have had a secondd operation by 10 years. Stopping smoking, high-dose mesalazine and azathioprine seem the best options to prevent postresection recurrence. Infliximab is useful in patients with refractory active CD to produce remission or to enable steroid dose reduction, and also in healing refractory fistulae.

SURGICAL MANAGEMENT OF ULCERATIVE COLITIS

The indications for surgery are the development of complications (e.g. perforation, haemorrhage, cancer) and the failure of medical treatment. Patients presenting with severe acute colitis for their first attack are the most likely to require colectomy (up to 25%).

Emergency surgery for severe acute colitis involves total colectomy and end ileostomy as a life-saving procedure. In the elective situation there are three surgical options:

- panproctocolectomy and end ileostomy
- total colectomy and ileorectal anastamosis
- panproctocolectomy and ileal pouch–anal anastamosis.

The choice of operation depends on patient fitness, sphincter function and a patient's wishes. All three elective procedures are now carried out with laparoscopic assistance in some centres.

In the emergency situation patients must be adequately hydrated before operation with a good urine output. A haemoglobin level of > 9 g/dL is usually acceptable in an otherwise fit patient without prior transfusion. Renal and hepatic function should be checked and significant electrolyte or clotting abnormalities corrected. In the elective situation more attention is directed at choosing the best time for surgery when nutritional status is optimized and the steroid dose is as low as possible.

OPERATION: EMERGENCY TOTAL COLECTOMY,
ILEOSTOMY WITH PRESERVATION OF THE RECTUM
The whole colon is removed from the caecum to the sacral pro-
montory. A terminal ileostomy is brought out in the right iliac
fossa. The rectum can either be closed and left inside the abdomen,
or brought out at the lower end of the wound, and then either left
open (as a mucous fistula) or closed just beneath the skin.

Procedure profile

Blood requirement	2 (more if significant anaemia)
Anaesthetic	GA
Operation time	2 hours
Hospital stay	10–14 days
Return to normal activity	6 weeks

Postoperatively the new ileostomy may take time to adapt and
high volumes of ileostomy effluent may cause dehydration and
electrolyte imbalance. Enteral nutrition can start straight away
and may be supplemented by a period of nasojejunal feeding.
Beware of a rectal stump leak causing peritonitis if there is no
mucous fistula.

Plans for a completion proctectomy or a restorative proctocolectomy with an ileal pouch can be discussed when the patient
has recovered from surgery.

OPERATION: PANPROCTOCOLECTOMY AND
TERMINAL ILEOSTOMY
Preoperative bowel preparation includes clear fluids for 2 days
plus two enemas.

The whole colon is removed from the caecum to the anus
using two incisions, one abdominal and the other perineal. The
terminal ileostomy is brought out at the right iliac fossa. The anal
canal is removed in the intersphincteric plane (compare this with
the abdominoperineal resection for cancer) to make as small a
perineal wound as possible. The empty pelvis is drained with
suction drains via the abdominal wall +/– the perineum.

Procedure profile

Blood requirement	2
Anaesthetic	GA
Operation time	3 hours
Hospital stay	10–14 days
Return to normal activity	6 weeks

Postoperative care is the same as for an abdominoperineal resection of the rectum and is described on p. 382.

OPERATION: TOTAL COLECTOMY AND ILEORECTAL ANASTOMOSIS

Preoperative bowel preparation includes clear fluids for 2 days plus two enemas.

This operation is as for the emergency total colectomy except the ileum is not brought out as a stoma but is anastomosed to the rectum by either a peranal stapling device or a hand-sewn anastomosis.

Procedure profile

Blood requirement	2
Anaesthetic	GA
Operation time	2.5 hours
Hospital stay	10 days
Return to normal activity	6 weeks

Early enteral feeding is now the norm after surgery. Temporary or permanent antidiarrhoeal drugs may be needed postoperatively. Be careful to avoid electrolyte imbalance and dehydration from diarrhoea. Remember the patient still has a rectum and therefore needs cancer surveillance postoperatively.

OPERATION: RESTORATIVE PROCTOCOLECTOMY

Bowel preparation includes clear fluids for 24 h +/− enema for rectum.

This is often done as a second-stage procedure after a previous total colectomy. The residual rectum is removed, the ileostomy taken down and fashioned into an ileal reservoir called a pouch. It is usually anastomosed to the top of the anal canal using a stapling device and the operation is covered with a temporary loop ileostomy. Male patients must be warned about potential injury to the nerves controlling erectile function.

Procedure profile

Blood requirement	2
Anaesthetic	GA
Operation time	2–3 hours
Hospital stay	10 days
Return to normal activity	6 weeks

Postoperative care is as for total colectomy and ileostomy. There is less concern about nutrition since it is an elective procedure and the patient would be well nourished before attempting this operation.

OPERATION: CLOSURE OF LOOP ILEOSTOMY

Bowel preparation includes clear fluids for 24 h.

This is usually a third-stage procedure after restorative proctocolectomy. After checking with a pouchogram that the pouch has healed and that there is no stenosis of the pouch–anal anastomosis, the loop ileostomy is mobilized around its site in the right iliac fossa, reanastomosed and the abdomen closed. There is rarely a need to open the midline abdominal wound.

Procedure profile

Blood requirement	Group and save
Anaesthetic	GA
Operation time	1 hour
Hospital stay	4–7 days
Return to normal activity	3 weeks

SURGICAL MANAGEMENT OF CROHN'S DISEASE

The management of Crohn's colitis is as for UC except the formation of ileal pouches in such patients is considered a contraindication by most surgeons.

Occasionally small bowel disease requires emergency surgery for obstruction, perforation or haemorrhage. Bowel preservation is important given that most patients require more than one operation. Operations are either small bowel resections and anastomosis or stricturoplasty. For CD found incidentally, for example ileocaecal Crohn's presenting as possible appendicitis, the management is debatable and depends upon the severity of the disease, the fitness of the patient and the experience of the surgeon.

OPERATION: ILEOCAECAL RESECTION (OPEN OR LAPAROSCOPIC)

The affected bowel is resected and the ends anastomosed. Mobilization can be achieved laparoscopically and the anastomosis formed either intra- or extracorporeally, the latter via a subumbilical incision.

Procedure profile

Blood requirement	2
Anaesthetic	GA
Operation time	Depends on number of strictureplasties
Hospital stay	7–14 days
Return to normal activity	6 weeks

OPERATION: STRICTUREPLASTY
Can be used for multiple discrete small bowel strictures and avoids resection of significant lengths of small bowel. The stricture is opened longditudinally and closed transversely creating a local dilatation in this area.

Procedure profile: as for ileocaecal resection

Following small bowel procedures for Crohn's most people now encourage early enteral feeding in uncomplicated cases. Multiple strictureplasties should be managed with more caution and perhaps wait for the patient to pass flatus. If the patient was on total parenteral nutrition preoperatively this should be continued initially postoperatively even if feeding enterally. The care of patients on steroids postoperatively is dealt with on p. 24. Beware of postoperative fistula formation, especially to the laparotomy wounds. Long-term follow-up will be needed, as there is a tendency for the disease to recur.

Rectal bleeding

Recognizing the pattern
This is an extremely common presentation to the colorectal clinic or surgical emergency take. The history has three vital questions (Fig. 9.1.1).

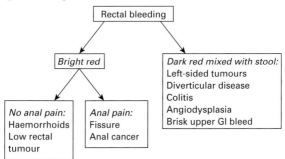

Fig. 9.1.1 Differential diagnosis of rectal bleeding.

- What colour is the blood?
- Is the blood separate from or mixed in with the stool?
- Is there any associated anal pain?

Examination should ensure that the patient is not hypovolaemic from significant blood loss.

Abdominal examination should look for tenderness indicating serosal inflammation (e.g. diverticulitis) or an abdominal mass (e.g. tumour, diverticular phlegmon). Perianal inspection is essential for anal cancers and the sentinel skin tag of anal fissures – the fissure can be seen usually in the midline by opening the anal canal slightly. However this is often extremely painful in patients with fissures. Rectal examination detects rectal tumours and occasionally sigmoid masses within the pelvis.

Proving the diagnosis
- FBC detects significant chronic blood loss.
- Proctoscopy allows visualization of the anal canal and treatment of haemorrhoids.
- Rigid sigmoidosocopy visualises the rest of the rectum and allows biopsy of mucosal inflammation (proctitis) or lesions.
- Either a barium enema or flexible sigmoidoscopy/colonoscopy to examine the colon. Even in the presence of haemorrhoids in those over 45 years old with fresh blood loss, a flexible sigmoidoscopy is advisable to rule out other causes of rectal bleeding.

Management
Following resuscitation where required, the management depends on the aetiology of disease. Any suspicion of significant blood loss should initiate active resuscitation before extensive history, examination or investigation. Large-bore i.v. cannulae, urinary catheterization and i.v. crystalloid or colloid whilst awaiting cross-matched blood are essential in the haemodynamically compromised patient.

Details of management of individual causes are given later in the chapter.

In patients bleeding rapidly (> 0.5 mL/min) a source in the upper GIT tract or small bowel should be considered. Arteriography and possible embolization by the radiologists should be considered.

Change in bowel habit

Bowel habit is very variable across individuals. A change in bowel habit is a change in the normal bowel habit for that individual. Although this happens to everyone at some point in their life it becomes concerning when the change persists for more than 4 weeks, especially when associated with other GI or constitutional symptoms or when occurring in those over 60 years of age. There are three major components to ask about.

- Change in stool frequency.
- Change in stool consistency including the passage of mucus.
- Evacuation or continence difficulties.

Recognizing the pattern

Causes are usually colonic or of small bowel origin but you need to consider pancreatic, biliary, endocrine and psychological causes. Always ask about new medication.

Abdominal examination may note tumours either arising from the colon or from other organs pressing onto the colon giving rise to the change in bowel habit. Check for any evidence of bowel obstruction. Examination should also include assessment of the thyroid.

Proving the diagnosis

Rectal examination and rigid sigmoidoscopy provide assessment of the rectum and any extrinsic pelvic mass. Colonoscopy or barium enema are used to rule out organic colonic disease.

Potential common causes of a change in bowel habit include:

- colorectal tumours
- diverticular disease
- inflammatory bowel disease
- coeliac disease
- irritable bowel disease
- hyper-/hypothyroidism.

Large bowel obstruction

This section should be read in conjunction with small bowel obstruction on p. 308.

Obstruction is a common surgical emergency. It is divided into large and small bowel obstruction. Except in cases of incarcerated hernias or volvulus, small bowel obstruction (SBO) usually has an outlet via the mouth and perforation is less common. Large bowel obstruction (LBO) is dependent on the competence of the ileocaecal valve. If the valve is competent, fluid and air can enter the colon but can't escape – 'closed-loop' obstruction. Perforation of the caecum (the thinnest part of the colon) is then a real risk. The majority of patients, however, have incompetent ileocaecal valves hence fluid can wash back into the small bowel.

Recognizing the pattern

The cardinal features are vomiting, abdominal pain and abdominal distension. In LBO, distension and discomfort predominate and precede vomiting. If the ileocaecal valve is incompetent then the vomit becomes faeculent and offensive. Constipation is common, but the evacuation of contents distal to an obstruction makes this feature unreliable. Further information in the history might point towards a large bowel cause. For example:

- A history of LBO in an elderly patient on constipating drugs and long-term laxatives might suggest a volvulus.
- A preceding history of a change in bowel habit with anorexia and weight loss in any type of bowel obstruction might point to a malignant aetiology.

On examination the patient may be tachycardic and even hypotensive. The abdomen should be distended and tympanitic but soft with minimal if any tenderness. The cause of obstruction may be palpable (e.g. a colonic tumour) or visible (e.g. an incarcerated inguinal or femoral hernia). Bowel sounds may be scarce but when heard sound obstructive ('tinkling'). Rectal examination may detect rectal or pelvic tumours causing obstruction by extrinsic compression. A capacious rectum with liquid stool is often evidence of pseudo-obstruction.

As with small bowel obstruction, signs that cause concern are:

- tachycardia +/– hypotension
- temperature > 38°C
- significant pain or localized peritonism over caecum
- peritonitis.

Proving the diagnosis

Having made a diagnosis of obstruction similar questions to those posed in the management of small bowel obstruction apply here.

- Is there any evidence of a closed loop obstruction or strangulation? If there is, the patient requires urgent resuscitation and definitive treatment.
- What is the clinical condition of the patient and how much resuscitation is needed?
- Is the level of obstruction in the large intestine? Look carefully at the X-ray.
- Is it mechanical or functional?
- What is the underlying cause of the obstruction?

These questions are answered with the help of the following investigations.

- Blood is taken for assessment of renal function given the significant fluid losses that can occur into the bowel lumen in obstruction.
- A raised WCC is suggestive of strangulation or perforation.
- Blood gases should be carried out in the haemodynamically compromised patient to assess the degree of metabolic acidosis.
- Plain X-ray shows obstruction and gives an idea of the level. It also demonstrates whether the ileocaecal valve is competent in LBO. Small bowel loops have transverse lines like a 'coiled spring' – the valvulae conniventes. Distended large bowel has haustra – transverse lines interrupted by the taeniae coli. Sigmoid volvulus has a characteristic 'coffee-bean' appearance with the sigmoid loop arising from the pelvis and extending to the right upper quadrant.
- A rigid sigmoidoscopy may demonstrate the obstructing lesion. It can also deflate the colon in cases of sigmoid volvulus or pseudo-obstruction.

Management

Resuscitation is the first priority. The patient has lost electrolyte-rich solution into the bowel lumen and so requires similar intravenous fluid to replace it. Beware of K^+ losses into the small bowel. The plasma K^+ can appear normal even when the total body K^+ is low if the patient develops renal failure. Place a urinary catheter to monitor urine output in all but the earliest stages of obstruction in the fittest patients. Regular clinical evaluation and assessment of fluid balance is vital.

LBO WITH INCOMPETENT ILEOCAECAL VALVE

A nasogastric tube is passed to stop vomiting and estimated fluid losses replaced intravenously. When the colon is involved in a hernia or in patients with colorectal tumours this allows appropriate and accurate fluid resuscitation before intervention to relieve the obstruction.

LBO WITH COMPETENT ILEOCAECAL VALVE

Bowel rest and i.v. fluid replacement are essential but there is less of a role for the nasogastric tube. In the absence of caecal tenderness, localized peritonism or significant colonic dilatation on the X-ray, careful resuscitation will reduce the perioperative morbidity and mortality. However if any of the above features are present, perforation is imminent and emergency surgery with simultaneous resuscitation is recommended. The obstruction can occasionally be relieved by an expandable mesh stent allowing more time for resuscitation and staging.

LBO WITH VOLVULUS

The commonest site is the sigmoid. These are by nature closed loop obstructions and as such require resuscitation and urgent treatment. The volvulus should be decompressed by a rigid or flexible sigmoidoscope and a flatus tube left in situ to splint the site of volvulus to prevent recurrence. Repeated recurrence or failure to decompress the volvulus makes laparotomy and sigmoid colectomy or a Hartmann's procedure inevitable except in those too unfit for surgery.

Benign and malignant colonic tumours

Colorectal cancer (CRC) is the second commonest cause of cancer-related death in the UK. Most if not all CRCs arise from pre-existing adenomas through sequential mutation in colonic cells – the adenoma–carcinoma sequence.

There are three major types of polyp in the colon: non-neoplastic (e.g. hyperplastic polyps, hamartomatous polyps in Peutz–Jeghers and juvenile polyposis, and inflammatory pseudopolyps in UC), benign adenomas and malignant adenocarcinomas. The risk of a polyp becoming malignant is based upon four factors:

- size
- number
- epithelial dysplasia
- histological type.

There are three major histological types of adenoma:

- tubular (65%)
- villous (10%)
- tubulovillous (25%).

Villous adenomas are the most likely to progress to malignancy. Ninety per cent of CRCs are sporadic with the remainder the result of inherited syndromes. The most common of these syndromes are hereditary non-polyposis colorectal cancer (HNPCC) caused by a mutation in the DNA mismatch repair genes, and familial adenomatous polyposis coli (FAP), caused by mutations in the APC gene.

Pathological staging

The purpose of pathological staging is to provide a guide to what if any postoperative treatment will be required and also gives a guide to prognosis. There are two commonly used staging systems for colorectal cancer. Both have their limitations but together, and with details of the tumour grade and the presence of lymphovascular invasion, a more complete picture is obtained.

Dukes' classification (Fig. 9.1.2)

A: tumour not penetrating beyond the muscle coat; no lymph node involvement.

B: tumour penetrating beyond the muscle coat; no lymph node involvement.

C: Lymph node involvement (occasionally described as C1 when apical node not involved and C2 when it is).

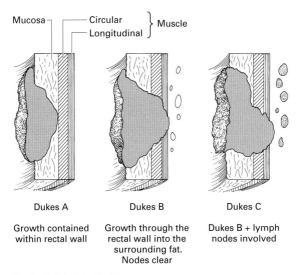

Fig. 9.1.2 Dukes' classification.

TNM classification

T1: tumour confined to the submucosa.

T2: tumour in the muscle coat but not through the bowel wall.

T3: tumour through the bowel wall into perirectal or colonic fat.

T4: tumour into an adjacent organ.

N1: fewer than five local nodes involved.

N2: more than five local nodes involved.

N3: tumour in the apical node.

M0: no metastases.

M1: metastases.

The tumour grade is classified as well, moderately or poorly differentiated.

Recognizing the pattern

The symptoms of CRC can be broken down to those arising from the GI tract and constitutional symptoms. The pattern of GI symptoms depends on the site of the tumour; 40% of tumours occur in the rectum, 30% in the sigmoid and 15% in the caecum. The symptoms can be divided into those arising from left-sided disease, from right-sided disease or from rectal disease.

Left-sided disease presents with a change in bowel habit or rectal bleeding passing altered blood. This is the most common site to present with large bowel obstruction.

Right-sided disease often presents innocuously with symptoms related to anaemia or less commonly with pain or a mass in the right iliac fossa. CRC should be strongly considered in anyone over 50 years with unexplained anaemia.

Rectal disease can often be misdiagnosed as more common causes of bright red rectal bleeding such haemorrhoids. However the blood is often mixed with the stool and not just on the paper. There may also be a feeling of tenesmus, and any involvement of the anal sphincters or canal may cause pain.

Proving the diagnosis

- A rectal examination is of ultimate importance in any patient with these symptoms. The fact that 40% of tumours occur in the rectum and 60% of these are palpable digitally serves to reinforce this view. A rigid sigmoidoscopy can pick up the remaining impalpable rectal tumours and allow biopsy.
- A double-contrast barium enema (DCBE) or colonoscopy is used to visualize the colon.
- If the symptoms suggest a left-sided tumour a flexible sigmoidoscopy can visualize up to the distal transverse colon and has a lower morbidity than a colonoscopy. It only requires an enema rather than full bowel preparation and does not require sedation.
- Biopsy is important for all rectal and any ambiguous lesions seen on DCBE. Histology from the biopsy will show adenocarcinoma with varying degrees of differentiation.

Management

Thirty per cent of patients present as emergencies and about half of these with large bowel obstruction.

The finding of any adenomatous polyp should instigate the investigation of the rest of the colon for further polyps. Further surveillance following the discovery of benign polyps following the initial colonoscopy is based upon the number and size of polyps found and whether the polyp was completely removed or destroyed. Colonoscopic polypectomy using cold snaring for smaller polyps and diathermy for larger polyps is usually successful.

Since 20–33% of patients with CRC have synchronous polyps at the time of diagnosis and 2–6% have a second colorectal malignancy, visualization of the remaining colon is essential.

Preoperative staging attempts to assess spread outside the bowel and any local invasion. A CT of chest, abdomen and pelvis allows assessment of regional lymph nodes, liver and lungs which are the common sites of metastasis. In rectal cancer, MRI of the rectum or endoanal ultrasound assess local invasion. Together with clinical examination these rectal assessments are helpful in evaluation of the height, fixity and position of rectal cancers as well as involvement of perirectal lymph nodes which aid in decisions regarding neoadjuvant treatment and type of operation.

Patients with liver metastases confined to a single lobe or with peripheral metastases in both lobes should be referred to a hepatobiliary surgeon for consideration of liver resection.

Preoperatively the following are required.

- FBC to assess the patient's haemoglobin given that bleeding is a common feature in this disease. An Hb > 9 g/dL is usually acceptable.
- Electrolytes should also be assessed, especially if bowel preparation has been given in elderly patients.
- Prophylactic broad-spectrum antibiotics (e.g. cefuroxime and metronidazole) are usually given as a single preoperative dose.
- Full bowel preparations are no longer common but are still useful in selected groups, such as laparoscopic resections and where on-table colonoscopy is planned.

Surgery for colorectal cancer follows oncological principles, namely that CRC spreads principally via the lymphatics which tend to run with the blood supply to the bowel. Thus to make a curative resection one must tie off the principal artery to the affected bowel to ensure that the maximum number of draining lymph nodes are removed with the specimen and therefore a long segment of bowel relying on that artery for its blood supply must be removed.

OPERATION: RIGHT HEMICOLECTOMY

The abdomen is opened and the terminal ileum, ascending colon and hepatic flexure of the colon are mobilized and excised. An anastomosis is made between the ileum and the transverse colon.

Procedure profile

Blood requirement	Group and save
Anaesthetic	GA
Operation time	1–2 hours
Hospital stay	5–7 days
Return to normal activity	4 weeks

OPERATION: LEFT HEMICOLECTOMY

The left side of the colon is mobilized and excised. An end-to-end anastomosis is usually performed. If the operation is carried out as an emergency for LBO, however, the proximal end of the bowel may be brought out as a colostomy (Hartmann's procedure; see p. 381) and the bowel may be rejoined later.

Procedure profile

Blood requirement	2
Anaesthetic	GA
Operation time	1–2 hours
Hospital stay	7 days
Return to normal activity	4 weeks

OPERATION: ANTERIOR RESECTION

This is a term applied to the operation to resect tumours in the rectum or rectosigmoid junction followed by a primary anastomosis. The left colon and splenic flexure are mobilized. Mobilization of the rectum within the pelvis is more difficult and time-consuming than operations within the abdomen. There is a risk of pelvic nerve damage and thus sexual and urinary dysfunction. There must be at least 1 cm of rectum distal to the tumour to ensure oncological clearance. The 'ultra-low' anterior resections for tumours in the middle and lower third of the rectum are possible due to circular stapling devices passed per anum and forming a stapled anastomosis with the descending colon which is brought down into the pelvis. Many surgeons advocate excising the whole mesorectum with the resected bowel in order to reduce the risk of local recurrence.

In a very low anastomosis a colon pouch can be created by turning back the distal left colon into a J configuration, and creating a common lumen. This attempts to replace the reservoir function that the resected rectum would normally provide. A protective loop ileostomy is frequently performed as part of the operation since anastomotic leakage is the most serious complication.

OPERATION: ABDOMINOPERINEAL RESECTION OF THE RECTUM

This operation is used for tumours where there is not an adequate length of bowel distal to the tumour or inadequate sphincter function to cope with a low anterior resection. In these circumstances the anus is removed with the rectum to maximize oncological clearance. A permanent colostomy is therefore unavoidable. The site of the colostomy is marked preoperatively with the patient in varying postures so that they have no problem seeing and changing the bag.

The anus is closed with a purse-string suture. The rectum is mobilized from above as in the anterior resection operation. In addition to this, the lower rectum and anus are also excised through a perineal incision around the anus and sphincters (extra-sphincteric dissection). The rectum is then removed and the subcutaneous fat and skin are closed, leaving a drain in the space left in the pelvis which is brought out through the abdomen.

The abdominoperineal operation may be performed by one surgeon doing both the abdominal and the perineal resections, or by two surgeons. The theatre staff will need to know whether one or two surgeons will be operating.

Procedure profile

Blood requirement	2
Anaesthetic	GA
Operation time	3 hours
Hospital stay	14 days
Return to normal activity	6 weeks

When the patient is too old or frail to withstand a major operation, or where there is an early tumour (T1) of the rectum that
is accessible in any patient, a local excision may be performed.
In the palliative setting this may need to be repeated a number of
times as malignant lesions always recur. Even in the attempted
curative procedure there is no guarantee that the patient has
no lymph node involvement (about 5–15% in T1 tumours) but
it does avoid the significant morbidity associated with major
abdominal surgery.

OPERATION: TRANSANAL RESECTION
This is used for low rectal cancers that can be reached by placing
a proctoscope to open the anal canal. The tumour is excised with
a surrounding disc of normal mucosa.

Procedure profile

Blood requirement	Group and save
Anaesthetic	GA
Operation time	30–60 minutes
Hospital stay	3–5 days
Return to normal activity	2 weeks

OPERATION: TEM PROCEDURE
More proximal rectal tumours can also be excised locally by
transanal endoscopic microsurgery (TEM). A large-diameter

operating proctoscope is placed in the rectum. A telescope attached to a video camera gives a good view of the rectal lumen and specialized instruments for manipulation, cutting and diathermy are inserted through ports in the proctoscope. Mucosal or full-thickness resections can be performed and the defect repaired by intraluminal suturing.

Procedure profile

Blood requirement	Group and save
Anaesthetic	GA
Operation time	30 minutes – 2 hours
Hospital stay	3 days
Return to normal activity	2 weeks

Common emergency operations for CRC include the following.

OPERATION: HARTMANN'S PROCEDURE

This operation is used most commonly in LBO from left-sided tumours or in perforated diverticular disease (see below) when a quick operation is necessary in frail patients. It is also used for unresectable rectal cancers. The lower end of the rectum is closed and left in situ. The upper end of the bowel is brought out as a colostomy. For perforated diverticular disease the perforated segment is resected if at all possible. In some cases continuity may be restored later.

Procedure profile

Blood requirement	2
Anaesthetic	GA
Operation time	2–3 hours
Hospital stay	10–14 days
Return to normal activity	6–8 weeks

OPERATION: TRANSVERSE LOOP COLOSTOMY

This operation is sometimes done on its own for acute colonic obstruction but it may also be part of a resection procedure. A transverse muscle-cutting incision is made in the right hypochondrium. The transverse colon is mobilized and the omentum separated from it. A loop of colon is brought out and maintained in position by passing it over a rubber tube or a plastic 'bridge'. The colostomy is opened by incising along the taenia. The edges of the colon are then sewn to the skin. Occasionally a loop colostomy is also formed from the sigmoid colon.

Other types of stoma are shown in Fig. 9.1.3. A 'double-barrelled' colostomy is formed where part of the colon has been resected and the two ends are brought out next to each other. An 'end' colostomy is formed when the lower bowel is closed off or removed, as in an abdominoperineal resection or a Hartmann's procedure (see above).

Postoperative management of patients having colorectal resections is very variable depending on the view of the consultant. There is gradually a move towards a multimodal accelerated recovery programme. Patients more frequently have epidural analgesia postoperatively and are mobilized from the first postoperative day. Nasogastric tubes are rarely necessary. Patients are often encouraged to take as much fluid as they will tolerate and to eat when they become hungry rather than waiting until they pass flatus. The belief is that this will reduce the period of ileus and allow quicker recovery of metabolic function and also protect the barrier function of the gut to microorganisms.

Encouraging deep breathing and stimulation of the calf pump is essential to avoid respiratory complications and DVTs. The main postoperative danger is an anastomotic leak. You should be aware of any deterioration of pain after day 3. The signs of a leak can be subtle, with pyrexia, tachycardia and oliguria associated with abdominal pain. Patients usually have a metabolic acidosis which may be compensated by tachypnoea. Faecal discharge from an abdominal drain may make the diagnosis obvious. An anastomotic leak requires resuscitation followed by urgent reoperation.

The patient commonly gets diarrhoea in the first few days after the bowel recovers and should be reassured that this will gradually settle down.

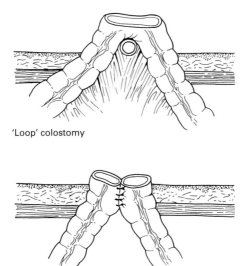

'Loop' colostomy

'Double-barrelled' colostomy

'End' colostomy

Fig. 9.1.3 Types of colostomy.

Abdominoperineal resections have a high risk of perineal wound complications and this must be inspected daily to ensure there is no infection or wound breakdown. Patients should avoid lying on their back or sitting for long periods for the same reason.

The care of a new stoma is crucial. Early feeding and mobilization should be encouraged. Stomas should have a clear bag over them in the first few days to check that they are well perfused and not retracting. Patients with ileostomies need to have the effluent measured from the ileostomy and care taken to avoid fluid and electrolyte imbalance.

If a temporary colostomy or ileostomy has been performed after an anterior resection then arrangements will have to be made to close it at a suitable time. Some surgeons request a water-soluble enema before the stoma is closed, to check there is continuity of the anastomosis without leakage.

OPERATION: CLOSURE OF COLOSTOMY OR ILEOSTOMY
The edges of the stoma are freed from the skin and the piece of colon or ileum is either resected or the defect closed, restoring continuity.

Procedure profile

Blood requirement	Group and save
Anaesthetic	GA
Operation time	1 hour
Hospital stay	7 days
Return to normal activity	3 weeks

OPERATION: REVERSAL OF HARTMANN'S
The previous midline wound is reopened. There are usually a lot of adhesions to divide before the two ends of the bowel are ready for anastomosis. The latter may be performed with sutures or a stapling gun. This procedure can be performed laparoscopically.

Procedure profile

Blood requirement	Group and save
Anaesthetic	GA
Operation time	3 hours
Hospital stay	7 days
Return to normal activity	3 weeks

NOTE ON LAPAROSCOPIC-ASSISTED COLORECTAL SURGERY

There are increasing numbers of laparoscopic colorectal procedures being performed. In malignant disease there is no evidence that it increases the risk of disseminating the tumour and adequate oncological resection is achievable. The same precautions and preoperative management are employed, except bowel preparation is used more frequently. Operating time is frequently longer. Any anastomosis can be performed either extraperitoneally through a small incision where both ends of the bowel are delivered through this incision or intracorporeally by endoscopic stapling devices. In laparoscopic anterior resection the head of the circular stapling device is fitted extracorporeally as the proximal colon is delivered along with the tumour through a small incision. The stapling device is passed per anum as normal and the two ends of the device are fitted together laparoscopically. The greatest advantages may eventually be in pelvic procedures where the view in open surgery is often obscured although there is no strong evidence that such procedures are superior to open procedures at the current time.

Diverticular disease

Diverticular disease is a common condition affecting the colon in the developed world. The condition is associated with muscle hypertrophy and raised intraluminal pressure. Mucosa-lined pouches are pushed out through the colonic wall, usually at the entry points of vessels (Fig. 9.1.4). These pouches are the diverticula. The condition is thought to arise because of a lack of fibre and fluid in the diet. Dietary fibre is not absorbed from the bowel lumen and so passes through the GI tract holding onto water. The moisture it retains makes the stool more bulky and soft, and more easily propelled along the colonic lumen. A diet poor in fibre and non-caffeinated forms of water results in the stool becoming dehydrated and harder and colonic pressures are raised. This lack of dietary fibre and fluid is also important in the pathogenesis of other colorectal conditions, especially haemorrhoids.

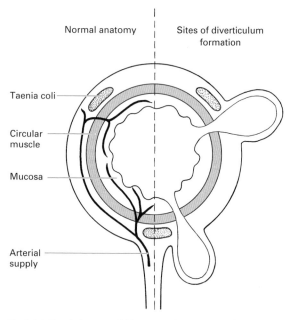

Fig. 9.1.4 Diverticula are usually blown out at the entry points of vessels.

Diverticular disease can affect any part of the colon but in the West 80% occurs in the left colon. Right-sided disease is uncommon in the West, but is the commonest site in South-East Asia.

Recognizing the pattern
Diverticular disease itself (diverticulosis) is essentially asymptomatic but presents with one of its complications. The most common of these are:
- inflammation (diverticulitis)
- bleeding PR (dark red and often painless rectal bleeding)
- perforation causing peritonitis (either abscess perforation causing purulent peritonitis or bowel perforation causing faecal peritonitis)

- fistula formation especially to bladder (65%) or vagina (25%)
- strictures (presenting as a change in bowel habit or LBO).

Patients are usually over 50 years old with the incidence increasing with age – more than 60% of 70-year-olds in the UK have diverticular disease. It is more common in women.

Diverticulitis usually presents with vague colicky lower abdominal pain which localizes to the left iliac fossa (for left-sided disease) and which becomes constant and worse on movement. The story is not unlike appendicitis but on the left with the prodromal pain in the hindgut area (suprapubic) instead of the midgut area (periumbilical).

On examination there is often a raised temperature and pulse rate with localized peritonism in the left iliac fossa. A tender mass in the left iliac fossa or palpable mass in the pelvis on PR, and a swinging high temperature would suggest a diverticular abscess. Generalized peritonitis obviously suggests perforation. A history of pneumaturia or passing faeculent material per urethra or per vaginum would suggest a fistula.

Proving the diagnosis

- Bloods show raised inflammatory markers – WCC, platelets, CRP.
- Microbiology may detect Gram-negative sepsis in urine or blood. Gram-negative septicaemia is a life-threatening condition.
- X-ray may show free gas under the diaphragm on an erect CXR in perforation but clinical examination is far more accurate than a CXR in diagnosing perforation of the colon.
- A contrast CT of the abdomen and pelvis is the investigation of choice for acute diverticulitis. It will also detect complications of the disease such as pericolic abscesses, fistulae and small amounts of free peritoneal gas.
- If imaging has not been performed during mild acute diverticulitis you should organize an outpatient barium enema when the attack has settled to confirm the likely diagnosis and assess the extent of the disease.

Management

Treat the acute attack with intravenous broad-spectrum antibiotics (e.g. cefuroxime and metronidazole). If the symptoms do not settle within 48 h the possibility of an abscess or an alternative diagnosis should be considered. Again a CT scan will be helpful and if an abscess is present CT-guided drainage may be possible. Intravenous antibiotics should be continued in this situation. There is varied opinion as to the degree of oral intake during an acute attack but most would agree that clear fluids should be taken as tolerated and some advocate any oral intake up to a low residue diet.

Once the acute attack has settled the patient should be advised on a high-fibre/fluid diet to reduce the incidence of further attacks.

Elective surgery should be considered in those who have frequent attacks of diverticulitis or those who have had a diverticular complication (e.g. stricture, abscess). The most common procedure is a sigmoid colectomy reflecting the prevalence of the condition in this segment of the colon. This should be organized at least 6 weeks after the acute attack has settled to allow the inflammation to settle.

The treatment of fistulae should ideally wait until any acute attack has been treated but the patient may need to continue a prophylactic dose of oral antibiotics until definitive surgery in the presence of a colovesical fistula to prevent recurrent urinary tract infections.

Perforated diverticular disease is one of the commonest causes of faecal peritonitis and calls for emergency surgery.

OPERATION: ELECTIVE SIGMOID COLECTOMY
As for left hemicolectomy (see p. 378) but the sigmoid is resected and the descending colon anastomosed to the upper rectum either by a sutured anastamosis or by a per anal stapling device. This operation has had good success laparoscopically.

Procedure profile: as for left hemicolectomy
OPERATION: EMERGENCY HARTMANN'S
PROCEDURE (see p. 381)
This is the commonest operation for perforated diverticular disease or an unresponsive diverticular abscess that cannot be drained radiologically. The area of perforation along with any attached segment of significant diverticular disease is resected if

at all possible and the rectum closed off. The proximal bowel is brought out as an end colostomy and, if the distal end is long enough and it is expected that the patient will be a candidate for reversal of the Hartmann's in the future, this too can be brought to the skin as a mucous fistula.

Procedure profile: as for left Hartmann's procedure
Postoperative care is as for other colonic resections.

Complete rectal prolapse

This is an intussusception of the upper rectum into the lower anal canal in which the whole bowel wall is inverted and passed out through the anus. It is associated with weakness of the pelvic musculature, often following multiple childbirth.

Recognizing the pattern
The patient is often an elderly multiparous woman. The four common complaints are:
- noticing the prolapse +/– difficulty reducing it
- faecal and mucus incontinence
- frequency and urgency of defecation
- pelvic discomfort.

Proving the diagnosis
The prolapse might be evident at the time of examination. Otherwise ask the patient to go to a toilet and strain. Whilst sitting on the toilet examine the anus for signs of the prolapse.

Management
Conservative measures should be used for those not fit for surgery, but they are of limited use. Stool softeners and pelvic floor exercises are the mainstay of this treatment.

Surgical management can be by the perineal (e.g. Delorme's or Altmeier's procedure) or abdominal approaches (e.g. abdominal rectopexy). There are advantages and disadvantages to both.

Three issues must be considered when deciding each operation:

- recurrence rate
- constipation and incontinence rate postoperatively
- morbidity of the procedure.

Details of the procedures themselves are beyond the scope of this chapter.

9.2 Perianal pain

This section deals with a number of related perianal conditions that present with pain in the perineum. In order to understand their aetiology, it is necessary to be familiar with the anatomy of the perianal structures and these are depicted in Fig. 9.2.1. The conditions include perianal abscesses, fistulae, fissures, haemorrhoids and perianal haematomas.

Perianal abscess

This is an extremely common condition seen on the surgical take. The most common cause of perianal abscess formation is infection arising in a perianal gland. These glands lie between the internal and external sphincters and open into the anal canal via the anal crypts at the pectinate line. If the opening of the gland becomes blocked or damaged, stasis can result and lead to infection. The resulting abscess lies between the anal sphincters and can track towards the skin at the anal margin (intersphincteric abscess) or spread laterally through the external sphincter into the ischiorectal fossa (Fig. 9.2.2). Occasionally the abscess tracks superiorly around or through the levator ani (suprasphincteric abscess). All of these can track out to the skin. If the infection in the anal glands simply tracts along its duct towards the anal canal and not out to the skin, it is called a submucous abscess.

Recognizing the pattern
Patients of any age including children may be affected. Sitting is often painful. On examination the abscess may be seen in the skin next to the anus, not the natal cleft. There is often surrounding

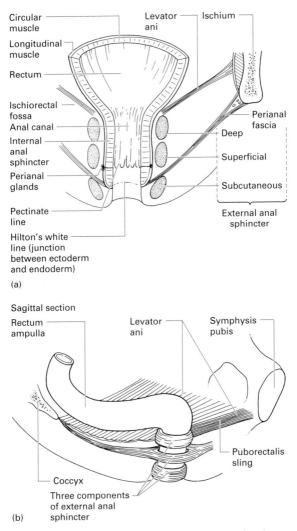

Fig. 9.2.1 (a) Anatomy of the anal canal. (b) Anal sphincters seen from the side.

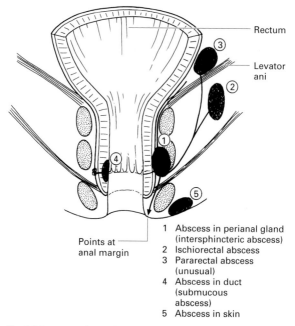

Fig. 9.2.2 Anatomical sites of abscess formation in the perianal region.

erythema and induration. Look for any pus from the anus that would give rise to suspicion of a fistula (see below). Suprasphincteric or submucous abscesses may not present with any swelling but the history of anal pain and evidence of a fever should make you suspect a perianal abscess. Have a high index of suspicion for an underlying predisposition in patients with multiple abscesses or evidence of previous abscesses of fistulae.

Conditions predisposing to perianal sepsis include:
- Crohn's disease
- immunosuppression including diabetes mellitus
- other infections e.g. TB
- neoplastic e.g. anorectal cancer.

Proving the diagnosis

The diagnosis is obvious on examination and no other tests are indicated. Ensure the abscess is not in the natal cleft associated with midline pits – this is a pilonidal abscess and has a different aetiology and postoperative treatment.

Management

Complex abscesses (e.g. secondary to Crohn's disease, suprasphincteric) should involve a senior surgeon. If there is evidence of surrounding cellulitis intravenous antibiotics should be started (e.g. flucloxacillin and metronidazole).

OPERATION: DRAINAGE OF PERIANAL ABSCESS

A rigid sigmoidoscopy and rectal examination are carried out to look and feel for internal openings of a fistula or other predisposing conditions. An incision is made over the abscess. The contents are evacuated and a sample sent for microbiological assessment. Loculi within the abscess are gently broken down with a finger but care must be taken not to extend the abscess upward through the levator ani or to create any false plane. If a low fistula is found some surgeons advocate laying open the tract at that time (see below) whilst others will wait for the inflammation to settle before dealing with the fistula at another time, as all would do for high fistulae. The cavity is usually left open and packed with an alginate dressing.

Procedure profile

Blood requirement	0
Anaesthetic	GA
Operation time	15 minutes
Hospital stay	Day case–1 day
Return to normal activity	1–2 weeks

After operation the abscess is re-packed daily with an alginate dressing so that the wound heals without closing over prematurely. Antibiotics may be indicated if there is significant cellulitis.

Check the microbiology even if the patient has gone home. Anaerobic cultures suggest a possible fistula.

Perianal fistula

A perianal fistula is an abnormal connection between the lumen of the anus or rectum and the skin. It occurs when a perianal abscess tracks to the skin. If the opening into the anus of the infected perianal gland remains patent a fistula results.

Various types of fistula are described according to the level at which they cross the anal sphincters. The important distinction is between those that open into the bowel below the deep part of the external anal sphincter ('low') and those that open above this ('high') (Fig. 9.2.3). The latter are less common and are often due to other disease such as Crohn's.

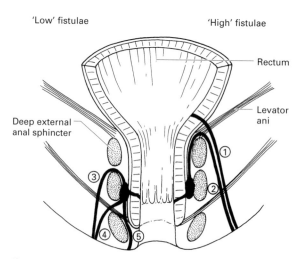

Fig. 9.2.3 The types of perianal fistula. High: 1, extrasphincteric; 2, suprasphincteric. Low: 3, high transphincteric; 4, low transphincteric; 5, intersphincteric.

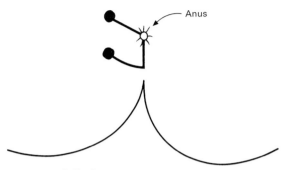

Fig. 9.2.4 Goodsall's rule.

Recognizing the pattern

The patient complains of persistent perianal discharge and recurrent abscesses. On examination the external opening is usually seen near the anus. The internal opening may be palpable on rectal examination or visible on proctoscopy or rigid sigmoidoscopy but is not always apparent. Goodsall's rule is a good guide but should not be relied upon. It states that a fistula lying in the anterior half of the anal area opens directly into the anal canal, while a fistula lying in the posterior half tracks around the anus and opens in the posterior midline (Fig. 9.2.4).

During rectal examination assess the tone of the anal sphincter. It may be weaker in the elderly, meaning that less muscle should be cut at operation.

Proving the diagnosis

The finding of an internal and external opening is evidence enough of the presence of a fistula. However any suggestion in the history or examination of secondary extensions or a complex tract should point towards preoperative evaluation with MRI.

Management

The treatment of a perianal fistula is to lay it open. However faecal continence is lost when major parts of the external and internal anal sphincters are divided. Therefore, low fistulae can be laid open, with only slight danger of minor incontinence due to damage to the internal anal sphincter.

When in doubt, however, fistulae should be managed with the use of a seton. This can be a suture or a rubber vascular sling, placed around the tract to act as a chronic drain or to mark the tract for future surgery (loose seton). Setons can be tightened (cutting seton) and used to divide the muscle slowly by pressure necrosis allowing fibrosis to occur as it cuts through but this can also cause problems with continence. The internal opening of a high fistula may need to be closed operatively with an advancement flap. Occasionally a covering colostomy may be required. Fibrin glue has been used in high fistulae following resolution of sepsis and this avoids any risk of incontinence.

Any predisposing cause of the fistulae such as Crohn's disease must also be treated.

OPERATION: LAYING OPEN OF LOW PERIANAL FISTULA
The patient is given a phosphate enema preoperatively.

A probe is passed into the external opening and carefully passed along the fistulous tract until it goes through the internal opening into the anal canal. Care must be taken not to create new tracts through injudicious use of the probe. A knife or diathermy is used to cut down on the probe and the tract laid open completely. Any lateral extensions of the tract must also be laid open.

Procedure profile

Blood requirement	0
Anaesthetic	GA
Operation time	15–30 minutes
Hospital stay	Day case–1 day
Return to normal activity	2–3 weeks

Postoperative care is as for perianal abscess drainage.

OPERATION: HIGH PERIANAL FISTULA
The whole tract cannot be laid open because too much muscle is involved and hence there is the danger of incontinence. The

lower part is opened and drained but care is taken to cut the least amount of external and internal sphincter necessary. A seton is passed through the tract to allow fibrosis and healing and a possible subsequent anal advancement flap.

Procedure profile: as for low fistula except full bowel preparation is often recommended

Anal fissure

Anal fissures are tears in the skin of the distal anal canal usually presenting with severe anal pain and fresh rectal bleeding. The traditional theory of the development of anal fissures involves a traumatic event in the anal canal in a susceptible patient with a hypertonic internal anal sphincter (IAS). This raised pressure reduces the blood flow that passes through the sphincters to reach the anal canal to the area of the fissure, preventing healing.

Recognizing the pattern
Although they can occur at any age they are more common in young adults and those occurring in older patients need to be treated with a higher level of suspicion. The pain is often characterized as being worst at the time of a bowel action and lasting for several hours following this. This distinguishes it from other causes of painful rectal bleeding.

On examination there may be a perianal skin tag ('sentinel pile') marking the site of the fissure. These are nearly always midline and about 90% are posterior. Multiple or non-midline fissures should again raise the possibility of an underlying anorectal process (e.g. Crohn's). Occasionally it is too painful even to part the buttocks to examine for a fissure and it is nearly always too painful to do a rectal examination.

Management
Acute fissures less than 6 weeks old may respond to conservative treatment such as stool softeners, bulking agents such as bran and local anaesthetic ointment. Once the fissure is chronic further treatment is required.

First-line treatment for chronic fissures is now medical. Topical ointments to reduce IAS pressures have reasonable success and are safe. The commonest used are glyceryl trinitrate and diltiazem. Botulinum toxin injected into the IAS has less experience but is very effective as a second-line treatment if topical ointments fail.

If the fissure persists surgery is considered. Essentially for classical idiopathic anal fissures associated with raised sphincter tone the lateral internal sphincterotomy is the treatment of choice although there is a small risk of incontinence. For those idiopathic fissures associated with normal or low-pressure sphincters or in the presence of a previous sphincter injury an anal advancement flap should be considered.

OPERATION: LATERAL SPHINCTEROTOMY
The lowermost fibres of the internal anal sphincter are divided usually in the 3 o'clock position up to the height of the level of the fissure. This weakens IAS pressure, allowing the fissure to heal.

Procedure profile

Blood requirement	0
Anaesthetic	GA
Operation time	15–30 minutes
Hospital stay	Day case
Return to normal activity	1–2 weeks

Postoperatively the patient should be put on a high-fibre diet and a short course of lactulose.

Haemorrhoids

Haemorrhoidal problems are extremely common. They are related to a combination of inadequate fibre and fluid intake and poor toileting habits. Haemorrhoidal cushions are normal submucosal structures lining the anal canal and are involved in the maintenance of continence. They contain:

- smooth muscle and fibroelastic tissue, which contribute to the support of the haemorrhoid
- arteriovenous fistulae which vary in size to contribute to continence.

Once the support structures are weakened by straining at stool and sitting on the bowl for long periods, and the mucosa is damaged by hard stool, the haemorrhoid bleeds, swells and prolapses into the anal canal, the latter increasing the likelihood of future injury by the anal sphincters.

Haemorrhoids are often classified into four groups:

- first degree: these piles remain within the anal canal
- second degree: these prolapse out of the anal verge but reduce spontaneously
- third degree: these prolapse and require manual reduction
- fourth degree: these are permanently prolapsed.

Recognizing the pattern

No specific age group but certain conditions such as pregnancy or an episode of acute diarrhoea or constipation may herald the onset of symptoms. Painless bright red rectal bleeding is the commonest presentation where the patient notices the blood on the tissue when wiping or dripping into the pan. Other symptoms include pain, itching (pruritus ani), mucus discharge and noticing the prolapsing haemorrhoid.

Proving the diagnosis

Examination of the anus may reveal skin tags which sometimes act as herald of anal disease. Fourth and sometimes third-degree haemorrhoids are obvious at the anal verge. Proctoscopy will reveal first- and second-degree haemorrhoids.

It is essential that anyone over 45 years old or those younger with an abnormal history are investigated for other causes of their symptoms since the condition is so common and more sinister conditions can therefore be overlooked. A rigid sigmoidoscopy in the clinic and a flexible sigmoidoscopy as a follow-up procedure are usually sufficient.

Management

Asymptomatic haemorrhoids do not require treatment. Patients with symptoms must be proactive in changing their diet and toileting habits by:

- increasing the fibre content of their diet
- increasing their non-caffeinated water intake
- avoiding straining at stool
- avoiding sitting on the toilet for long periods of time.

First-degree haemorrhoids should settle with the above conservative treatment. If they don't they should be treated as for second-degree haemorrhoids.

Second-degree haemorrhoids are treated with local procedures administered in the outpatient department. These include injection sclerotherapy with Phenol or banding of haemorrhoids.

For third- and fourth-degree haemorrhoids local treatments can be tried and may have success in rendering the patient asymptomatic. However they often require some form of operative intervention (see below).

Strangulated haemorrhoids occur when a prolapsed haemorrhoid has become incarcerated by the sphincters outside the anal canal causing loss of blood supply to the tissue and intense pain. It is treated by bed rest, elevating the foot of the bed, ice packs to the perianal area, analgesia, stool softeners and GTN ointment. Some advocate haemorrhoidectomy the same day, others only if conservative measures are not successful after 3 days.

OPERATION: MILLIGAN–MORGAN
HAEMORRHOIDECTOMY

Bowel preparation is with a phosphate enema. Intravenous cefuroxime and metronidazole are given with the premedication.

The haemorrhoid and its associated external component are dissected off the internal sphincter up to the apex of the anal cushion. The blood supply pedicle is ligated at this point (or occasionally diathermied which may reduce postoperative pain) and the haemorrhoid excised. Adequate skin bridges must be left between each excised haemorrhoid to avoid anal stenosis postoperatively. The operation is extremely painful and the area is infiltrated with local anaesthetic. Ideally stool softeners should be started 2 days before surgery.

Procedure profile

Blood requirement	Group and save
Anaesthetic	GA
Operation time	30 minutes
Hospital stay	Day case–1 day
Return to normal activity	2–3 weeks

Postoperatively the patient should be placed on regular and varied analgesia (e.g. paracetamol, NSAID, opioid) but limiting constipating drugs (e.g. opioids) as much as possible. In addition topical GTN for 2 weeks and oral metronidazole for 1 week both contribute to a reduction in pain. Stool softeners should be continued for 1 week.

Reactionary haemorrhage may occur in the first few hours after the operation. There is often a slight secondary haemorrhage at 7–10 days after the operation and the patient should be warned about this.

OPERATION: STAPLED HAEMORRHOIDECTOMY
Bowel preparation is with a phosphate enema. Intravenous cefuroxime and metronidazole are given with the premedication.

This operation essentially involves excising redundant rectal mucosa above the haemorrhoids so hitching up the anal cushions and preventing prolapse. After dilatation of the anal canal, a purse string suture is placed 4 cm above the dentate line. A circular stapler is introduced transanally. The anvil of the device is positioned proximal to the purse-string and the suture is tied down on to the anvil. Retraction of the suture pulls the attached rectal mucosa into the stapler. Closure of the anvil and firing of the stapler simultaneously excises a ring of mucosa proximal to the haemorrhoids, thus interrupting the blood supply, but maintaining continuity of the rectal mucosa. It does not involve any excision of the sensitive anal or perianal skin and as a result seems to result in considerably less postoperative pain. However it does leave behind the external component of the haemorrhoid.

Procedure profile: as for Milligan–Morgan

Perianal haematoma (thrombosed external pile)

This is due to a ruptured superficial perianal vein, which gives rise to a subcutaneous haematoma.

Recognizing the pattern
The patient may be of any age. There is frequently a history of straining at stool. The condition presents with a sudden onset of severe perianal pain. Left untreated the pain gradually settles over a week or so and the haematoma resolves.

On examination there is a cherry-like, rounded, blue haematoma in the subcutaneous tissue next to the anal verge. It is exquisitely tender.

Management
In the first 2–3 days the treatment is to evacuate the haematoma after infiltrating with local anaesthetic. This gives immediate relief. If the haematoma has been present for longer than a week, it is probably best left to resolve naturally.

10 Hernias

10.1 Hernias and other groin lumps

ANATOMY OF THE GROIN

A wide variety of interesting conditions can present as a lump in the groin. Students are often confused about the anatomy of this area and hence uncertain of the interpretation of physical signs and the surgical approach to a hernia. The femoral sheath is usefully described as a gap between the anterior abdominal wall and the posterior abdominal wall where these two structures meet in the groin. Through this gap pass the main vessels to the leg ('pulling the sheath' around them as they leave the abdominal cavity) and, medial to them, is the femoral canal. This part of the anterior abdominal wall consists of the external oblique, internal oblique and transversus abdominus muscles. These are thin sheet-like muscles which end anteriorly and inferiorly as thin but strong tendinous sheets (aponeurosis). The inguinal ligament is a thickening of the external oblique aponeurosis along its lower border. The ligament is attached to the pubic tubercle medially and the anterosuperior iliac spine laterally. Behind the inguinal ligament are the muscles of the posterior abdominal wall running into the anterior thigh (psoas and iliacus) and also the pectineus. The femoral vessels lie on top of these muscles behind the inguinal ligament (Fig. 10.1.1).

Inguinal hernias occur through the inguinal canal in the lower part of the anterior abdominal wall and therefore originate above the inguinal ligament. Femoral hernias occur down the femoral canal and are therefore posterior to the inguinal ligament and appear in the thigh below and lateral to the pubic tubercle. Obturator hernias occur from within the true pelvis and they can be palpated within the adductor compartment of the thigh. They are rare in comparison to inguinal and femoral hernias.

Surgery: Diagnosis and Management, 4th edition. Edited by N. Rawlinson and D. Alderson. © 2009 Blackwell Publishing, ISBN: 978-1-4051-2921-3

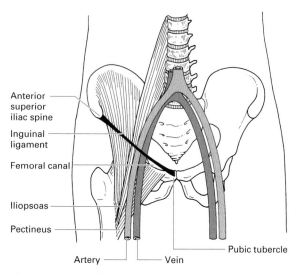

Fig. 10.1.1 Anatomy of the inguinal ligament.

GENERAL ASSESSMENT

In approaching a patient with a groin lump it is necessary to define the anatomical landmarks. It is particularly important to define the line of the inguinal ligament by palpating the bony points from which it arises (Fig. 10.1.2).

A list of possible groin lumps and their relationship to the inguinal ligament is given in Table 10.1.1.

Inguinal hernia

Inguinal hernias result from a weakness of the transversalis fascia, a normally strong fibrous sheet which covers the posterior wall of the inguinal canal between the inguinal ligament below and the arching fibres of the anterior abdominal wall muscles above (internal oblique and transversus). The transversalis fascia condenses as a ring (the internal or deep inguinal ring) lateral to

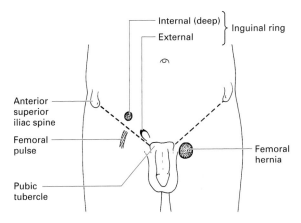

Fig. 10.1.2 Landmarks in the groin.

the inferior (deep) epigastric vessels and through this ring is transmitted the spermatic cord in the male (and the round ligament in the female) on its passage from the posterior abdominal wall via the inguinal canal to the scrotum (labia majora). The deep ring is naturally wider in the male. Medial to the inferior epigastric vessels the posterior wall of the inguinal canal is also 'filled in' by the transversalis fascia. In the female this space is non-existent.

In men inguinal hernias can be either indirect or direct. Indirect hernias follow the path of the spermatic cord and originate, therefore, lateral to the inferior epigastric vessels. Direct hernias originate medial to these vessels. Both types are a result of a weakness in the transversalis fascia in the posterior wall of the inguinal canal but because this weakness is either congenital or acquired the different varieties of inguinal hernia occur in men of different ages.

Strangulated hernias are described on p. 424.

Recognizing the pattern
Indirect inguinal hernias occur in babies and young infants as a consequence of a failure of the processus vaginalis (the

Table 10.1.1 Lumps in the groin.

Anatomical structure	Pathology	Above or below the inguinal ligament	Pitfalls
In the skin/subcutaneous tissue	Lipoma, fibroma, haemangioma, etc.	Either	Simple subcutaneous lumps may have a transmitted cough impulse or pulsation
Deep to the skin			
Femoral vein	Saphena varix (see Varicose veins, p. 527)	Below	May also have a cough impulse
Femoral artery	Aneurysm (see Vascular disorders, p. 513)	Below	An aneurysm of the external inguinal iliac artery would be above the inguinal ligament
Lymph nodes, inguinal or femoral	Primary or secondary neoplasia or infection	Either	
Hernias	Inguinal, direct or indirect	Above	Large inguinoscrotal hernias lie in front of and obscure the pubic tubercle
	Femoral	Below	Arise below and can then turn upwards and medially

embryonic peritoneal tube which allows the testis to descend from the posterior abdominal wall into the scrotum) to close and obliterate. A similar structure develops in the female infant to allow the passage of the round ligament but because it has nearly always obliterated by birth these hernias occur much less frequently in females. The occurrence of bilateral inguinal hernias in a female infant should alert the clinician to the possibility of testicular feminization syndrome. See chapter 14 for further management of inguinal hernias in this age group.

Later in life inguinal hernias can develop in the line of the spermatic cord or round ligament (indirect), again exploiting a potential weakness in the transversalis fascia at the deep ring. Direct hernias can also occur in males (never in females) through the weak triangular-shaped area of the posterior wall of the inguinal canal medial to the inferior epigastric vessels. Classically these occur in older men, often associated with conditions which regularly raise intra-abdominal pressure such as chronic cough, constipation and straining to pass urine in chronic bladder outflow disease.

The patient presents with a swelling in the groin that may cause some discomfort or restrict activity. In both types of hernia there may be a family history of the condition and there may also be an immediate precipitating cause such as an episode of heavy lifting or severe coughing, due for example to chronic bronchitis.

On examination there is a bulge in the groin above the line of the inguinal ligament. In the early stages the hernia is lateral to the pubic tubercle and as it enlarges it may protrude over the pubic tubercle (above and medial) and down into the scrotum or vulva. The lump has a cough impulse over it unless it is incarcerated. After reduction an indirect hernia is controlled during coughing by pressure over the deep inguinal ring (see Fig. 10.1.2). On relieving the pressure the hernia runs obliquely down the canal. A direct hernia is not so controlled and bulges straight forward.

Management
Not all inguinal hernias are symptomatic and not all require surgical correction. If an inguinal hernia is painless and doesn't restrict activity particularly in frail and elderly patients, treatment is not

required. In frail patients with symptomatic hernias in whom surgical treatment is considered to be high risk a correctly fitted truss may be helpful. This works by compressing the inguinal canal from front to back and thus preventing the hernia from protruding. A truss is not suitable for treatment of a large hernia because they tend to bulge round the sides of the truss before long.

If the hernia is painful surgical correction is advised in all but the frailest patients. Inguinal hernia repair is one of the commonest surgical procedures in modern practice.

Preoperatively the patient should be advised to stop smoking for at least 2 months before surgery. Patients who continue smoking up to the time of a hernia repair are at risk of chest infection after the operation and this puts added strain on the repair in the early stages. Obesity also makes the operation more difficult, puts more strain on the repair postoperatively and increases the risk of postoperative chest infection and thromboembolic complications (DVT/pulmonary embolism).

Surgery should be postponed in patients with active chest infections to allow treatment with physiotherapy and antibiotics.

Patients with recurrent inguinal hernias may have to be warned that a satisfactory repair of the abdominal wall may only be possible if the testicle and spermatic cord are removed. Their consent must be obtained if this is being considered. This is not necessary if a recurrent hernia is being repaired laparoscopically. All patients should be warned, however, that testicular ischaemia and atrophy is a rare and unpredictable sequel of inguinal hernia repair occurring in approximately 1 : 5000 primary cases.

OPERATION: OPEN REPAIR OF INGUINAL HERNIA
The key to successful open inguinal hernia repair is identification of the hernia's anatomy before correction or repair of the anatomical defect. In an indirect hernia repair the sac must be separated from the structures of the spermatic cord taking great care not to damage the testicular vessels or vas deferens. The whole sac can then be reduced or, after ensuring the sac is empty (often by twisting it round), it can be transfixed at the level of the deep ring and the excess excised. In large inguinoscrotal sacs the distal

(scrotal) portion of the sac should be left open to prevent the formation of a postoperative hydrocoele. The testis should not be delivered from the scrotum into the groin during inguinal hernia repair as this increases the risk of ischaemia.

Direct sacs can sometimes be densely adherent to the spermatic cord making it initially difficult to differentiate from an indirect hernia. The key is the position of the inferior (deep) epigastric vessels to the neck of the hernia sac (lateral to a direct sac, medial to an indirect sac).

Two operations have proved reliable in the management of inguinal hernia using open techniques. In the Shouldice operation the transversalis fascia is opened from the deep ring to the pubic tubercle. The hernia sac (indirect, direct or sliding) is reduced into the preperitoneal space after which the transversalis fascia is repaired (using a double breasting suture) to produce a firm posterior wall and a new deep ring. In the Lichtenstein repair a prosthetic mesh (usually prolene) is sutured over the posterior wall of the canal between the inguinal ligament and the conjoint 'tendon' (fused internal oblique/transversus abdominis) again forming a new deep ring around the emergent spermatic cord.

Both these procedures can be performed under local anaesthetic and both give consistently excellent results (recurrence rates of less than 1% at 5 years) in expert hands. The Lichtenstein (often called tension-free) repair has gained popularity over the Shouldice technique because it is easier to teach and learn and gives more consistent results in the hands of less experienced surgeons.

Recurrent hernias pose a particularly difficult problem, especially when several previous attempts at repair have failed. For these cases the Stoppa operation has proved very useful. In this procedure a higher incision (above the groin) is made and the preperitoneal plane dissected (space between the peritoneum and the layered anterior abdominal wall muscles). A large prolene mesh is then inserted to line the lower anterior abdominal wall and pelvis thus covering all possible hernia defects and forming a strong and impenetrable lamina to further recurrence.

Procedure profile

Blood requirement	0
Anaesthetic	General, regional, spinal, local
Operation time	30–45 minutes
Hospital stay	Day case or planned overnight stay
Return to normal activity	2–3 weeks

Postoperatively the patient is mobilized early and can leave hospital as soon as he or she can walk independently. Hernias are increasingly repaired as day-case procedures. When a general anaesthetic is chosen it is useful to infiltrate the wound area with local anaesthetic to reduce postoperative pain. Pain may increase when the local anaesthetic wears off. Warn the patient to expect this. Strong analgesia may be required for the first 48 h but non-steroidal anti-inflammatory agents such as diclofenac or ibuprofen are very effective. Mild analgesics such as aspirin or paracetamol will suffice thereafter. The patient is usually advised to take things gently for 2 weeks from the operation date. Thereafter they should undertake gradually increasing exercise in order to regain muscular fitness. There is no evidence that early return to work increases the recurrence rate. Rather, the evidence is that prolonged inactivity increases the risk of recurrence and prolonged postoperative pain.

OPERATION: LAPAROSCOPIC REPAIR OF INGUINAL HERNIA

In this approach a prosthetic mesh is placed in the preperitoneal space (between peritoneum and anterior abdominal wall muscles) to cover the defect in the inguinal canal. The mesh must be large enough to overlap the margins of the weakness of the posterior wall of the inguinal canal with a wide (3 cm or greater) margin. Two methods have been described: a transabdominal preperitoneal repair (TAPP) or a totally extraperitoneal (TEP) repair. The TEP repair is rapidly gaining popularity because the laparoscopic ports do not need to traverse the peritoneal cavity (removing the risk of injuring intra-abdominal structures such as intestine).

Instead of an incision in the groin (painful) only three or four very small (5–10 mm) stab wounds are required for insertion of the laparoscopic ports. With infiltration of local anaesthetic around these at the end of the procedure, most patients require no additional postoperative analgesia. Return to full activity is quicker than after traditional open techniques. The operation is, however, more costly to the health service and is only effective and safe when the surgeon is specially skilled in laparoscopic surgical techniques. It is likely, therefore, that for many years to come the open repair will remain the standard technique for unilateral primary inguinal hernia repair with the laparoscopic technique reserved for patients with bilateral or recurrent hernias.

Procedure profile

Blood requirement	0
Anaesthetic	GA
Operation time	30–60 minutes
Hospital stay	Day case or overnight
Return to normal activity	7–10 days

Femoral hernia

Femoral hernias protrude down the femoral canal, which is medial to the femoral vessels and lateral to the pubic tubercle. From a knowledge of the anatomy of the femoral canal, it can be understood that femoral hernias always have a narrow neck. It is constricted by the inguinal ligament anteriorly; the pubic bone and reflected part of the inguinal ligament (lacunar ligament) medially; the pectineal part of the pubic bone posteriorly; and the femoral vein laterally (Fig. 10.1.3).

Consequently, the risk of strangulation is high. As the angle between the inguinal ligament and the pectineal part of the pubic bone is greater in females than males, the femoral canal is wider

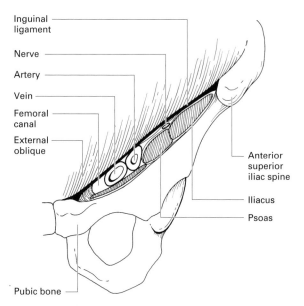

Fig. 10.1.3 The femoral canal lies behind the inguinal ligament medial to the femoral vein.

in females. Femoral hernias are far more common in females and are in fact quite rare in men.

Recognizing the pattern

The patient is nearly always female and middle aged or elderly, although femoral hernias can occur in either sex and at any age. The patient is nearly always thin or has lost weight recently, the hernia exploiting the 'weakness' in the femoral canal which is normally filled by fat to allow expansion of the femoral vein during times of increased blood flow. The history is of a lump appearing in the groin, which is frequently painful. Femoral hernias often present with an episode of strangulation and small bowel obstruction is not uncommon. A strangulated hernia will be missed if the groin is not adequately exposed during the

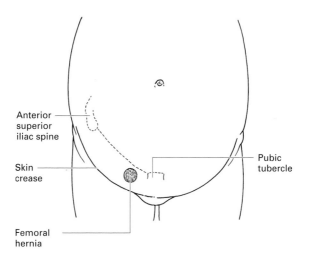

Fig. 10.1.4 Groin crease is not a guide to the position of the inguinal ligament. Always define the bony landmarks, especially in obese patients and children.

general examination of a patient with intestinal obstruction or abdominal pain.

On examination there is a rounded swelling tucked in medially in the groin. Its neck is below and lateral to the pubic tubercle. It may be of any size but is usually 2–3 cm in diameter. It is irreducible. If the hernia enlarges sufficiently, it tends to spread upwards over the inguinal ligament and pubic tubercle and at this stage can be confused with an inguinal hernia. If the groin is carefully palpated, however, its origin can be determined. Definition of a femoral hernia from an inguinal one is important as the former are much more likely to strangulate and should therefore be managed surgically without undue delay even in frail and elderly patients (Fig. 10.1.4).

Management

The management of a femoral hernia is surgical repair. A truss should never be prescribed. Two main approaches are possible:

- below the inguinal ligament
- above the inguinal ligament.

A strangulated hernia should always be approached from above in order to deal with possible bowel infarction.

OPERATION: FEMORAL HERNIA REPAIR – APPROACH FROM BELOW (LOCKWOOD'S OPERATION)

This approach is only used for the elective repair of non-strangulated femoral hernias. An incision is made in the groin below the inguinal ligament and the hernia found in the sub-cutaneous tissue. Its neck is isolated, the contents reduced back into the abdomen and the sac excised or fully reduced. The femoral canal is closed at its lower end by suturing the inguinal ligament to the pectineal fascia posteriorly. This operation is very minor and can be done under a local anaesthetic but great care must be taken to ensure the deep (pectineal) sutures are correctly placed. If they are placed too inferiorly they will cut out with inevitable recurrence.

Procedure profile

Blood requirement	0
Anaesthetic	GA or LA
Operation time	15–30 minutes
Hospital stay	Day case or planned overnight
Return to normal activity	2–3 weeks

OPERATION: FEMORAL HERNIA REPAIR – APPROACH FROM ABOVE THE INGUINAL LIGAMENT

This is the preferred approach when the hernia is painful or the patient has abdominal pain or vomiting indicating the possibility of bowel strangulation. It allows a simultaneous exploration of the peritoneal cavity (laparotomy) when bowel resection is required. The approach to the femoral ring is essentially preperitoneal exploiting the anatomical space between the peritoneum (and intra-abdominal contents) deeply and the anterior abdominal layers in front. Several variations have been described e.g.

Henry (midline between rectus abdominis) McEvedy (lateral to rectus abdominis) and Lotheissen (through posterior wall of inguinal canal). The latter is not recommended unless a coexistent inguinal hernia is also suspected or the surgeon cannot differentiate the site of the hernia.

The most satisfactory (simplest) method is a modification of the Henry operation. The patient is placed supine on the operating table under a general anaesthetic with 15° head-down tilt. The bladder is catheterized and emptied. An incision is made suprapubically (Pfannensteil). The external oblique is incised in the line of the skin incision and the rectus muscles retracted laterally to expose the preperitoneal space. Working downwards (usually from the opposite side of the table to the hernia) the surgeon dissects below the inguinal ligament to expose the neck of the hernia which can then be reduced with traction from above and pressure from below. If the hernia will not reduce (due to a tight neck) the lacunar ligament can be incised medially under direct vision thus avoiding injury to any vessels. Once reduced the sac can be opened to inspect any contents (and resect infarcted/strangulated intestine if necessary). The sac (peritoneum) is then closed and the hernia defect closed (repaired) with a series of interrupted non-absorbable sutures between the inguinal and pectineal ligaments taking care not to narrow the femoral vein.

It is very easy during this procedure to inspect the contralateral femoral ring at the same time and perform a bilateral repair if necessary.

Procedure profile

Blood requirement	0
Anaesthetic	GA
Operation time	30–60 minutes
Hospital stay	5–7 days
Return to normal activity	Up to 4 weeks

Postoperative care is much the same as for an open inguinal hernia repair. If a urinary catheter is used it is taken out on day 1.

Where a femoral hernia has been repaired electively with no bowel resection, the recovery is rapid for either surgical approach.

10.2 Other hernias

Incisional hernia

An incisional hernia occurs where there has been breakdown of the muscle closure in a previous abdominal wound. There is often a history of postoperative wound haematoma or sepsis but the hernia itself may not appear for several weeks or months after the initial operation.

Recognizing the pattern
The patient is often obese and elderly. The initial operation was commonly an emergency procedure and complicated by wound infection, haematoma and prolonged recovery.

The patient notices a bulge at the site of the previous operation scar often associated with discomfort. They may also suffer from more generalized abdominal pain associated with obstruction of loops of bowel within the hernia.

On examination the incisional hernia is easily visible when the patient stands up or strains but it may be invisible when they lie flat. It can usually be demonstrated by asking the patient either to cough or to tense their abdominal muscles by straight leg raising. The margins of the muscular defect are palpable beneath the skin and the size of the defect should be determined. Note whether the contents of the incisional hernia are fully reducible or not.

Management
Once the muscle layers of a laparotomy wound have separated, it is difficult to be certain of obtaining a sound repair at a second closure. Frequently the tissues are poor anyway, and the patient's obesity, age and poor health mitigate against obtaining a good result.

In the absence of obstructive symptoms conservative management is advised while attempts are made to improve the patient's general condition. The patient is strongly advised to lose weight and a surgical belt is provided to control the worst of the bulging. Preoperatively the patient should also stop smoking.

Significant discomfort or symptoms of obstruction are indications for surgery. The theatre staff frequently regard an incisional hernia repair as a minor operation and do not realize that its repair may entail a full laparotomy. The hernia cannot be repaired until the adherent loops of bowel have been freed and the edges of the muscle clearly defined. Deep instruments may therefore be necessary. It is essential that the anaesthetist and theatre staff be fully informed of the potential for operative complexity and a prolonged procedure. Epidural anaesthesia is often helpful for postoperative pain relief in difficult cases. Most surgeons cover this operation with prophylactic antibiotics to prevent would infection. Antiembolic measures should be used. The patient should be warned that the operation carries a significant failure rate for the reasons noted above.

OPERATION: OPEN REPAIR OF INCISIONAL HERNIA
The stretched scar in the skin is excised. The muscle edges are defined and adhesions divided. Often it is necessary to open the peritoneal cavity and great care should be taken to avoid intestinal injury. Several repairs have been described. Direct suturing is only recommended for defects less than 3 cm diameter. In this type of closure continuous or interrupted sutures are inserted taking wide bites of tissue. A large incisional hernia is best closed using a piece of mesh which is placed on the inner aspect of the abdominal wall and considerably 'underlaps' the previous defect placing it between the peritoneum and the abdominal wall muscles at the rim of the defect. It has been clearly demonstrated that any tension in the repair carries a high risk of recurrence. Specifically deep tension sutures are no longer recommended as they inevitably cut out and predispose to wound infection and recurrent weakness.

Procedure profile

Blood requirement	Group and save (or 2)
Anaesthetic	GA +/– epidural
Operation time	1–2 hours
Hospital stay	1–7 days
Return to normal activity	4–6 weeks

OPERATION: LAPARASCOPIC REPAIR OF INCISIONAL HERNIA

An increasing number of incisional hernias are being repaired using an intraperitoneal mesh. After establishing a pneumoperitoneum, adhesions are divided and the contents of the sac reduced. The laparascopic approach allows clear identification of all defects and these are covered by a mesh of appropriate size that extends about 2 cm beyond the margins of the hernia. In order to prevent adhesion to underlying bowel the deep surface of the mesh is coated with material such as Gore-Tex.

Procedure profile

Blood requirement	Group and save
Anaesthetic	GA
Operation time	1–2 hours
Hospital stay	1–3 days
Return to normal activity	2–4 weeks

Postoperatively, following repair of large defects, the patient may develop chest problems and chest physiotherapy will be important. An external binder can sometimes be used to take the tension off the wound.

Umbilical hernia

Hernias in this region are umbilical in infants, and paraumbilical in adults. Umbilical hernias in infants are dealt with on p. 594.

Paraumbilical hernia in adults
Recognising the pattern
A hernia in this site in adults occurs just adjacent to the umbilicus through a weakness in the linea alba. It is commoner in older women, and obesity, multiparity and weak abdominal muscles are predisposing causes. The sac may contain both omentum and bowel and in this age group gastrointestinal symptoms of subacute obstruction are more common. The hernia may become quite large and irreducible. Strangulation may occur. These hernias are increasingly seen following laparoscopic procedures and are therefore technically incisional hernias (sometimes called port-site hernias).

Management
The patient should be encouraged to lose weight where appropriate. Operation is usually advised because of the risk of strangulation although this remains small unless the hernia becomes large.

OPERATION: PARAUMBILICAL HERNIA REPAIR
For small to medium-sized hernias an incision is usually made along the lower lip of the umbilicus. The sac is dissected clear and then opened. The adhesions holding the bowel and omentum are freed and the bowel returned to the abdomen. The defect is then closed in one of several ways. Very small defects can be closed by direct sutures (non-absorbable) or figure of eight sutures. Larger defects require overlapping of the external oblique ('vest in pants' Mayo repair) or the use of a prosthetic mesh as for incisional hernias.

Procedure profile

Blood requirement	0
Anaesthetic	GA or LA
Operation time	30–45 minutes
Hospital stay	Day case or overnight (longer if extensive dissection is required)
Return to normal activity	1–3 weeks

Postoperative care is similar to that for an incisional hernia.

Epigastric hernia

This is a midline hernia through a defect in the linea alba above the umbilicus. The initial weakness may be at the site of a penetrating vessel. It usually contains extraperitoneal fat only, although if it enlarges a true peritoneal sac may protrude. In this case it may contain omentum. However, it hardly ever contains intestine.

Recognizing the pattern
The hernia presents as a small painless swelling in the epigastrium. It may be painful on exercise. Occasionally it causes episodes of severe epigastric pain and vomiting. These episodes may have been extensively investigated but no cause found previously.

On examination the small epigastric mass is palpable and more prominent when the patient coughs or tenses the abdominal muscles. If the defect is small the hernia (which can be quite large) may not have a cough impulse (similar to femoral hernias).

Management
These hernias usually require operative repair.

OPERATION: REPAIR OF EPIGASTRIC HERNIA
A transverse skin incision is made over the hernia. The fatty hernia is excised and the defect in the linea alba closed with non-absorbable sutures. There may be other epigastric hernias present which should also be removed.

Procedure profile

Blood requirement	0
Anaesthetic	GA or LA
Operation time	15 minutes
Hospital stay	Day case
Return to normal activity	3–7 days

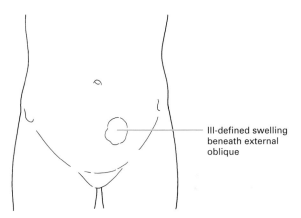

Fig. 10.2.1 Spigelian hernia.

Spigelian hernia (interstitial hernia)

In these quite rare hernias the sac protrudes through the linea semilunaris (the lateral edge of the rectus sheath), at the level of the semi-circular fold of Douglas (Fig. 10.2.1). It usually lies underneath the external oblique, between it and the internal oblique. These hernias often have a narrow neck and strangulation may occur.

Recognizing the pattern

They are usually seen in obese people over the age of 50 years and present as a swelling below and lateral to the umbilicus. They may cause some discomfort, which is worse on exertion, and occasionally cause nausea and vomiting when intestinal contents become strangulated.

Management

The management is by surgical repair.

OPERATION: REPAIR OF SPIGELIAN HERNIA

The skin incision is placed transversely over the hernia. It is useful to mark the site with the patient awake and standing as these hernias often reduce when anaesthesia is induced making identification of the site of the hernia impossible. The sac is isolated, emptied and ligated, and the defect closed in layers. The operation can be performed laparoscopically when a piece of mesh is placed internal to the defect in the preperitoneal space. In the open operation mesh is also favoured to minimize the risk of recurrence.

Procedure profile

Blood requirement	0
Anaesthetic	GA
Operation time	30–45 minutes
Hospital stay	Day case or planned overnight
Return to normal activity	2–3 weeks

Obturator hernia

This is a very rare hernia that protrudes from the pelvis out through the obturator canal. It lies beneath the adductor muscles of the floor of the femoral triangle in the upper thigh.

Recognising the pattern
These hernias are commoner in women. The swelling is usually hidden, although it may be more obvious if the leg is laterally rotated, abducted and flexed. Pain is often referred along the obturator nerve to the knee. These hernias are often not recognized until they present with intestinal obstruction or strangulation. As with femoral hernias a Richter's type of strangulation/partial obstruction can occur (see Fig. 10.2.2a).

Management
The management is by surgical repair.

OPERATION: REPAIR OF OBTURATOR HERNIA
The hernia is repaired from above, usually through a lower midline laparotomy incision performed in a patient with bowel obstruction.

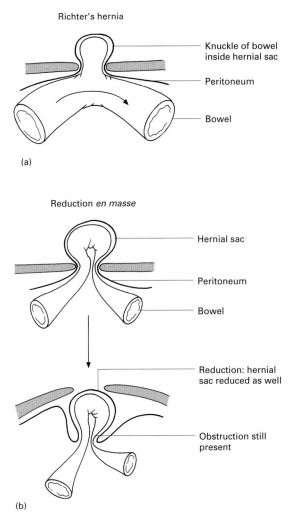

Fig. 10.2.2 Some terms used for special types of strangulation. (a) Richter's hernia; (b) reduction *en masse*.

Procedure profile

Blood requirement	Group and save if laparotomy planned
Anaesthetic	GA +/− epidural
Operation time	30–60 minutes
Hospital stay	1–7 days
Return to normal activity	4 weeks

Strangulated hernia

Most types of hernia may become irreducible and are at risk of strangulation and obstruction. The following text should be read in conjunction with p. 308, covering small bowel obstruction in general.

  Various stages are recognized.

- In a simple irreducible hernia, the contents cannot be reduced but the blood supply is intact and there are no symptoms of intestinal obstruction. The usual cause is adhesions between the sac and its contents and a neck tight enough to prevent reduction but not compromise blood supply. At this stage the hernia is usually not painful.
- In an obstructed hernia, the sac contains bowel which has become obstructed.
- In a strangulated hernia, the blood supply of the contents is compromised and there is a danger of, or actual, necrosis of the tissues enclosed in the hernia. Both the preceding types of irreducible hernia predispose to strangulation.
- Richter's hernia. A knuckle of the sidewall of the bowel is caught in the sac but the continuity of the bowel is maintained (Fig. 10.2.2a). In this case the bowel wall is strangulated but there is no intestinal obstruction at least in the early stages. This is seen most commonly in femoral hernias but can also be seen in obturator hernias.
- Reduction *en masse*. If an irreducible/obstructed hernia is forcibly reduced it is possible to reduce the visible mass of the hernia but for the sac and its neck to be reduced as well. In this

case the contents remain potentially strangulated even though the external hernia has disappeared (Fig. 10.2.2b). Any clinician attempting to reduce a strangulated hernia must be aware of this possibility. If the patient's symptoms (e.g. of bowel obstruction and abdominal pain) persist after reduction of the hernia, early operation is indicated.

Recognizing the pattern

Either a pre-existing hernia suddenly becomes irreducible, painful and tender or the patient presents with a new tender mass at a hernia site. There may be accompanying symptoms of intestinal obstruction. Occasionally patients present only with general abdominal symptoms and have not themselves noticed the hernia. Examination of potential hernia sites is mandatory in such patients.

The hernia is irreducible and tender. A distended abdomen and obstructive bowel sounds may confirm suspicions of intestinal obstruction. A supine abdominal X-ray may be helpful showing dilated bowel loops.

Management

A strangulated hernia must be explored surgically, the hernia reduced and the contents examined and resected if non-viable.

Patients with intestinal obstruction will be dehydrated even if the initial serum urea and electrolyte measurement is normal. They require a good quality intravenous drip. If the hernia cannot be reduced, urgent operation is required. The serum electrolytes should be within the normal range before the anaesthetic is given. The operative site should be shaved before the operation starts. A strangulated hernia is often infected and antibiotics should be given on induction of anaesthesia. A wide-bore nasogastric tube should be positioned and aspirated before induction. If this is not possible a rapid sequence induction will be used with cricoid pressure on intubation (with a cuffed endotracheal tube).

OPERATION: FOR STRANGULATED HERNIAS

The details are given under individual hernias and small bowel resection. In general, the sac is opened and the contents inspected and then the strangulation released. The affected bowel is wrapped in a warm saline swab. It may be necessary to wait several minutes in order to be sure that it is viable. If it is not, it is resected. If there is gross contamination, the wound will need to be drained. Such a drain can be removed when its contents are clear, serous or slightly serosanguinous and the patients pulse and temperature have been normal for 24 h.

Procedure profile

Blood requirement	Group and save (or 2)
Anaesthetic	GA +/− epidural
Operation time	69–90 minutes
Hospital stay	About 7 days, depending on extent of resection and degree of ileus
Return to normal activity	4 weeks

Postoperatively the patient may have an ileus for 1–2 days and should continue on intravenous fluids and restricted oral intake. Apart from this the postoperative course is as for any other hernia.

11 Urinary tract surgery

11.1 Disorders of the upper urinary tract

Renal pain is felt in the loin between the twelfth rib and the iliac crest. The pain is usually more or less constant. Ureteric pain is colicky and radiates down and forwards from the loin to the groin, vulva or scrotum. Common surgical causes of renal pain are stones, pyelonephritis, ureteric obstruction and, rarely, renal tumours.

Renal tract stones

Stones form in the renal tract due to increased concentration of solutes in the urine such as calcium, uric acid or oxalic acid during periods of dehydration. Rarely a specific biochemical abnormality (such as hyperparathyroidism) is the cause. Roughened areas within the renal pelvis and calyces may act as focal points for the formation of stones (Randall's plaques). Other predisposing factors include stasis and pooling of urine due to obstruction and urinary infection.

The commonest type of stone is composed of calcium and magnesium phosphates and carbonates. These precipitate in alkaline urine and are soft and friable. The commonest pure stones are calcium oxalate. They are hard and rough and may cause haematuria. The formation of both calcium oxalate and uric acid stones is favoured by acid urine. Oxalate stones are radio-opaque and cystine and uric acid calculi are radiolucent.

The stones are usually formed in the renal calyces or pelvis. They may continue growing to fill the whole of the renal pelvis (staghorn calculus). Alternatively, they may remain small and

Surgery: Diagnosis and Management, 4th edition. Edited by N. Rawlinson and D. Alderson. © 2009 Blackwell Publishing, ISBN: 978-1-4051-2921-3

pass down the ureter into the bladder causing ureteric colic. The stone may become stuck at any point in this passage, but particularly at the:

- pelviureteric junction
- crossing point of the ureter and iliac artery
- entrance of the ureter into the bladder.

Infection may develop proximal to an impacted stone, and if the upper tract is obstructed, a pyonephrosis may develop. This condition, in which the renal pelvis and proximal ureter are filled with pus, constitutes a surgical emergency, since it requires urgent decompression and drainage to prevent septicaemia, shock and renal damage.

Recognizing the pattern

The patient may be of any age, although stones are unusual before adolescence. Males are more commonly affected than females in a ratio of 2 : 1.

Stones within the kidney give rise to pain in the loin and often present with episodes of urinary infection. If a stone passes down the ureter, the patient experiences excruciating bouts of severe colic starting in the loin and radiating round into the flank and groin. The pain is so severe that the sufferer tends to roll around in agony unable to find a comfortable position.

On examination there may be tenderness in the renal angle but the physical signs are minimal compared with the severity of the pain. Constitutional upset with fever and malaise indicate secondary infection.

Proving the diagnosis

The presence of red cells in the urine on microscopy is a helpful finding. In the early stages these may be absent and in that case the examination should be repeated after 24–48 h. Evidence of infection should also be sought (midstream urine, MSU).

A plain abdominal X-ray taken in the kidneys, ureters and bladder (KUB) may show the stone lying in the kidney substance or along the line of the ureter (Fig. 11.1.1). Ninety per cent of urinary stones are radio-opaque (compared with 10% of gall-stones). If a stone is seen, its diameter should be measured, since this will indicate whether it is likely to pass spontaneously.

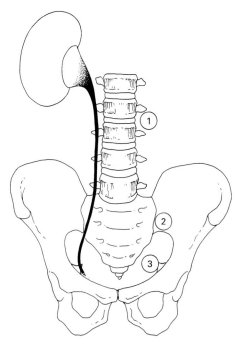

Fig. 11.1.1 The landmarks for the ureter on an abdominal X-ray. 1, lumbar transverse processes; 2, sacroiliac joint; 3, ischial spine.

An emergency CT scan (CT-KUB) or intravenous urogram (IVU) will confirm the diagnosis and show the position of the stone.

Screening tests for raised serum calcium and uric acid should always be performed.

Management

This is either conservative or operative, the choice depending on the size and position of the stone. Try to decide whether the stone will pass spontaneously. The critical size is 0.5 cm.

If it is clearly too large to travel down the ureter, then it must be removed. If, however, natural passage is possible, then the initial management is usually conservative. If there is infection in an obstructed upper tract, drainage must be established. This is usually achieved by means of a percutaneous nephrostomy tube, inserted by a radiologist under ultrasound guidance.

The patient is put on a regular non-steroidal analgesic (e.g. diclofenac suppository), although pethidine may be required in severe colic. The patient will often require admission. The urine should be sieved to detect the passed stone. Patients are usually discharged when pain free and followed up by KUB to ensure the stone has gone. If the stone is still present after a reasonable time (2–4 weeks) then consider surgical treatment.

The surgical management of urinary calculi has advanced rapidly in the last decade. Using percutaneous renal surgery a track can be created between the skin and the intrarenal collecting system. A nephroscope can then be passed and the stone removed with forceps. If the stone is too large, it can be disintegrated by ultrasound or shattered by an electrohydraulic discharge. The fragments are then removed.

Extracorporeal shock-wave lithotripsy (ESWL) was first developed in Germany. In the early lithotriptors, a shock wave was created by an underwater spark generator and the energy was focused onto the stone by positioning the patient in a bath, using X-ray screening to locate the stone. A general anaesthetic was often necessary. More modern lithotriptors use electromagnetic or piezoelectric-generated shock waves and are preferable because they require minimal analgesia.

Surgical intervention is indicated for renal stones if lithotripsy is not available or fails, or if the stone is too large (e.g. some staghorn calculi). The surgical management of the stone depends on whether it lies in the kidney or ureter and, if in the ureter, at what level.

Management of stones in the kidney

Ninety per cent of renal stones can be treated by endoscopic surgery (the technique is similar to that described in the ureter although a flexible ureteroscope is required), percutaneous renal surgery and/or ESWL. For the rest, open surgery may be required. Occasionally a nephrectomy is required for a staghorn calculus if a preoperative radionuclide scan has demonstrated that the kidney contributes less than 15% of the overall renal function.

If the urine is infected, antibiotics are commenced preoperatively. The stone or stones must be adequately demonstrated radiologically. The timing of the surgery should be coordinated with the radiologist if percutaneous surgery is planned. The radiographers should also be warned that they will be required during the operation.

OPERATION: PERCUTANEOUS NEPHROLITHOTOMY (PCNL)

A cystoscope is passed and a ureteric catheter inserted into the ureteric orifice on the appropriate side. Radio-opaque contrast solution is introduced. Under X-ray-screening a trocar needle is inserted into the renal pelvis via a percutaneous puncture in the flank. The tract is then dilated over a guide wire, so that it will admit a larger sheath, through which a rigid nephroscope is inserted. Calculi in the renal pelvis are extracted. It may be necessary to fragment larger stones using a lithoclast or other technique. The renal pelvis is irrigated and an X-ray obtained to confirm that all the stones have been removed. A nephrostomy drain is inserted, via the tract, into the renal pelvis. Staghorn calculi may require more than one percutaneous puncture for removal or a combination of PCNL and ESWL.

Procedure profile

Blood requirement	Group and save
Anaesthetic	GA
Operation time	1–3 hours
Hospital stay	3–5 days
Return to normal activity	2 weeks

Postoperatively a nephrostogram is performed when the urine draining through the nephrostomy tube is clear to ensure that there is free passage of urine down the ureter, before the nephrostomy is removed.

The patient should be encouraged to drink as much fluid as possible and ideally over 2.5 L/day. Any cause of renal stones found on screening must be treated.

Management of stones in the ureter

Stones in the mid- and lower ureter may be treated either by ESWL or by endoscopic surgery when a rigid or flexible instrument is passed into the ureter and the stone fragmented using one of many available energy sources (laser, pneumatic drill, electrical spark). The fragments are removed using grasping forceps and a stent is usually placed at the end of the procedure.

Stones in the upper ureter may also be treated by ESWL, or they may be pushed into the renal pelvis and treated as a renal stone by percutaneous renal surgery or by ESWL. Rarely, if non-invasive methods fail, open or laparoscopic surgery is performed.

OPERATION: ENDOSCOPIC TREATMENT OF URETERIC STONE

Stones in the lower third of the ureter may be removed by passing a cystoscope into the bladder through which a flexible guide wire is passed into the ureteric orifice in question and manipulated beyond the stone. A rigid or flexible ureteroscope is exchanged for the cystoscope and the guide wire used to give passage of the scope into the ureter. X ray image intensification is used throughout. With the stone visualized a Holmium laser fibre is passed down the working channel of the ureteroscope and the stone is slowly disintegrated with the laser energy. Larger stone fragments are removed from the ureter by passing forceps or baskets down the scope. Small fragments are left to pass spontaneously. A double pigtail stent is usually passed at the end of the procedure along the course of the ureter to facilitate fragment and blood clot passage. A date is set to remove the stent within 2 weeks of the procedure.

Procedure profile

Blood requirement	0
Anaesthetic	GA
Operation time	Variable
Hospital stay	1–3 days
Return to normal activity	Variable – 4–6 weeks of open procedure

Pyelonephritis

This is due to parenchymal infection of the kidney secondary to either ascending infection from the bladder or problems in the kidney itself such as renal stones or pelviureteric obstruction. Occasionally the kidney may become infected as a complication of septicaemia. The organism is usually a Gram-negative bacillus. Pyelonephritis with urinary tract obstruction is an emergency and should be diagnosed without delay. Rapid progression to septicaemia and shock can occur.

Recognizing the pattern

The patient is of any age but more frequently female and of child-bearing age.

There is a sudden onset of illness with a high fever and vomiting. The systemic symptoms are often dominant and the patient may not complain of any symptoms referable to the urinary tract in the early stages. On questioning, however, there may be pain in the loin and this can be severe. The patient may describe symptoms of a urinary tract infection, such as frequency and dysuria, and may give a past history of similar episodes.

On examination there may be a tachycardia and a high fever (up to 39.5°C) often with rigors. There is localized tenderness over the affected kidney.

Proving the diagnosis

The diagnosis is confirmed by finding bacteria and pus cells in the urine. Pus cells may be absent in the early stages if the affected kidney shuts down and fails to excrete infected urine into the bladder. One negative midstream urine specimen (MSU) should not therefore be taken as excluding the diagnosis but must be repeated.

An ultrasound is performed to exclude pyonephrosis. A plain abdominal X-ray may show an associated calculus in the position of the kidney or ureter, which should subsequently be confirmed on a CT-KUB or IVU.

Management

It is important to arrange urinary and blood cultures before treatment is commenced. If the kidney is obstructed it is urgently decompressed by inserting a percutaneous nephrostomy tube. Antibiotics are given in high dosage, intravenously if necessary. Analgesia (opiates or non-steroidal anti-inflammatories) may be needed. If a perinephric abscess forms, it is drained through a loin incision.

Renal tumours

Renal tumours may be either benign or malignant. Benign tumours include cysts and true benign neoplasms. Malignant tumours may be primary or secondary. Primary renal tumours arise either from the urothelium of the calyces and pelvis (pelvi-ureteric transitional cell cancers) or from the kidney substance itself (renal cell cancer, clear cell cancer or hypernephroma).

Pelviureteric transitional cell cancers

Urothelial tumours can arise anywhere where there is transitional cell epithelium. They are associated with the ingestion of carcinogens such as noxious chemicals in tobacco smoke and some industrial carcinogens.

Recognizing the pattern

The patient is usually over the age of 40 years. They present with a history of painless haematuria or occasionally ureteric colic associated with the passage of a clot. There are usually no physical signs.

Proving the diagnosis

An IVU or CT scan will show either a filling defect in the renal tract, evidence of obstruction, with hydronephrosis, or a non-functioning kidney. If the filling defect is not demonstrated, a retrograde ureteropyelogram, via a ureteric catheter inserted at cystoscopy or a ureteroscopy may be performed. Urinary cytology may show carcinoma cells.

Management

As a urothelial tumour represents instability in the epithelium of the renal tract, it is usually considered necessary to remove the whole of the renal tract on the affected side. The need for this must be explained to the patient. Occasionally two incisions are necessary, one in the loin to remove the kidney and a second in the lower abdomen to remove the pelvic part of the ureter. The procedure is increasingly performed by laparoscopic surgery.

OPERATION: NEPHROURETERECTOMY
The kidney is explored and its vessels isolated and ligated via loin, anterior or midline incisions, or via a laparascopic approach. The kidney is removed and the ureter is followed down into the pelvis and excised together with a cuff of the bladder mucosa. The bladder muscle is repaired. A urinary catheter is left in situ and the renal bed drained.

Procedure profile

Blood requirement	2
Anaesthetic	GA
Operation time	2–3 hours
Hospital stay	5–10 days
Return to normal activity	4–6 weeks (open), 2–4 weeks (laparoscopic)

Postoperatively there is a danger of haemorrhage into the renal bed and the vital signs must be carefully monitored. The urinary catheter should not be removed until it is clear that the bladder repair has healed. This usually occurs within 7 days. If there is any doubt, a cystogram is helpful.

The patient should be followed up by cystoscopy and with regular review of the other kidney by IVU. This is in order to detect the development of further tumours.

Renal cell cancer (hypernephroma, clear cell cancer or the kidney)

Renal cell cancer is an adenocarcinoma arising from the substance of the kidney. The tumour may grow very large. It tends to spread along the renal vein and grow into the inferior vena cava.

It may even extend into the right atrium of the heart. Metastasis occurs via the lymphatics to para-aortic lymph nodes and via the bloodstream to the lungs, brain and bone. It may be clinically silent until it has grown to a large size, and systemic symptoms often divert attention away from the local disease.

Recognizing the pattern

The patient is usually over 50 years old and more commonly male. However, the disease can also affect young people and can present with a wide variety of symptoms. The typical triad is a palpable mass, loin pain and haematuria.

It may present in less typical ways such as with a pyrexia of unknown origin associated with night sweats. The tumour may bleed into the renal tract, producing 'clot colic' or anaemia. Patients may also present with symptoms from metastases (e.g. pathological fracture). A tumour spreading along the renal vein sometimes obstructs the testicular vein on the left, causing a varicocoele. Finally, hormonal secretion from the growth may cause hypertension (renin), polycythaemia (erythropoietin) or hypercalcaemia (parathormone). Renal cell cancers are increasingly noted incidentally on imaging for other symptoms.

On examination the lump in the loin may be palpable. It is usually only possible to feel the lower pole, which may be ballotted and moves down on respiration. It is resonant to percussion due to the overlying colon.

Proving the diagnosis

Investigation of the urine will often show microscopic haematuria. An ultrasound of the renal area shows a solid mass arising from the kidney. The ultrasound may also be used to investigate whether or not there is growth in the renal vein and vena cava. An IVU will show a renal mass distorting the calyces and will also demonstrate contralateral renal function. A CT scan, with intravenous contrast, is performed to assess the degree of local spread, the exact size of the tumour and the presence of para-aortic lymph node metastases. This will also demonstrate a normal functioning contralateral kidney, which is crucial if a total nephrectomy is contemplated. Bilateral cancers are occasionally demonstrated on a CT scan and may be associated with a familial condition called von Hippel–Lindau disease.

Management

During the preoperative work-up, a careful search should be made for the presence of metastases. A chest X-ray should be performed. A biochemical profile and full blood count are helpful in detecting metabolic or haematological complications of the tumour.

The standard treatment for patients with hypernephroma is radical nephrectomy by open operation. A laparoscopic approach is increasingly being used for smaller tumours. Even if metastases are present, this operation will control symptoms related to the primary tumour, such as haematuria and pain and may be a prerequisite for adjuvant chemotherapy or immunotherapy with interleukins and interferons. Partial nephrectomy is considered when the tumour is small or it is important to preserve normal renal tissue.

OPERATION: RADICAL NEPHRECTOMY

The tumour may be very bulky and this can make the operation difficult and increase the blood loss. Occasionally it is necessary to open the chest and divide the diaphragm in order to get adequate exposure.

The kidney is usually exposed via either anterior, transperitoneal or loin incisions, or via a laparascopic approach. You should determine which approach the surgeon intends and inform the theatre staff and anaesthetist. When the approach is through the bed of a rib, a pneumothorax is not uncommon. A chest drain may be needed postoperatively.

If the tumour is invading the inferior vena cava, then the surgeon will have to control that vessel in order to effect an adequate removal. The chest may be opened to achieve this. The renal vessels are ligated and the kidney, together with the adrenal, the surrounding fat and fascia and the upper ureter are removed. A drain may be left in the renal bed.

Procedure profile

Blood requirement	2–6
Anaesthetic	GA
Operation time	2–3 hours
Hospital stay	5–10 days
Return to normal activity	4–6 weeks (open), 2–4 (laparoscopic)

Where a pneumothorax has occurred, a postoperative chest X-ray should be carried out in the erect position in the first few hours after the operation to check that the lung has fully re-expanded.

There is a danger of haemorrhage in the first 24 h and careful monitoring of pulse, blood pressure and fluid balance is necessary during this period. There may be an ileus but this is not usually prolonged beyond 48 h. Very occasionally surrounding organs are damaged during the removal of a large tumour. Examples of this are damage to the tail of the pancreas on the left side (risking a pancreatic fistula) and damage to the stomach, colon or spleen.

Haematuria

Haematuria is a common presenting complaint and a routine series of investigations is undertaken. There are three important points to establish in the history.

Is it true haematuria?
Other causes of red urine include the following:
- drugs, e.g. rifampicin, para-aminosalicylic acid (PAS), nitrofurantoin and phenindione
- foodstuffs such as beetroot
- porphyria
- haemoglobinuria
- factitious haematuria.

The differentiation can be made on the history and on urine microscopy. Ward testing 'stix' for blood are also helpful, though they may also be positive in porphyria and haemoglobinuria.

It is also important to make certain that the blood is not coming from the vagina or rectum. This can be discovered by a careful history and examination.

The causes of true haematuria are listed in Table 11.1.1.

What is the timing of the bleeding in the urinary stream?
Blood at the start of the urinary stream suggests a urethral lesion. Blood at the end of the urinary stream suggests a localized

Table 11.1.1 Causes of haematuria.

General
Bleeding disorders
Anticoagulants
Haemoglobinopathy

Local
Kidney
Glomerulonephritis
Carcinoma
Trauma
Infarction
Papillary necrosis

Ureter
Tumours
Stones

Bladder
Cystitis
Trauma
Foreign body
Stones
Tumours

Urethra
Benign prostatic hypertrophy
Prostatic carcinoma
Urothelial tumours

bladder lesion. Blood showing throughout micturition suggests a renal, ureteric or diffuse bladder disorder.

Is the haematuria painful or not?

In painful haematuria the bleeding is usually secondary to a cystitis, which may itself be secondary to other problems such as bladder neck obstruction or stones (see p. 441). You have to remember, however, that infection is a common complication of urothelial tumours.

In painless haematuria further investigation is mandatory to exclude a carcinoma.

Proving the diagnosis
- Microscopy and culture of MSU. Red cell casts or protein indicates glomerular disease. Pus cells are present in an acute infection. If they are present and the urine is sterile, the possibility of tuberculosis, tumour or calculi must be considered.
- Exfoliative cytology of a fresh specimen of urine may show tumour cells.
- An ultrasound or IVU is mandatory in all cases of painless haematuria and in most cases of painful haematuria.
- Cystoscopy is mandatory in adults (usually flexible cystoscopy under local anaesthetic).

Management
The treatment of cystitis is with antibiotics, and, if it is the first episode in a young woman, no further investigation may be needed providing the haematuria settles. If it persists, if the infection recurs or if the patient is male, further investigation of the urinary tract by cystoscopy and IVU is required. This is in order to exclude causes such as urothelial tumours, calculi or prostatic hypertrophy.

The management of renal cell cancer is dealt with on p. 437, pelviureteric tumours on p. 434 and bladder tumours on p. 446.

Recurrent bleeding due to enlarged veins on a benign prostate may necessitate prostatectomy or the use of 5-α-reductase inhibiting drugs.

Ureteric obstruction

The ureters may be obstructed by intrinsic (stone, clot, tumour) or extrinsic (compression) lesions. Either may cause hydronephrosis and ultimately, if unresolved, renal impairment. Pain may be colicky or persistent. Occasionally the pelviureteric junction may be extremely tight (PUJ obstruction). The pain with PUJ obstruction is typically made worse after drinking excessive volume.

Recognizing the pattern
Pain may or may not be a feature. Haematuria may be present. Suspect ureteric obstruction in all cases of unexplained renal failure. Hydronephrosis is often detected incidentally.

Proving the diagnosis

Ultrasound is effective at demonstrating hydronephrosis. Other imaging (CT scan, IVU) may be required. Retrograde studies are helpful to determine the exact level of ureteric obstruction.

Management

Tailor the management to the cause. In cases of PUJ obstruction the tight ureteric segment is excised and the ureter is reformed over a stent. This is increasingly performed as a laparoscopic operation. External compression is most often due to cancers of the colon, rectum, bladder, prostate or cervix. If the ureter cannot be easily separated from the cancer then the kidney may need to be removed or drained externally. Occasionally the ureter can be rerouted and anastomosed to the opposite ureter (transureteroureterostomy).

11.2 Conditions of the lower urinary tract

Bladder stones

Bladder calculi have the same aetiology as renal calculi. A stone in the bladder may have originated in the renal pelvis, although if a stone can pass down the ureter it usually manages to pass out through the urethra. In most cases bladder stones form primarily in the bladder. Stone formation is favoured by urinary stasis (e.g. bladder diverticulum, bladder outflow obstruction), infection or the presence of a foreign body.

Recognizing the pattern

Bladder stones can occur in any age group. Males are more commonly affected than females.

The typical pattern of symptoms is pain, frequency and haematuria. The pain is felt in the suprapubic area, perineum and tip of the penis or labium majus. It is worse when the patient is upright and the stone is lying on the trigone. The pain increases with any jolting movements or at the end of micturition. Urinary frequency is also more troublesome during the day and there may be a feeling of incomplete emptying after micturition. Haematuria commonly occurs at the end of the stream. Occasionally there may be intermittent obstruction to urinary flow.

On examination the prostate may be enlarged. In women it may be possible to feel a bladder stone on bimanual vaginal examination.

Proving the diagnosis
- Test the urine for blood, pus cells and evidence of infection.
- Request a plain abdominal X-ray; 90% of bladder stones are radio-opaque.
- Cystoscopy enables you to see the bladder stone and also to look for any predisposing pathology (e.g. prostatic hypertrophy or bladder diverticulum).

Management
Stones in the bladder should be removed either by endoscopic surgery or by open bladder surgery (cystolitholapaxy).

OPERATION: ENDOSCOPIC REMOVAL OF BLADDER STONE (LITHOLAPAXY)
The stone is visualized, using a rigid cystoscope. It must be fragmented prior to removal by using a lithoclast, or alternatively by crushing it with a lithotrite. The smaller pieces of the stone are then washed out from the bladder. If there is a urethral stricture or enlarged prostate, this is usually treated at the same time, e.g. by dilatation or transurethral resection of the prostate (TURP) (see p. 458).

Procedure profile

Blood requirement	0
Anaesthetic	GA
Operation time	30–60 minutes
Hospital stay	2–5 days
Return to normal activity	1–2 weeks

Litholapaxy is not suitable for larger or particularly hard stones, or for stones that have formed around a foreign body. In these cases, or if there is another lesion which will require open operation (e.g. a very large prostate or a bladder diverticulum) the stone is removed via an open cystostomy.

OPERATION: CYSTOLITHOLAPAXY
The bladder is approached by either a transverse suprapubic (Pfannenstiel) incision or a vertical midline incision. The rectus muscles are retracted and the bladder opened between stay sutures. The stone is removed and any predisposing cause also treated. A suprapubic catheter is left in the bladder, and a urethral catheter inserted if a prostatectomy has been performed. The bladder is closed in two layers. A drain is left in the wound.

Procedure profile

Blood requirement	Group and save
Anaesthetic	GA
Operation time	1–2 hours
Hospital stay	7 days
Return to normal activity	4–6 weeks

The bladder wound heals in 5–7 days and the catheter is then removed. It is important to avoid urinary infection and prophylactic antibiotics are given over the early postoperative course.

Bladder tumours

Virtually all bladder tumours are malignant and of these, 95% are transitional cell carcinomas (TCCs). The remainder are rare and are either squamous cell carcinomas (associated with chronic irritation and squamous metaplasia due to bilharzia, bladder stones or indwelling urinary catheters) or adenocarcinomas (associated with ectopia vesicae or persistent urachal remnants).

The majority of TCCs have no known aetiology. However, there is an increased incidence in those who have worked in the dye, rubber and printing industries. Beta-naphthylamine and benzidine have been implicated as the carcinogens. Smokers have an increased risk of developing TCCs, as have those who have had pelvic irradiation or who have been treated with cyclophosphamide.

TCCs are staged according to the TNM classification (T = tumour, N = nodes, M = metastases; Fig. 11.2.1). The tumour staging is as follows.

- Cis: in situ carcinoma affects multiple areas in the bladder and has a tendency to progress to anaplastic and invasive disease.
- Ta: papillary, no invasion of lamina propria.
- T1: invades lamia propria.
- T2a: invades superficial muscle.
- T2b: invades deep muscle.
- T3: invades perivesical tissue.
- T4: invades adjoining organs such as prostate, uterus and pelvic side wall.

If the tumour is staged by the pathologist, then the stage is prefixed by 'p' (i.e. Ta becomes pTa).

Tumours are also graded on histological appearance:

- G1: well differentiated
- G2: moderately differentiated
- G3: poorly differentiated.

Recognizing the pattern

Ninety per cent of patients present with painless haematuria, occasionally passing clots which may lead to clot retention; 15% have frequency and dysuria due to carcinoma in situ or to associated infection. Obstruction of the bladder neck may cause the symptoms of retention of urine. Involvement of the ureteric orifices can cause hydronephrosis and loin pain. Nerve involvement causes continuous suprapubic pain radiating to the groin and perineum.

Usually there are no signs. The patient may be anaemic secondary to prolonged or severe blood loss. In advanced cases abdominal examination may reveal a palpable mass in the pelvis, enlarged lymph nodes in the groin or a palpable liver.

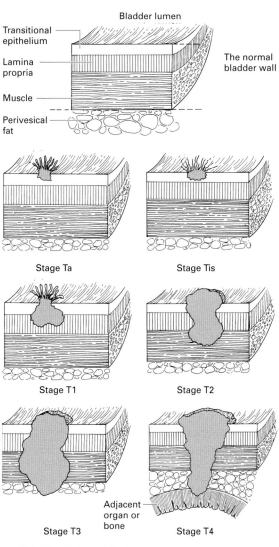

Fig. 11.2.1 The staging of bladder tumours.

Proving the diagnosis

- Urine microscopy and culture. This will demonstrate the presence of red cells due to bleeding and white cells due to infection, or occasionally sterile pyuria due to the tumour.
- Urine cytology. This may show the presence of malignant cells, particularly if there is carcinoma in situ.
- IVU. The tumour may appear as a filling defect in the bladder and the function of both kidneys can be assessed.
- Flexible cystoscopy. This is the gold standard investigation, since it allows the tumour to be visualized.

Staging

Bladder tumour staging is a combination of pathological assessment (see above) taken together with the impression of the examining surgeon (at the time of tumour resection) and the results of a CT scan performed for all tumours thought to be invading deep muscle. Tumours fall into two broad categories – superficial (non-invasive) bladder cancer and invasive (into muscle and beyond).

Management

Carcinoma in situ may be treated with a course of intravesical immunotherapy (bacille Calmette–Guérin or BCG), following which a further cystoscopy is performed and biopsies taken. If there is evidence of residual disease, then cystectomy should be considered.

Superficial TCCs (stages Ta and T1) are treated initially by transurethral resection. For multiple tumours, a course of intravesical chemotherapy (mitomycin C or epirubicin) or immunotherapy (BCG) is appropriate. All patients with superficial bladder tumours need to be followed up with regular check cystoscopies, initially after 3 months, as recurrence is likely. Recurrences are treated by cystodiathermy. Five per cent of superficial tumours become invasive.

Invasive TCCs (stages T2, T3 and T4) are treated by removal of the bladder (cystectomy) and subsequent diversion of the ureters to either a 'neo bladder' formed from small intestine or a conduit to the skin (usually formed from ileum and called an ileal conduit). An alternative to surgery is radical radiotherapy.

Radiotherapy may also be used to palliate non-curable tumours that bleed and cause pain. Chemotherapy for advanced disease is partially effective.

OPERATION: TRANSURETHRAL RESECTION OF BLADDER TUMOUR (TURBT)

The tumour is excised completely, including the superficial layer of bladder wall muscle in its base, using the resectoscope. The specimens are sent for histological staging. The main danger of this procedure is bladder wall perforation.

Procedure profile

Blood requirement	Group and save
Anaesthetic	GA
Operation time	30–60 minutes
Hospital stay	3–4 days
Return to normal activity	1–2 weeks

OPERATION: RADICAL CYSTECTOMY

If the patient is to have an ileal conduit, the site of this should be established preoperatively and the skin marked. If the patient is to have a neobladder then they should still be marked and counselled about an ileal conduit. A lower midline incision is made and a full laparotomy performed. The bladder is removed en bloc with the iliac and obturator lymph nodes. In males, the prostate is also removed and in females, the uterus, fallopian tubes and ovaries. The urethra is only excised if there is evidence of urethral disease.

Following the cystectomy, one of several procedures is performed in order to provide a means of draining the urine.

- Ileal conduit. The ureters are sutured to a segment of isolated ileum, which drains the urine continuously via an ileostomy, into a bag on the patient's abdomen.
- Continent ileal pouch. The principle is the same as above, except that the urine is stored in a pouch fashioned from a

segment of ileum and/or caecum. This is catheterized intermittently by the patient through a small abdominal stoma.
- Neobladder. A 'new bladder' is fashioned from a segment of ileum or colon, sutured to the internal urethral meatus and the ureters are implanted into this.

Procedure profile

Blood requirement	4–6
Anaesthetic	GA
Operation time	3–4 hours
Hospital stay	2 weeks
Return to normal activity	3 months

There may be much blood loss during this procedure, so the patient must be monitored carefully postoperatively, for signs of haemodynamic instability or evidence of further bleeding. Often these patients are kept in the intensive care or high-dependency unit for the first 24 h. The urine output must be watched closely, as must the patient's renal function. Breakdown of the urinary anastomosis may result in a urinary fistula. If there is an ileostomy, it should be checked regularly for signs of ischaemia (oedema, dusky blue colour). The long-term sequelae of diverting the ureters into a segment of bowel include chronic urinary infections and pyelonephritis.

Cystitis

Cystitis is the term used to describe inflammation of the bladder. There are several causes (see Table 11.2.1) although infection is the commonest and is dealt with in section 1.8.

Recognizing the pattern
The typical symptoms of cystitis are frequency of micturition and burning dysuria. The patient may also complain of suprapubic pain, haematuria, urgency, urge incontinence and nocturia.

Table 11.2.1 Causes of cystitis.

Infective
Idiopathic
Secondary to:
    diabetes mellitus
    pregnancy
    residual urine
    stone
    foreign body (e.g. catheter)
    enterovesical fistula

Interstitial cystitis

Radiation cystitis

Drugs (e.g. cyclophosphamide)

On examination there are often no physical signs, although there may be suprapubic tenderness. There is often an associated pyrexia.

Proving the diagnosis

- MSU. White cells are characteristically found. There may also be red cells in the urine. If there is infection, the organisms may be seen on direct microscopy or may be grown in culture. This is often the only investigation that is required.
- Cystoscopy is required for recurrent infective cystitis as well as for persistent symptoms without evidence of infection. The appearance of radiation cystitis is typical, showing multiple areas of friable mucosa and telangiectasia. The bladder capacity is often very small. In interstitial cystitis the bladder capacity is often very small also, and on filling, an ulcer (Hunner's ulcer) may appear.
- Bladder biopsy is indicated if interstitial cystitis is suspected, and also to exclude carcinoma in situ which may present is a similar way.
- Ultrasound of the urinary tract is indicated if there is recurrent infective cystitis in a female, or a single episode in males and

children, or persistent infection despite adequate antibiotic treatment.
• Urinary flow tests are indicated in men who have had one proven urinary tract infection to ensure adequate bladder emptying and to exclude bladder outflow obstruction.

Management

Infective cystitis is treated with the appropriate antibiotic. Prophylactic antibiotics (e.g. trimethoprim 200 mg nocte) may help prevent infections.

Radiation cystitis may require repeated cystoscopies and diathermy of bleeding vessels. If the bleeding is persistent or excessive, a cystectomy is sometimes performed.

Interstitial cystitis (cause unknown, but may be related to an autoimmune aetiology) is also difficult to treat. Various treatments have been tried, including bladder distension to increase capacity, oral steroids or antihistamines and intravesical dimethyl sulphoxide or heparin. As with radiation cystitis, cystectomy may be the final solution for these patients.

Incontinence

This is the involuntary loss of urine. It occurs when the pressure in the bladder exceeds the resistance in the outflow tract. There are two types of incontinence.
• Urge incontinence occurs when the bladder muscle is overactive.
• Stress incontinence occurs when the outflow tract (urethra and pelvic floor) are weakened.

Recognizing the pattern

The patient may be of any age but the prevalence of incontinence increases with age. Patients with urge incontinence will describe urgency, frequency and nocturia (the desire to pass urine during the night). Patients with stress incontinence will describe urinary leakage on coughing, sneezing, running etc. Often the pattern is mixed. Recording the pad usage and the effect on the patient's quality of life are essential. Consider the aetiology whilst taking a history – enquire about vaginal deliveries and assisted births, previous surgery and symptoms that may suggest neurological disease (often a cause of urge incontinence).

A neurological examination should be performed. In females, a vaginal speculum examination may show the impression of the bladder (cystocoele) or rectum (rectocoele) in the vagina and indicate the degree of urethral descent on straining.

Proving the diagnosis

- An MSU should be examined, since urinary tract infection often causes bladder irritability and urge incontinence, especially in the elderly.
- An ultrasound of the bladder may reveal chronic retention of urine in patients with neurological disease.
- Urodynamic studies are the definitive examination. Fluid is instilled into the bladder, while the intravesical pressure is monitored. In urge incontinence, characteristic rises in intravesical pressure are found as a result of abnormal detrusor muscle contractions. Any loss of urine associated with stress incontinence can also be noted.

Management

Infection is treated with the appropriate antibiotic. If there is neurological disease causing incontinence, the bladder may be emptied by intermittent self-catheterization or an indwelling catheter.

Urge incontinence may be treated by drugs that reduce the contractions of the bladder – anticholinergics. Some operations have been described for severe urge incontinence where the bladder is bivalved and small intestine is sutured into the bladder (clam ileocystoplasty).

Stress incontinence should be treated initially by pelvic floor exercise. More severe stress incontinence, which is not helped by these techniques, may be treated surgically by supporting the bladder neck using a transvaginal tape or internal sutures (colposuspension). Other methods of increasing urethral resistance include topical application of estrogen in postmenopausal women and injection of bulking agents around the urethra. In some men with incompetent sphincters, it may be possible to insert an artificial sphincter. Duloxetine, a drug that acts to increase the urethral sphincter pressure, may be used in conservative management.

OPERATION: TENSION FREE TRANS VAGINAL TAPE
Preoperatively the patient is encouraged to consider the complication of hypercontinence (inability to pass urine naturally) and taught intermittent self-catheterization.

In a lithotomy position a small incision is made inside the anterior wall of the vagina in the axis of the urethra. A manmade tape is passed around the urethra like a hammock and brought up the skin of the suprapubic region using long needles. A cystoscopy demonstrates that the bladder has not been breached by the needles and the tape is cut flush with the skin. The vagina is repaired using absorbable sutures. The tape is left loose – 'tension free'.

Procedure profile

Blood requirement	Group and save
Anaesthetic	GA (LA for some infirm patients)
Operation time	40 minutes
Hospital stay	24 hours
Return to normal activity	1 week

Acute retention of urine

This is painful complete inability to pass urine of sudden onset. It is most commonly due to an enlarged prostate in an elderly man. Other causes include urethral stricture, prostatic carcinoma, stones or blood clot in the urethra, urinary tract infection, constipation, neurological disease (e.g. cauda equina compression and multiple sclerosis), pregnancy, pelvic tumour and drugs (e.g. alcohol and anticholinergics). Trauma causing acute retention is considered on p. 644. Postoperative retention of urine is considered on p. 59.

Recognizing the pattern

The patient presents complaining of an inability to pass urine, and suprapubic pain, which characteristically comes in spasms. There may be a history of chronic symptoms secondary to bladder outflow obstruction.

On examination the bladder is enlarged and tender. The urethra should be palpated for stones or stricture and a rectal examination should be performed to assess the size of the prostate and to exclude constipation (particularly in the elderly).

Proving the diagnosis

The diagnosis is proved by catheterization (see below). Further investigations should be arranged to try and discover the cause.

- Test the urine for blood or signs of infection.
- Perform a white cell count and haemoglobin.
- Measure the urea and electrolytes to assess renal function.
- Arrange an ultrasound of the renal tract if the renal function is abnormal.

Management

The patient should be admitted and a catheter placed without delay. The options for catheterization include urethral and suprapubic catheter placement. Both techniques should be familiar to medical students.

PROCEDURE: URETHRAL CATHETERIZATION

A 12- to 16-gauge Foley catheter is inserted with strict, aseptic technique. An assistant should be available. Firstly, prepare the trolley and make sure that everything you require is there. After cleansing the penis or vulva, squeeze plenty of local anaesthetic lubricant gel into the urethra. Poor lubrication is a frequent cause of failure to catheterize. After allowing time for the anaesthesia to work, pass the catheter gently but firmly. If resistance occurs, maintain this gentle firm pressure. Do not force the catheter as this may cause further spasm and oedema, and could create a false tract. As the bladder is entered, urine flows. This may take a few seconds as the lubricant is cleared from the inside of the catheter.

Pass most of the catheter up into the bladder and then inflate the balloon (if present). Connect the catheter to a bag. If you encounter difficulty passing the catheter, call someone with more experience before you damage the urethra. After catheterizing a male, pull the foreskin over the glans again or a paraphimosis may result. After catheterization the urine is drained into a bag. Record the residual volume and character of the urine.

Failure to pass a catheter may be evidence of a urethral stricture.

PROCEDURE: SUPRAPUBIC CATHETERIZATION
If urethral catheterization is not successful, suprapubic catheterization is required. Local anaesthetic is infiltrated two finger breadths above the symphysis pubis in the midline and a catheter is inserted through a small incision via a trocar. Make sure that you can feel the bladder and that you can aspirate urine with the needle used for infiltrating the local anaesthetic. Once the catheter is in the bladder, inflate the balloon (if present) to secure it. Remember to push enough catheter into the bladder to allow it to remain inside once the bladder has emptied. If the catheter does come out, it must not be reintroduced when the bladder is empty as the trocar may enter the peritoneum and damage the bowel.

Postoperative or bed-ridden patients who have gone into acute retention can have the catheter removed once they are mobile. If acute retention recurs, the catheter is reinserted for 24–48 h. Once the patient is up and in less pain, the problem usually resolves. Similarly, following acute retention secondary to constipation or urinary tract infection, the catheter may be removed once the condition has been treated.

Patients with acute retention due to prostatic enlargement and who are fit can be treated by early prostatectomy. With 'acute on chronic' retention time must be allowed for a general assessment and the detection and treatment of any chronic renal failure before a prostatectomy can be undertaken. Catheterization of a patient who has been in retention for a long period (chronic retention) may result in a diuresis. Monitor the urine output, fluid input and blood pressure in such patients.

In a very elderly patient who is quite clearly unfit for operation, the only solution may be long-term catheter drainage.

Small, soft, silastic catheters are available for this and the patient may either change this himself or have it done by a district nurse at home.

Give patients oral antibiotics is there is suspicion or proof of urinary tract infection at the time of catheterization. Oral ciprofloxacin 500 mg bd for 5 days is usually sufficient.

Bladder outflow obstruction

This is usually due to disease of the prostate (benign prostatic hyperplasia (BPH) or carcinoma) or urethra.

Recognizing the pattern
It usually affects men, who may present with either obstructive symptoms (hesitancy, poor flow and terminal dribbling) or irritative symptoms (frequency of micturition, urgency and nocturia) or a combination of both.

Proving the diagnosis
As with the investigation of incontinence, bladder outflow obstruction can be investigated by carrying out urodynamic studies, which should include measurement of the urinary flow rate. Bladder outflow obstruction is a combination of reduced urinary flow rates and symptoms. A postmicturition ultrasound scan will indicate if the bladder is retaining urine.

Management
The management of the patient with bladder outflow obstruction will depend on the specific cause of the blockage. The commonest cause is benign enlargement of the prostate, called BPH.

Benign prostatic hyperplasia (BPH)
This is a benign nodular or diffuse proliferation of both the musculofibrous and glandular elements in the prostate gland. It involves the inner zone of the gland, unlike carcinoma. The rest of the gland is compressed to form a capsule. It occurs to a varying degree in all men over the age of 50 years. The cause is uncertain but possible factors are an imbalance between androgens and estrogens

in later life or a benign neoplastic process. The enlargement causes elongation, narrowing and kinking of the prostatic urethra.

There is no relation between the size of the prostate on examination and the degree of obstruction. The obstruction results in hypertrophy of the detrusor muscle, producing a trabeculated appearance of the bladder wall. The mucosa may protrude between bands of muscle, forming saccules or diverticula. Eventually the muscle may become atonic, leading to chronic urinary retention, infection and stone formation. Alternatively, the muscle may become unstable, leading to abnormal contractions. Engorged veins at the base of the bladder may burst and cause haematuria. Back pressure may eventually cause obstruction of the upper tracts with hydronephrosis and eventually renal failure. Acute retention may occur at any stage.

Recognizing the pattern
The patient is usually aged between 55 and 75 years.

The history is of a poor urinary stream with hesitancy and terminal dribbling. Micturition is incomplete, resulting in a gradually increasing volume of residual urine. As the bladder hypertrophies, the detrusor becomes unstable, resulting in urinary frequency and nocturia. There may be associated urgency of micturition and urge incontinence. The patient may present with an episode of acute retention, commonly precipitated by drinking, bed rest or being trapped in a situation where he has to hold on too long due to lack of toilet facilities.

The prostate is examined through the rectum. Make sure the patient's bladder is empty. Assess the following:
- shape
- symmetry
- surface
- size
- sulcus of the prostate.

The sulcus is the median groove on its posterior surface. It is preserved in BPH but may disappear in malignant disease. In a normal prostate it is possible to slide the finger forward round each side of the convex surface of the gland. It is 2–3 cm across. In BPH the gland is smooth but symmetrical, the surface is flattened and it is difficult or impossible to get the examining finger forward round each side.

There may be general evidence of chronic renal failure and uraemia, e.g. dehydration, anaemia, skin pallor or hypotension. Abdominal examination may reveal a palpable bladder.

Proving the diagnosis
Investigations performed to confirm the diagnosis of BPH are as follows.

- An ultrasound of the urinary tract. This looks for hydronephrosis secondary to back pressure, postmicturition residual urine in the bladder and the size of the prostate gland. Increasingly a trans rectal ultrasound scan of the prostate is undertaken to accurately size the prostate.
- Test MSU for blood, protein and glucose and to exclude infection.
- Send blood for urea, creatinine and electrolytes to assess renal function, prostate-specific antigen (PSA) to screen for prostate cancer and full blood count in case of anaemia secondary to blood loss or renal failure. Patients should be counselled prior to PSA testing, some may wish not to proceed with a test that is rarely diagnostic.
- Urinary flow studies.

Management
If the symptoms are mild and renal function is normal, a policy of 'watchful waiting' may be undertaken. Otherwise, medical or surgical treatment should be considered.

Medical therapy includes 5-α-reductase inhibitors (e.g. finasteride and dutasteride) which reduce the volume of the prostate gland by preventing the conversion of testosterone to the active compound dihydrotestosterone. Alpha-blocker drugs provide good symptomatic relief for patients by relaxing the smooth muscle of the bladder neck and prostate. The two classes of drugs may be used in combination. Alternative therapies such as plant extracts (Saw Palmetto) are often used by patients with some success.

The usual treatment of this condition is surgical removal of the obstructing part of the prostate gland via the following procedures:

- transurethral resection of the prostate (TURP)
- retropubic prostatectomy (open prostate removal)
- alternative energy sources to destroy the prostate (laser, heat, cold, microwave etc).

The indications for prostatectomy for proven BPH include the following:

- severe symptoms secondary to BPH
- complications of BPH (acute retention, renal failure, bladder stone formation, recurrent infection, heavy haematuria, detrusor instability)
- failed medical therapy.

If the urine is infected, this must be sterilized with antibiotics before operation. Any uraemia is improved by a few days of catheter drainage. Dehydration and anaemia must also be corrected.

The patient should be told that one result of prostatectomy is retrograde ejaculation, resulting in a reduction in the quantity of ejaculate on sexual intercourse. In younger patients this may mean a reduction in fertility and this should be discussed with them preoperatively.

OPERATION: TRANSURETHRAL RESECTION OF THE PROSTATE (TURP)

The operation is a specialist procedure requiring experience with a resectoscope. The whole of the lateral and middle lobes of the prostate are resected. On completion a urethral catheter is inserted and the bladder is irrigated with fluid to prevent blood clots forming within the bladder. The prostatic chippings must be sent for histology to exclude a prostatic carcinoma.

Procedure profile

Blood requirement	Group and save
Anaesthetic	GA or spinal
Operation time	30–90 minutes
Hospital stay	3–5 days
Return to normal activity	4 weeks

Postoperatively ensure that the catheter drains satisfactorily. A bladder irrigation system is usually maintained for 24 h.

Should clot retention occur, it is relieved by syringing the bladder with 50–100 cm³ of normal saline (do not withdraw the syringe too forcefully as this causes the catheter to collapse). Occasionally it may be necessary to take the patient back to theatre to control severe bleeding.

The catheter is removed once the urine is clear of blood. Do not remove it too soon as it may be difficult to reintroduce in the early postoperative period.

Early postoperative complications include primary and secondary haemorrhage, urinary tract infection, septicaemia, the 'TUR syndrome' (which is due to absorption of irrigation fluid and may cause hyponatraemia or hypotension if extreme), failed trial without catheter and deep vein thrombosis. Long-term complications include retrograde ejaculation and urethral stricture. Incontinence is a rare but much feared complication.

Prostatic carcinoma

This is an adenocarcinoma. There is no known aetiological factor, although it often coexists with BPH. The tumour is usually androgen dependent. The incidence is increasing.

It arises in the outer zone of the gland (unlike BPH). It can still occur therefore after a transurethral prostatectomy for BPH. Local direct spread may involve the bladder, the ureters or the urethra. Direct invasion posteriorly is hindered by the fascia of Denonvilliers and involvement of the rectum is unusual.

Blood-borne spread occurs to bone, particularly the pelvis, lumbar vertebrae or greater trochanter of the femur via the communications of the prostatic venous plexus. Bony secondaries are characteristically osteosclerotic and appear on X-ray film as areas of increased density.

The stages of the tumour's development are shown in Fig. 11.2.2.

Recognizing the pattern

The patient is usually over the age of 65 years, though the condition is being diagnosed more frequently in younger men. Prostatic carcinoma usually presents with a disturbance of flow

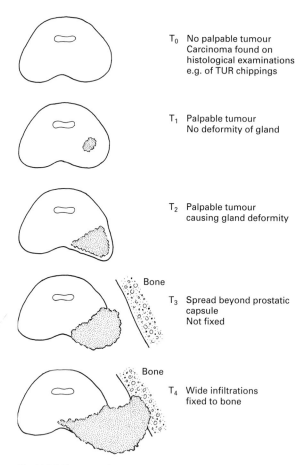

T_0 No palpable tumour
Carcinoma found on
histological examinations
e.g. of TUR chippings

T_1 Palpable tumour
No deformity of gland

T_2 Palpable tumour
causing gland deformity

Bone

T_3 Spread beyond prostatic
capsule
Not fixed

Bone

T_4 Wide infiltrations
fixed to bone

Fig. 11.2.2 The stages of prostatic carcinoma.

similar to BPH. The history of flow disturbance is usually
shorter. Other presentations are with back pain or bilateral sciatica (due to vertebral secondaries), neurological lesions due to
compression of the spinal cord or the general symptoms of carcinomatosis. Increasingly early, asymptomatic prostate cancer is
being discovered by screening and the use of PSA testing.

Rectal examination characteristically shows asymmetrical, nodular enlargement of the prostate, which feels hard and irregular with obliteration of the posterior median sulcus. Metastases in bone may cause areas of tenderness, particularly in the pelvis, femur and lumbar region of the back.

Proving the diagnosis

The diagnosis is proved by the following investigations.

- Prostatic-specific antigen (PSA) is the most specific tumour marker for prostatic carcinoma. It may also be raised in some patients with BPH, prostatitis and following TURP. In prostatic carcinoma, its level correlates to a degree with the stage and grade of the tumour. In metastatic disease it may be elevated to a level more than 10 times normal. It is also used as a follow-up investigation in patients with prostatic carcinoma, since an increase in levels may herald the development of metastases. A raised PSA is never on its own diagnostic of prostate cancer.

- Histology. A trucut biopsy needle is passed via the rectum into the prostate usually under ultrasound control. Several prostate cores are sampled. Antibiotics are administered to prevent serious sepsis.

Other investigations to assess and stage the disease are as follows.

- Test the urine for signs of infection.
- Full blood count.
- Urea and electrolytes to assess renal function.
- Alkaline phosphatase (raised if there are bony secondaries).
- Technetium bone scan. This will demonstrate the presence of bony metastases. It is sometimes necessary to supplement this with plain X-rays of suspicious areas.
- CT or MRI of the pelvis. This is useful to indicate whether the prostate cancer is organ confined or spreading outside of the gland. Enlarged lymph nodes may be also seen.
- Pelvic lymph node sampling may be undertaken laparoscopically to detect lymph node metastases in some cases.

Management

The principles of management of prostate cancer are complex. It is a common diagnosis but it is an uncommon cause of death. Many men will die with prostate cancer rather than of prostate cancer. Nevertheless there are some men who will develop aggressive prostate cancer and require curative or palliative treatment. Because there are so many treatments available the patient needs to be well informed and their choice is important.

Prostate cancer which is confined to the prostate may be removed by surgery (radical prostatectomy) or destroyed by radiotherapy. New methods of destroying prostate cancer include brachytherapy (radiation seed placement) and cryotherapy (freezing of the prostate). All of these techniques carry risks of incontinence and impotence.

Prostate cancer that has spread beyond the prostate may be treated by hormone manipulation, radiotherapy and chemotherapy. Hormone manipulation exploits the fact that the cancer is usually extremely sensitive to the effects of testosterone. By reducing the active testosterone in the bloodstream then the prostate cancer effectively stops growing and enters a period of remission. Antiandrogens are often used in combination with a gonadotrophin-releasing hormone agonist which exhausts the pituitary gland of trophic hormones. Traditionally men were offered bilateral orchidectomy to reduce testosterone production.

OPERATION: RADICAL PROSTATECTOMY

This operation may be performed either open or by a laparoscopic approach. The prostate gland is removed by dividing the bladder neck above the prostate and the urethra below the prostate. The bladder is then re-anastomosed onto the urethra using multiple sutures. A catheter is placed and remains in the bladder for several weeks. Bleeding may be extensive due to the large pelvic veins that encircle the prostate and pelvic floor.

Procedure profile

Blood requirement	2–6
Anaesthetic	GA
Operation time	2–3 hours
Hospital stay	5–7 days (less for laparascopic operation)
Return to normal activity	1–2 months

Postoperatively it is imperative that the catheter is well secured to the patient as it is protecting a delicate anastomosis. Should the catheter become displaced then the most senior doctor available should be requested to replace it, often with the guidance of a cystoscope. The catheter is left for an average of 2 weeks and removed. The patient is encouraged to develop pelvic floor exercises to improve his continence. Patients with erectile problems after surgery may benefit from oral therapy (e.g. Viagra).

Acute prostatitis

This is acute inflammation of the prostate gland. It may follow bacteraemia or urinary tract infection. The organisms commonly involved are *Escherichia coli*, *Streptococcus faecalis*, *Staphylococcus aureus* and *Neisseria gonorrhoeae*.

Recognizing the pattern
The patient may be an adult of any age but is usually over 35 years.

The history is of symptoms of general infection including malaise, fever, rigors and muscle pain. There is pain in the perineum and frequency of micturition, dysuria or occasional haematuria. An abscess may cause acute retention or pain on defaecation.

On examination the patient is pyrexial and rectal examination reveals a very tender, swollen and occasionally 'boggy' prostate.

Proving the diagnosis
An attempt should be made to isolate the causative organism from the urine. The patient is asked to micturate and the first urine passed is collected separately from the rest and examined.

Management
Prostatitis is a difficult infection to eradicate completely so antibiotics are continued for at least 6 weeks. Oral ciprofloxacin and occasionally intravenous broad-spectrum antibiotics are required.

If an abscess is present, it must be drained – usually via the perineum.

Chronic prostatitis

This is a condition characterized by recurrent mild episodes of acute inflammation of the prostate gland or by constant pain in the perineum. It may be due to persistent infection, usually with *Chlamydia trachomatis*, or there may be an apparently sterile chronic inflammation. It is sometimes referred to as chronic pelvic pain syndrome in the absence of infecting organisms.

Recognizing the pattern
The patient may be of any age.

The history is one of intermittent episodes of perineal pain varying in severity and frequency and often causing great distress. Other symptoms include low backache, mild bouts of fever and dysuria.

On examination the prostate may be enlarged, firm and irregular.

Proving the diagnosis
This is essentially clinical with laboratory confirmation of the infective organism if possible. It is important to collect specimens carefully and to isolate the first-pass urine, the secretion from the urethra obtained on massaging the prostate per rectum and the urine passed after prostate massage.

Management
Treatment is with antibiotics, especially doxycycline and ciprofloxacin, but the condition is difficult to eradicate. Resection of the prostate does not usually help. In some patients with refractory chronic prostatitis α-blocker drugs may be used. Complimentary therapies can be helpful.

Urethral stricture

This is narrowing of the urethra causing obstruction to urine flow followed by back pressure on the bladder, ureter and kidney. The signs are similar to those discussed under BPH.

It may be caused by inflammation following infection, usually with *Neisseria gonorrhoeae*, or following instrumentation (e.g. transurethral surgery or catheterization). It may also follow traumatic injury to the urethra. Distal stenoses at the meatus are usually caused by condyloma accuminata or by balanitis xerotica obliterans.

Recognizing the pattern

The patient can be of any age and is usually male.

There may be a history of catheterization, prostatectomy, trauma or urethral infection. The patient presents with flow problems including a poor stream and dribbling. The flow can often be increased by abdominal straining. Fibrosis and narrowing may cause painful ejaculation and very occasionally distortion of the erect organ (chordee) which may make intercourse impossible.

On examination the external genitalia should be inspected for meatal stenosis. The urethra should be carefully palpated along its length and the stricture may be felt. Abdominal examination may reveal a palpable bladder.

Proving the diagnosis

The diagnosis is confirmed by the following.
- Urinary flow rate. The flow curve is characteristically flat.
- Urethroscopy. This is usually achieved with the flexible cystoscope and the stricture is visualized directly.
- Urethrography. The use of contrast medium to outline the urethra in detail.

Management

A stricture is usually a chronic condition requiring regular follow-up. The initial treatment is commonly by internal urethrotomy and this is followed by regular self-dilatation. A urethroplasty (excision of the scarred segment and re-anastomosis or grafting of the urethra) is an alternative.

If the urine is infected, antibiotics should be given before operation and bladder washouts performed. Prophylactic antibiotics are given at induction.

OPERATION: INTERNAL OPTICAL URETHROTOMY

A urethrotome is passed under direct vision. This is a special instrument that allows a small knife to be passed from the end of a modified cystoscope. The stricture is viewed and incised to the required depth. Often a guide wire is passed through the stricture prior to cutting the stricture.

Procedure profile

Blood requirement	0
Anaesthetic	GA
Operation time	30 minutes
Hospital stay	2–3 days
Return to normal activity	1 week

Evidence suggests that for some strictures regular self-dilatation postoperatively with disposable rigid catheters may reduce the frequency of recurrence. The patients are often followed up by regular flow rates.

Avoidance of excessive instrumentation of the bladder, care at prostatectomy and the use soft catheters for as short a time as possible will all help in cutting down the incidence of strictures. The prevention and rapid treatment of sexually transmitted infection is equally important.

11.3 Male genitalia

Conditions of the foreskin

The care of the foreskin remains a mystery to most parents. Generally speaking it should be left alone for the first year or two of life. Thereafter it can be gently but firmly retracted, usually at bath time. Adhesions gradually separate and the glans becomes fully visible. This process is usually complete by the age of 1–5 years.

In young boys the foreskin is often relatively long and the tip tends to be slightly tight causing a groove as it is retracted on to the penile shaft. This will stretch up by natural processes as development occurs. It must be distinguished from a scarred stricture which can result in a paraphimosis, non-retractile foreskin or even a 'pinhole meatus'.

Non-retractile foreskin
Recognizing the pattern
The patient is usually brought along by his parents, who are concerned that the foreskin does not retract. There may be a history of recurrent balanitis.

On examination the foreskin is adherent. Check how far it can be retracted and whether there is any stricturing at the tip.

Management
There is no need for surgical treatment until after the age of 4 years unless complications such as recurrent balanitis or phimosis occur. Before this time the only management is to reassure the parents and give advice about the care of the foreskin as above. After the age of 4 years examination under an anaesthetic is performed (see below). The preputial adhesions are separated and a circumcision performed only if there is a phimosis.

Balanoposthitis (balanitis)
This is acute inflammation of the glans and foreskin, usually caused by pyogenic organisms (*Staphylococcus*, *Streptococcus* and coliforms) or fungal infection (*Candida*). It occurs commonly in young boys with a non-retractile foreskin. In elderly patients there may be a predisposing cause such as carcinoma or diabetes.

Recognizing the pattern
The patient with acute balanitis may be of any age and presents with either irritation or pain in the penis, and a discharge from beneath the foreskin. Recurrent balanitis may cause a phimosis with disturbance of micturition.

On examination the inflammation is visible and pus may be seen oozing from the meatus.

Management

The management is to give antibiotics and treat the cause. Frequently this means a circumcision once the inflammation has settled down. In older patients the urine should be tested for glucose.

Phimosis

This is a narrowing of the opening of the foreskin. It can follow trauma or recurrent infection. In adults a chronic skin condition called balanitis xerotica obliterans is a common cause of phimosis.

Recognizing the pattern

The patient is usually young and there is a history that the foreskin balloons out on micturition, causing a spraying stream. Adults often complain of pain and splitting of the foreskin on intercourse.

On examination the foreskin is tight and cannot be easily rolled over the glans penis. In balantis xerotica obliterans the foreskin may be thickened and pale.

Management

Management is by circumcision. In some cases it is possible to preserve the foreskin by treating balanitis xerotica obliterans with steroid cream.

Paraphimosis

This condition occurs when a tight foreskin is forcibly retracted back off the glans and cannot be pulled forwards again. The tight band causes obstruction of venous return followed by swelling of the distal foreskin and glans. It can occur at any age. It is especially common in the elderly patient who after catheterization has not had his foreskin pulled forwards again.

Management

Unless reduced quickly the distal foreskin rapidly becomes so swollen that reduction is impossible. The swollen glans and foreskin are wrapped in a swab and squeezed gently to reduce the oedema. This may be facilitated by the application of ice to the glans and by the use of local anaesthetic gel. Once the oedema has reduced, pressure is applied to the glans to push it back through the tight band. This procedure can, if necessary, be carried out with a dorsal penile nerve block. In some cases a dorsal slit may be required to obtain reduction. Circumcision is performed at a later date when the oedema has settled.

Trauma to the foreskin

A torn frenulum is usually seen in young men following intercourse. Occasionally the foreskin may be caught in the zip of trousers resulting in tears or superficial lacerations.

Management

A torn frenulum usually requires no treatment other than reassurance to the patient and advice about intercourse. A catgut stitch may be required if there is bleeding from the torn frenular artery. A lubricant such as KY jelly may be helpful. If the problem becomes recurrent, a circumcision may become indicated.

OPERATION: CIRCUMCISION

The indications for circumcision are as follows:

- phimosis
- recurrent balanitis
- balanitis xerotica et obliterans
- carcinoma of the foreskin.

Balanitis should be treated with antibiotics before surgery.

If there is a phimosis, this is stretched and preputial adhesions are separated.

A dorsal split is made in the foreskin down to the predetermined level and the foreskin then carefully removed, preserving sufficient epithelium next to the glans (5 mm). Following haemostasis, the preputial layer of skin is sutured to the skin of the penile shaft using absorbable sutures. Care is taken to align the skin correctly. A penile nerve block is useful postoperative analgesia. The foreskin is always sent for histological analysis.

Procedure profile

Blood requirement	0
Anaesthetic	GA
Operation time	15–30 minutes
Hospital stay	Day case
Return to normal activity	Up to 1 week

Postoperative the patient must avoid sexual activity for 2 weeks until the skin has healed. In cases of confirmed balanitis xerotica obliterans it is necessary to counsel the patient that the condition may recur on the glans penis itself causing narrowing of the external urethral meatus.

Carcinoma of the penis

This is a squamous cell carcinoma. It is rare in the UK but occurs more frequently in the Far East and Africa. Carcinoma of the penis is associated almost exclusively with an intact foreskin and may be related to previous infection with the human papilloma virus. It may start as leucoplakia of the glans. Erythroplasia of Queyrat is the name given to carcinoma in situ of the penis. It consists of a persistent red, raw area on the glans. This precancerous condition usually responds to local radiotherapy or application of 5-fluorouracil cream.

With advanced disease the whole penis may be engulfed with malignant growth and the urethra may be invaded. Lymphatic spread occurs to the inguinal nodes. Blood-borne spread is late and rare.

Recognizing the pattern
The patient is usually but not exclusively elderly. The presenting complaint is one of a lump or discharge and irritation. Later the discharge becomes bloody and offensive. The foreskin is usually non-retractile. Advanced disease presents with an ulcerated, fungating lesion destroying the whole penis or a mass in the groin. Urethral obstruction with retention of urine is rare.

On examination the lesion is visible if the foreskin can be retracted. If not, it is usually possible to feel it beneath the foreskin. In 60% of cases the nodes in the groin are enlarged but only half of these are malignant. The rest are due to reactive changes secondary to the inflammation and infection.

Proving the diagnosis

The diagnosis is proved by taking a biopsy, and a circumcision may be required to reveal the growth.

A CT scan of the pelvis may be useful to assess lymphatic spread, if block dissection is contemplated.

Management

Even in the presence of enlarged nodes in the groin, it is usual to treat the primary growth first and then only treat the nodes if they are still enlarged after 3–4 weeks.

Lesions of the distal penis may be treated with either radiotherapy or surgery. Surgery may involve partial removal or the penis or full amputation of the penis in which case the urethra is diverted to the perineum and the patient sits to pass urine.

Persisting enlarged lymph nodes in the groin are often removed by block inguinal lymph node dissection whereby all the lymph tissue of the groin is removed. Deep inguinal lymph nodes in the pelvis may be involved and surgically removed in some cases. A combination of chemotherapy and radiotherapy may be required.

Erectile dysfunction

Difficulty in achieving and maintaining an erection causes severe distress to men and their partners. The physiology of erection is complex and many factors such as psychological stress, arterial disease, diabetes, smoking and venous leakage may be to blame.

Management

The cause is usually obvious and in the majority it is psychological. The opportunity should be taken to exclude diabetes and to check serum cholesterol. Hormone screening is rarely indicated. Counselling can be useful. Oral therapies which assist arterial smooth muscle relaxation (e.g. sildenafil) are very helpful. Rarely men will require the insertion of an inflatable or rigid prosthesis.

Scrotal conditions

The following conditions in the scrotum commonly present.
- Absent testis.
- Lumps in the scrotum.
- Painful testis.

Absent testis (cryptorchidism)

The testis may be absent from the scrotum either because it is undescended or because it is retractile. The testis develops as a retroperitoneal organ at the lower pole of the kidney and during development descends caudally through the inguinal canal and into the scrotum. Its descent may be either incomplete (arrested at any site along the course of its descent) or abnormal. If it is abnormal the testis is ectopic and can lie in a pubic, inguinal, femoral or perineal site.

A retractile testis has descended normally but is pulled up into the inguinal canal by an active cremasteric muscle reflex.

A true undescended testis is frequently abnormal and may never undergo spermatogenesis. There is evidence, however, that bringing the testis down into its correct place early in life can improve the chances of fertility. There is also an increased danger of malignant change in an undescended testis. Neither of these problems occurs with a retractile testis.

An undescended testis should be spotted early in life at a routine medical examination. This will enable plans to be made to bring the testis into the scrotum before the age of 2 years. Frequently, however, the condition is first diagnosed later than this. The longer the testis remains undescended, the greater the danger of infertility. There is also an increased risk of malignancy in the undescended testis. Though this risk does not appear to be affected by bringing it into the scrotum it does make testicular self-examination easier.

Less common presentations of the undescended testis include torsion and trauma.

Recognizing the pattern

The patient can present at any age from newborn to between 20 and 30 years old, although in the UK boys usually present in infancy.

On examination the scrotum is underdeveloped and flattened. The condition may be unilateral or bilateral and the position of both testes should be determined. The undescended testis may be palpable in the groin or inguinal canal and should be located if possible.

Management

The undescended testis should be brought into the scrotum by performing an orchidopexy, preferably before the age of 2 years. At this age the operation must be undertaken by an expert as damaging the delicate testicular vessels will bring about infertility. This is exactly what the operation is designed to prevent. Orchidopexy ensures optimal conditions for subsequent development of the testis, as well as making it easier to examine in later years. It also renders it less prone to traumatic injury and torsion.

If the testis is impalpable, it may be located intra-abdominally, or it may be in an inguinal position where it is atrophied and hence impalpable. An ultrasound of the groin may be helpful in locating an undescended testis, as may an abdominal CT scan or laparoscopy. It may be possible to bring an intra-abdominal testis into the scrotum, employing microvascular anastomotic techniques in order to supply it with an adequate blood supply, since the length of the testicular artery will probably be insufficient. If an undescended testicle is discovered later in life then orchidectomy may be preferable depending on the age of the patient and the site of the testis.

OPERATION: ORCHIDOPEXY (DARTOS POUCH PROCEDURE)

An incision is made in the groin and the testis found and mobilized together with its vessels. The latter are freed right up into the deep inguinal ring, and further into the abdomen if necessary. They are separated from the processus vaginalis and any small inguinal hernial sac. A subcutaneous pouch is then made in the scrotum between the skin and the dartos muscle. The testis

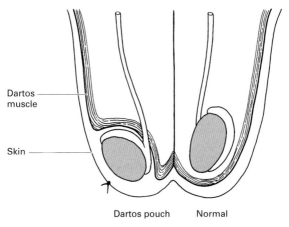

Fig. 11.3.1 Dartos pouch orchidopexy.

is pulled down through a small hole in the dartos muscle (Fig. 11.3.1). Once the bulk of the testis is through this hole it is unable to retract back and hence it becomes fixed in the scrotum. The scrotal and inguinal wounds are closed with a soluble suture.

Procedure profile

Blood requirement	0
Anaesthetic	GA
Operation time	30 minutes per side
Hospital stay	Day case
Return to normal activity	2 weeks

Postoperatively the scrotum may be bruised and swollen for a while and the parents may need some reassurance that this will settle down. When a dartos pouch has been made and where the testicular vessels are short the scrotum will be pulled well up into the groin. This should not cause concern providing the testis remains within the scrotal tissues.

Lumps in the scrotum

Patients with lumps in the scrotum are common cases in surgical examinations. It is important to develop a disciplined technique for examining them as there is frequently embarrassment on the part of both the patient and the student, making logical thought more difficult.

A routine should be established as follows.

- Can you get above it? That is to say, is the lump truly scrotal or is it a continuation of a lump in the groin which descends into the scrotum (e.g. an inguinal hernia)?
- What is its relation to the testis? Which anatomical structure does it arise from?
- Is the lump tender or not?
- Does it transilluminate? Scrotal lumps lend themselves to the technique of transillumination. Use a good torch with a narrow beam and observe the other side of the swelling in a darkened environment.
- Define the characteristics of the lump:
  - shape
  - size
  - surface
  - consistency
  - mobility.

The features of individual types of lump will be dealt with below.

Hydrocoele

A hydrocoele is a collection of fluid in the tunica vaginalis. Hydrocoeles may be either primary or secondary. In the primary type there is no predisposing cause in the scrotum, but there may be a persistent processus vaginalis (congenital or infantile hydrocoele) (see Fig. 14.2.2).

Secondary hydrocoeles represent a reaction to some pathology in the testis or its covering (e.g. testicular infections, tumours, torsion of the testis or hydatid of Morgagni). In adults the possibility that a hydrocoele is secondary to an impalpable tumour of the testis must always be considered.

Recognizing the pattern

The patient may be of any age. Primary hydrocoeles are common in young boys; secondary hydrocoeles are more common in adults. They may be of significant size in older men. The patient usually presents because he has noticed a swelling in the scrotum. Occasionally the hydrocoele is large enough to cause discomfort.

On examination you can get above the swelling. It has a smooth surface and is of any size. It transilluminates well. The testis is within it and not palpable separately. It is usual to obtain an ultrasound to document the diagnosis and observe a normal underlying testicle.

Management

Hydrocoeles in children are treated as a patent processes vaginalis and should be dealt with operatively in the same way as an inguinal hernia (see p. 594).

A hydrocoele in an adult is usually corrected surgically although asymptomatic hydrocoeles in elderly men may be managed conservatively.

OPERATION: REMOVAL OF HYDROCOELE

An incision is made in the scrotum, and the hydrocoele and its immediate coverings are separated by gentle finger dissection. If this is carried out in the correct layer, very little bleeding occurs. The hydrocoele is then delivered out of the scrotum and incised, releasing its fluid. The testis is inspected for abnormalities. The coverings of the tunica fall behind the testis and cord and can be fixed there with sutures. In this way the hydrocoele cannot refill. The testis plus the everted coverings are then replaced in the scrotum and the skin is closed over them with absorbable sutures. Accurate haemostasis is essential. A scrotal support may be applied.

Procedure profile

Blood requirement	0
Anaesthetic	GA or LA
Operation time	15–30 minutes
Hospital stay	Day case
Return to normal activity	1–2 weeks

Postoperatively the patient should rest quietly for 12–24 h. Haematoma formation is the main complication to be avoided. If a haematoma does occur, convalescence will be prolonged and there is a danger that it may become infected. Large haematomas should be evacuated under sterile conditions in theatre.

Epididymal cysts

Epididymal cysts are very common and often multiple. They may be of any size and contain either clear or milky fluid.

Recognizing the pattern

The patient is usually postpubertal and the condition seems to be more common in the middle aged and elderly.

He has usually noticed a lump which may have become large enough to cause trouble by its size. Occasionally the cyst is painful or the patient may be experiencing pain on direct pressure over it.

On examination it is possible to get above the swelling, which is situated above and behind the testis in the epididymis. The testis is palpable and separate from it. Cysts are frequently multiple and several cysts next to each other give rise to a lobulated swelling. The condition is often bilateral. The cysts are fluctuant but only transilluminate if they contain clear fluid.

Management

Conservative management may be prescribed for small asymptomatic cysts. Larger and symptomatic cysts may be excised but there is a significant risk of recurrence in all cases.

OPERATION: EXCISION OF EPIDIDYMAL CYST
The testis is exposed within the tunica vaginalis and delivered out of the scrotum. Either the individual cysts or the affected part of the epididymis can then be excised. The epididymis has a good blood supply and a lot of time must be spent securing full haemostasis.

Procedure profile

Blood requirement	0
Anaesthetic	GA or LA
Operation time	15–30 minutes
Hospital stay	Day case
Return to normal activity	1–2 weeks

Postoperative care is much the same as for a hydrocoele.

Painful testis
Pain from the testicle is severe and may be caused by trauma, infection (epididymo-orchitis), testicular torsion or testicular tumour.

Testicular trauma
The testes frequently take the brunt of footballs, hockey balls and rugby scrums. Mostly minor bruising occurs but it is associated with significant pain. Occasionally the testicle is shattered and is some cases removal is required to stop bleeding and ease pain.

Epididymo-orchitis
Epididymo-orchitis is an inflammation of the epididymis and testis due to bacterial, chlamydial or viral infection. The most common viral cause is mumps and it may then be associated with the characteristic parotitis.

Bacterial infections may be gonococcal or due to other bacteria such as coliforms. Chlamydial infection is becoming more common. The infection is thought to arise through reflux of infected urine or prostatic fluid along the vas. The epididymis alone may be infected or the inflammation may occasionally spread to involve the testis as well.

Recognizing the pattern

Bacterial infection usually occurs in the elderly whereas viral and chlamydial infections are more common in the younger sexually active men.

The typical picture is of an acute onset of very severe pain in the testis. There is swelling of the scrotum and the epididymis and testis become hard and very tender. The patient is ill with a fever, and rigors are not uncommon. There may or may not be associated dysuria and frequency.

Proving the diagnosis

The main differential diagnosis is torsion of the testis. The presence of a urinary infection, demonstrated by examination of an MSU, may be helpful, although it does not, of course, rule out a torsion. The large, hot, swollen testis of epididymo-orchitis is characteristic, as are the systemic signs of infection. When there is difficulty in deciding whether or not the testis is twisted, the scrotum should be explored. No harm is done by exploring an infection but much harm can follow conservative treatment of a torsion.

Management

The treatment is to give antibiotics, a scrotal support and bed rest. The epididymis frequently remains very hard and indurated for several weeks.

Torsion of the testis

The testis and epididymis are normally fixed within the scrotum by a 'bare area' which is outside the tunica vaginalis. Part of the epididymis and testis are involved in this 'bare area'. Torsion of the testis can occur when this attachment is minimal and the organ is on a 'mesentery' (Fig. 11.3.2). Occasionally the epididymis and testis are more separated than usual and in this case torsion can occur between the two. The actual twist occurs due to the action of the cremaster muscle. The fibres of this muscle run from the inguinal region downwards and medially across the

(a)

Normal

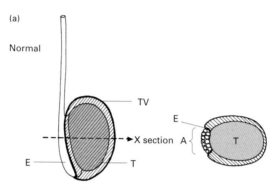

Tunica vaginalis (TV) enveloping testis (T) and anterior half of epididymus (E). Broad bare area (A)

(b)

Testis prone to torsion

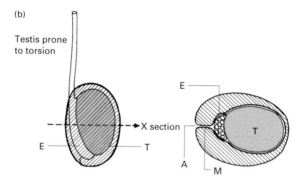

Tunica vaginalis includes epididymis. Small bare area (A) and mesentery (M).

Fig. 11.3.2 The anatomy of testicular torsion.

front of the testis. When they contract the testis tends to rotate with its medial side moving forwards, giving rise to the classically described 'bell-clapper' testis. Torsions not infrequently occur at times of excessive strain, exercise or during sexual intercourse.

Undescended testes have a higher incidence of torsion than those that are fully descended.

Recognizing the pattern

Torsion can occur at any age but is more common between the ages of 15 and 25 years.

There is a sudden onset of very severe scrotal pain, often associated with right iliac fossa pain radiating into the loin. The patient may feel ill and faint and experience nausea and vomiting. He may give a history of previous episodes of testicular pain, which have resolved, when the testis has twisted and untwisted spontaneously.

On examination the patient looks pale and ill and is in pain. The testis is swollen and hard and exquisitely tender. Because of this tenderness the twist in the cord may not be palpable.

The contralateral testis may lie horizontally (bell-clapper testis). Elevation of the twisted testis does not relieve the pain in contrast to the findings in epididymo-orchitis.

Proving the diagnosis and management

Where torsion is suspected the scrotum should be explored under a general anaesthetic without delay. Further investigation is inappropriate. If the testis is twisted far more than 4 h irreversible damage is likely to occur. At operation the diagnosis is confirmed by seeing the twist in the spermatic cord. As these abnormalities are usually bilateral the opposite testis should usually be fixed when torsion has occurred on one side.

Preoperatively the patient or his parents must be warned of the slight possibility of the testis needing to be excised and consent obtained for this, as well as fixation of the contralateral testis.

OPERATION: CORRECTION OF TORSION OF THE TESTIS

The scrotum is incised through the midline septum and the tunica on the affected side is opened. If this is done carefully, the testis is not rotated and the twist may be demonstrated. It is corrected and the colour of the testis observed. It may help to wrap it in a swab soaked in warm water. If the testis is necrotic, it should be removed. For fixation, the tunica is sutured behind the cord, as in a hydrocoele. A non-absorbable suture is passed through the upper and lower poles of the testis and it is secured in the scrotum, with its long axis running vertically. The contralateral testis is then approached, via the same incision, and fixed in the same way. The scrotal skin is closed with a soluble suture.

Procedure profile

Blood requirement	0
Anaesthetic	GA
Operation time	30–60 minutes
Hospital stay	2–3 days
Return to normal activity	2 weeks

Where the testis has proved viable a scrotal support is supplied. This and bed rest for 24 h will assist the testicular swelling to settle.

Torsion of testicular appendage

The testis may have a vestigial appendage, such as a hydatid of Morgagni, which is the remains of the Müllerian duct. This arises on a pedicle from the junction of the upper pole of the testis and the epididymis. Torsion of this pedicle leads to ischaemia and infarction of the appendage.

Recognizing the pattern

The patient may be of any age, although torsion of a testicular appendage is commoner in preadolescent boys. The presentation is very similar to that of testicular torsion, with acute onset of severe testicular pain. It may be difficult to distinguish from testicular torsion on examination, although it may be possible to palpate the appendage, which will be exquisitely tender.

Proving the diagnosis and management

In view of the fact that the clinical presentation mimics that of testicular torsion, the diagnosis is usually made at operation, when the scrotum is explored. If a twisted appendage is found, the pedicle should be ligated and the appendage excised. There is no need to proceed with fixation of the testes.

Varicocoele

A varicocoele is a collection of varicose veins in the pampiniform plexus of the cord and scrotum. It carries a higher than average incidence of infertility and this is thought to be due to the higher scrotal temperature associated with the abnormality. A left-sided varicocoele can be secondary to lesions causing obstruction to the testicular vein such as a renal cell cancer growing along the renal vein.

Recognizing the pattern

The patient is usually a young adult. The varicocoele may have been spotted at a routine medical examination.

The usual complaint is of a dull ache, especially at the end of the day or after exercise. The varicose veins themselves may also have been noted and caused the patient concern.

The varicocoele is usually plainly visible when the patient stands up. On palpation the typical 'bag of worms' feel is easily recognized. The left side is more commonly affected than the right. The swelling diminishes or even disappears when the patient lies flat.

Management

The patient is reassured that no harm is likely to come from this lesion. It is routine to obtain a renal ultrasound in cases of left-sided varicocoele. Indications for operation are if the pain is persistent in spite of adequate support or if there is associated infertility. A varicocoele may be dealt with by either laparoscopic or open clipping of the testicular veins at any level or by percutaneous embolization.

Testicular neoplasms

Ninety-two per cent of testicular neoplasms are malignant but they only account for 1 or 2% of all male malignancies. They are therefore uncommon. The incidence is rising perhaps as a result of environmental carcinogens.

Benign neoplasms are more rare. Leydig (interstitial) cell tumours account for 7% of testicular tumours and they may secrete androgens. In young boys they may produce early puberty and the 'infant Hercules' syndrome. Sertoli cell adenomas (< 1%) secrete estrogens and produce feminization.

Malignant neoplasms of the testis are commonly either seminomas (40% of testicular tumours) or teratomas (30%); 15% are of a mixed type. Undescended testes have approximately a 10-fold increased risk of neoplastic change and these patients represent about 8% of those with a malignant testicular tumour.

Seminomas probably arise from the primordial germinal cells in the testicular tubule. This is a solid tumour and tends to be slow growing. It is usually very radiosensitive.

Teratomas may have solid or cystic components and are less radiosensitive than seminomas; 90% of teratomas will secrete human chorionic gonadotrophin and/or α-fetoprotein, which can be measured in the serum and used as a tumour marker.

The prognosis of seminomas and teratomas depends on the stage of the growth and in the case of a teratoma its degree of differentiation. Five-year survival for organ-confined disease is in excess of 95% and still greater than 75% for patients who present with metastases.

Staging of testicular tumours is as follows.
- Stage I: disease confined to the testis.
- Stage II: abdominal lymph node involvement.
- Stage III: supra- and infradiaphragmatic lymph node involvement.
- Stage IV: extralymphatic spread (e.g. lung and liver).

Spread of these tumours is usually via the bloodstream and the lymphatics. Local spread to the scrotum is rare. Bloodstream spread occurs earlier in teratomas and metastases appear in the lungs and the liver. Lymphatic spread is common in both seminomas and teratomas. The lymph drainage of the testis follows its arterial supply and spread therefore occurs to the para-aortic lymph nodes at the level of the umbilicus. Inguinal lymph node involvement is rare and occurs when the scrotal skin is invaded.

Lymphomas comprise a further 7% of testicular tumours. They are more common in the elderly and are usually of the non-Hodgkin's type. Treatment is by combination chemotherapy but the overall results are poor.

Recognizing the pattern

Seminomas tend to occur between the ages of 25 and 45 years, whereas teratomas occur in a slightly younger age group, between 15 and 30 years.

The patient or his partner may notice a small painless lump in the testis or that one testis is larger than the other. Alternatively, these findings may be noted at a routine medical examination. Other presenting symptoms are unexplained pain in one testis, haemospermia or the development of a secondary hydrocoele. Some patients present with symptoms of metastatic disease (weight loss, haemoptysis, abdominal mass).

On examination a hard swelling is felt within the testis, and it is possible to get above it. The tumour does not transilluminate. The examination should include the abdomen, liver, chest and left supraclavicular fossa, feeling for evidence of metastatic spread.

Proving the diagnosis

All solid lesions arising in the testicle deserve to be removed for histological evaluation. Ultrasound is helpful in confirming that the mass is truly testicular in origin.

Management

A chest X-ray is performed and blood taken for a-fetoprotein and β-human chorionic gonadotrophin levels before the operation. Other investigations may be performed in the postoperative period. These include a CT scan of the chest, abdomen and pelvis in order to stage the disease.

Explain to the patient that the testicle is to be removed through a groin incision. Counsel the patient that removal of one testicle is unlikely to affect hormone levels and that fertility is only moderately affected.

OPERATION: RADICAL ORCHIDECTOMY

The groin is explored through an oblique incision as for an inguinal hernia and the spermatic cord isolated. A soft vascular clamp is placed on the cord at the deep inguinal ring. This prevents the venous spread of malignant cells while the testis is being manipulated. The testis is delivered into the groin and double ties placed around the cord at the level of the deep inguinal ring.

The cord structures are cut and the testis sent for histology. The inguinal canal is closed and the skin closed with absorbable sutures.

Procedure profile

Blood requirement	0
Anaesthetic	GA
Operation time	30–60 minutes
Hospital stay	2–3 days
Return to normal activity	Varies according to need for further treatment

The patient requires a scrotal support and his recovery is much the same as far an inguinal hernia.

Further treatment then depends on the histology and the clinical staging. Serum tumour markers are measured 1 week postoperatively and if they remain elevated this indicates the presence of metastases. In patients who have had a teratoma excised, the tumour markers should also be measured at 3-monthly intervals, since a rise generally indicates recurrent tumour. A testicular prosthesis may be inserted at a later date.

Patients with seminomas receive inguinal and para-aortic radiotherapy, including those with stage I disease. Those with metastases may also given chemotherapy.

Patients with teratomas receive combination chemotherapy postoperatively for stage II and above. Retroperitoneal lymph node dissection may be considered if there is evidence of persistent disease, with elevated tumour markers, following chemotherapy. Stage I patients can be offered either prophylactic chemotherapy or close surveillance. Chemotherapy and radiotherapy will impact on the spermatogenesis within the remaining testicle. Sperm banking is advisable.

RETROPERITONEAL LYMPH NODE DISSECTION
This is a major operation that aims to remove enlarged lymph nodes within the field of lymphatic tissue that is found in the para-aortic region. Depending on the side affected the para-

aortic lymph nodes and nodes between the aorta and inferior vena cava are excised en bloc from the level of the renal vessels to the aortic bifurcation. Retrograde ejaculation is a common side-effect of such surgery.

Procedure profile

Blood requirement	4–6
Anaesthetic	GA
Operation time	2–6 hours
Hospital stay	7 days
Return to normal activity	4–6 weeks

12 Vascular surgery

12.1 Assessment of chronic ischaemia of the leg

Chronic leg ischaemia is a result of atherosclerosis in the majority of patients.

In the initial assessment, five questions have to be answered before decisions about management can be made.

- Is the leg ischaemic?
- What is the site of the lesion?
- How severe is the ischaemia?
- Which risk factors for atherosclerosis are present?
- What is the full extent of the atherosclerotic process?

The answers are first found by clinical assessment and confirmed by investigation.

Clinical assessment

Is the leg ischaemic?
Recognizing the pattern
The patient is more often male than female and is usually beyond middle age.

The main complaint is of pain in the limb and this may be as follows:

- intermittent claudication
- rest pain
- painful ulceration.

Mild to moderate ischaemia is associated with intermittent claudication, which is a cramp-like pain in the muscles of the leg that occurs on walking a certain distance (known as the

Surgery: Diagnosis and Management, 4th edition. Edited by N. Rawlinson and D. Alderson. © 2009 Blackwell Publishing, ISBN: 978-1-4051-2921-3

claudication distance). It is relieved by rest and recurs on walking the same distance. Intermittent claudication needs to be differentiated from the pain associated with sciatica, cauda equina syndrome, musculoskeletal conditions (specifically osteoarthritis) and venous claudication.

Rest pain is associated with more severe ischaemia. Typically, it occurs at night when the patient is in bed and affects the toes or the dorsum of the foot and may wake the patient. The pain may be relieved by hanging the leg over the edge of the bed or by walking around the bedroom. Rest pain needs to be differentiated from night cramps, gout and peripheral neuropathy.

Trophic changes are associated with extreme ischaemia. These changes consist of discoloration of the foot with scaly skin, painful ulceration over bony prominences and gangrene. Ulceration and gangrenous changes need to be differentiated from those associated with venous hypertensive disease, neuropathies, infections and malignant ulcers.

On examination, the features of ischaemia depend upon its severity and usually include the following.

- Absent pulses. Feel carefully for the femoral, popliteal and foot pulses. In mild to moderate disease this may be the only abnormal finding. Absent pulses indicate disease at or proximal to the site examined. The presence of blood flow in an artery can be detected with a hand-held Doppler ultrasound probe even when pulses are not palpable.
- Audible bruits. Auscultate over the aorta, iliac, common femoral and superficial femoral vessels. The presence of a bruit indicates a stenosis at or proximal to the site examined.
- Cold extremity. Compare the temperature of the good side to that of the symptomatic side.
- Postural colour change (Buerger's test). With the patient supine, raise both legs in the air. If the leg is severely ischaemic, there is insufficient pressure to perfuse the elevated limb and the foot becomes pale. After a minute, ask the patient to sit up and hang the legs over the edge of the couch. The colour returns slowly to the ischaemic leg and the skin will develop the rubor of reactive hyperaemia.
- Persistent venous guttering. This sign can be elicited at the same time as postural colour change. As the legs are elevated the

foot veins empty. When the legs are placed in the dependent position, the veins remain 'guttered'. The time taken for the venous gutter to fill is an indication of the severity of the ischaemia.
- Ulcers or gangrene. Ischaemic gangrene is usually dry (unless infected) and well demarcated. Arterial ulcers have pale granulation tissue and show little sign of active healing.

What is the site of the lesion?

This can usually be diagnosed with accuracy before imaging is undertaken. Knowledge of the normal anatomy of the vascular tree is necessary (Fig. 12.1.1).

Recognizing the pattern

The level of the lesion may be determined from the history. Claudication commencing in the calf, progressing to the thigh and finally involving the buttock is usually caused by common iliac or coincident external and internal iliac disease. If this occurs bilaterally and is associated with impotence in the male and absent femoral pulses it is indicative of aortic occlusion and is known as Leriche's syndrome. External iliac, common femoral or coincident superficial femoral and profunda femoral disease gives rise to calf claudication progressing to the thigh. Superficial femoral, popliteal or crural (calf) vessel disease tends to give rise to calf claudication only.

In patients with rest pain and or trophic changes, disease is invariably present at more than one level.

On examination the level of the pulse deficit will usually be diagnostic of the level of the block. An absent femoral pulse indicates disease in the iliac system or above, and so on. The presence of a bruit indicates a narrowing at or proximal to that site.

How severe is the ischaemia?
Recognizing the pattern

Intermittent claudication represents the least severe symptom of ischaemia and the longer the claudication distance, the more minor the problem. Rest pain indicates more severe ischaemia. The onset of trophic changes and ulceration are signs that the limb is at risk. Poor cardiac output or the presence of anaemia will exacerbate any symptoms of peripheral vascular disease.

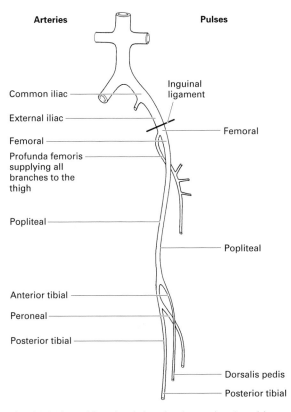

Arteries

Common iliac

External iliac

Femoral

Profunda femoris
supplying all
branches to the
thigh

Popliteal

Anterior tibial

Peroneal

Posterior tibial

Pulses

Inguinal
ligament

Femoral

Popliteal

Dorsalis pedis

Posterior tibial

Fig. 12.1.1 The arterial supply to the lower leg: the named arteries and the palpable pulses.

On examination, normal appearance of the leg indicates mild ischaemia. The presence of postural colour change and venous guttering indicates a more severe degree of ischaemia. Trophic changes such as ulceration and gangrene indicate that the leg is at risk.

Which risk factors for atherosclerosis are present?

Atherosclerosis is a generalized disease process affecting all the large and medium-sized arteries in the body. Risk factor management is an integral part of the management of the patient presenting with an ischaemic leg.

Recognizing the pattern

Cigarette smoking is the major risk factor for developing atherosclerosis. The patient may be diabetic. The patient may have treated or untreated hypertension. Hyperlipidaemia should be excluded. A strong family history of cardiovascular disease should be noted.

On examination the following should be considered.

- Nicotine staining of the fingers should be sought.
- Brachial systolic and diastolic blood pressure should be measured.
- Xanthelasmas should be sought.
- Dipstick urinalysis for glucose should be performed.

What is the full extent of the atherosclerotic process?

Atherosclerosis is a generalized disease process affecting the arteries of the heart and the brain as well as those of the legs.

Recognizing the pattern

Any history of myocardial infarction or angina pectoris should be noted. Recent infarction or unstable angina are significant risk factors if operative intervention is being considered. Look for a previous history of stroke, transient ischaemic attack or amaurosis fugax. Note any history suggestive of mesenteric angina or of deteriorating renal function.

On examination the presence of carotid artery bruits, renal artery bruits and aortic bruits should be noted. An asymptomatic abdominal aortic aneurysm may be present in up to 15% of patients presenting with peripheral vascular disease, and therefore abdominal palpation is necessary.

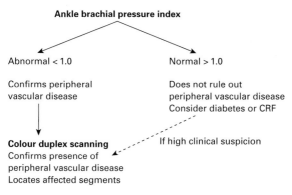

Fig. 12.1.2 Algorithm to determine the presence and site of disease.

Investigations

Non-invasive vascular assessment

Clinical assessment as outlined above should give a reasonable indication of the presence, site and severity of leg ischaemia. It should then be possible to confirm the diagnosis of leg ischaemia, locate the haemodynamically significant arterial lesions and plan the intervention (if indicated) using non-invasive vascular assessment (Fig. 12.1.2).

ANKLE BRACHIAL PRESSURE INDEX (ABPI)
This test may be performed in the outpatient clinic. It confirms the diagnosis of peripheral vascular disease, gives a good indication of the severity of the disease and forms the baseline for future evaluation of the disease. With the patient supine, a sphygomanometer cuff is placed above the elbow, flow through the brachial artery is detected using a hand-held Doppler ultrasound probe and the cuff is inflated to suprasystolic pressure. The cuff is deflated slowly and the point at which audible flow is re-established is the brachial systolic pressure. This is repeated on the opposite arm. The cuff is then placed around the leg just above the level of the ankle. Systolic blood pressure is measured

in the dorsalis pedis and the posterior tibial arteries using the Doppler in the same manner. The ratio of the highest systolic blood pressure measured at the ankle to the higher brachial systolic pressure, is the ABPI for that leg and is normally 1. The ABPI is of limited value in patients with diabetes mellitus or chronic renal failure where artificially high values may be a reflection of the incompressibility of calcified arteries. A normal ABPI does not exclude peripheral vascular disease.

COLOUR DOPPLER IMAGING (COLOUR DUPLEX)
This is a combination of B-mode ultrasound imaging with computed colour-coded Doppler ultrasound. It is possible to visualize the vessels using the B-mode imaging component and to focus the ultrasound beam on the vessel lumen to determine the flow velocity through the vessel. The investigation depends on a highly trained individual and it can be time-consuming to visualize the whole arterial tree. It can confirm the presence of peripheral arterial occlusive disease and identify the sites affected.

OTHER INVESTIGATIONS
• Full blood count – for anaemia, blood dyscrasia.
• Plasma viscosity – for collagen diseases, inflammatory condition.
• Coagulation screen – for coagulopathy.
• Urea and electrolytes and creatinine – for renal disease (possibly renovascular).
• Blood sugar – for diabetes mellitus.
• Blood lipids – for hyperlipidaemia.
• Electrocardiogram (ECG) – for ischaemic heart disease.
• Ultrasound of aorta – for abdominal aortic aneurysm.

Arteriography
Arteriography should be reserved for those patients in whom surgical or radiological intervention is being considered. There are a number of techniques for obtaining arteriograms.

TRANSFEMORAL ARTERIOGRAPHY
Under sterile conditions and local anaesthesia, a needle is placed into the femoral artery. A guide wire is passed through the needle

into the artery. A dilator covered by a sheath is placed over the guide wire and passed into the lumen of the artery. The guide wire and the dilator are now removed leaving the sheath accessing the arterial lumen. A longer guide wire is now passed through the sheath proximally into the aorta and a fine-bore catheter is passed over the guide wire into the aorta. The guide wire is removed. Radio-opaque contrast material may be injected to acquire the images.

TRANSBRACHIAL/TRANSAXILLARY ARTERIOGRAPHY

The sheath is placed in the brachial artery or the axillary artery. It is usually used when the femoral pulses are impalpable as a result of aortoiliac occlusive disease.

DIGITAL SUBTRACTION ARTERIOGRAPHY

With this technique, an initial image is taken and stored in a computer. The contrast material is injected and a series of images taken in rapid succession and stored on the computer. The initial image with bone and soft tissue shadowing is then subtracted from each of the subsequently obtained images leaving only the contrast material visible. Each of these images is superimposed on one another, building up high-resolution images of the arteries. The advantage of this technique is that high-quality arteriograms are obtained with the minimal use of contrast material. It is possible to inject the contrast material intra-arterially or intra-venously. The resolution of the images is not as good using the latter technique.

MAGNETIC RESONANCE ANGIOGRAPHY

It is possible to obtain angiographic images of arterial flow using a magnetic resonance imaging technique. It is becoming more readily available and is undergoing refinement to improve the quality of the images.

Hazards

There are hazards associated with arteriography. These include haemorrhage, haematoma formation and bruising at the arterial puncture site. False aneurysm formation may also occur.

Arterial intimal dissection may result in detachment of a segment of plaque which embolizes causing distal ischaemia. Thrombosis at the site of puncture or of plaque disruption may also occur resulting in acute ischaemia.

Allergic reaction to the contrast material may also occur. The contrast materials used are nephrotoxic and may cause acute renal failure. In patients with impaired renal function a renal protective regime should be used.

12.2 Management of the ischaemic limb

- All patients with chronic ischaemia should be advised to stop smoking. The prognosis is worse if they continue.
- Diabetics should be encouraged to obtain tight control of their diabetes and this should be monitored using glycosylated haemoglobin estimations.
- Patients with hyperlipidaemias should be encouraged to adopt a lipid-lowering diet and should be commenced on a statin. There is evidence that patients presenting with peripheral vascular disease should be commenced on a statin, regardless of cholesterol level, as it may decrease the risk of significant cardiac and cerebrovascular events.
- Hypertension should be controlled.
- Patients who are overweight should be encouraged to lose some, as excess weight requires the leg muscles to do more work, increasing oxygen demand.
- Foot care is important, and bacterial and fungal infections should be treated. Chiropody should be strongly advised in patients unable to care for nails, calluses or bunions. Advice on foot hygiene and sensible footwear is important.
- Other underlying conditions such as cardiac failure or anaemia should be treated. Atherosclerosis is a generalized disease process and the majority of patients presenting with leg ischaemia will die as a result of coronary or cerebrovascular disease.
- There is strong evidence that treatment with antiplatelet agents will decrease the risk of these events and therefore patients should be prescribed aspirin 75 mg daily (or clopidogrel 75 mg daily if they are sensitive to aspirin).

Management of intermittent claudication

The treatment is conservative in the majority of cases. As well as the general measures outlined above, the patient should be advised to commence a walking exercise programme. Ideally this should be supervised with regular monitoring. The patient should be advised to walk at a steady pace until the initial claudication distance is reached, and advised to walk into the pain as far as is possible (ideally 75% of the distance between the initial and the maximal claudication distance) before resting. When the pain has gone the patient should repeat the exercise three or four times, on a daily or twice-daily basis if possible. It is thought that there is an alteration in the metabolic process in the muscle fibres allowing them to function in a state of anaerobic respiration. Over a period of time the claudication distance may increase until ultimately the patient should be able to walk as far as they wish without pain.

Indications for intervention are relative and include the following.
- Decreasing claudication distance.
- Short claudication distance (< 100 m and proximal disease).
- Persisting symptoms, which interfere with the patient's work or quality of life to an intolerable degree.
- The development of rest pain or ulceration.
- Low risk for intervention.

Management of rest pain and/or trophic changes

The presence of true rest pain and or ulceration and gangrene is a definitive indication for intervention. After the relevant clinical and non-invasive vascular assessment has been performed and a management plan formulated, an arteriogram is performed. Arterial reconstruction should be considered in terms of risk/benefit to the patient's life and limb. Factors to be considered include the following.
- The fitness of the patient for the procedure
- The outcome if the patient does not have the procedure
- The success/failure rate associated with the procedure. This frequently depends on the state of the distal arterial tree (run-off).

The preoperative care of the arteriopath is more complex than that of most other surgical patients and includes the following.

- Assessment of coronary artery disease, diabetes and chronic renal failure are important. Vascular patients with a high risk of cardiovascular complications may benefit from perioperative β-blocker therapy (if there are no contraindications). This includes patients with a history of MI or angina, evidence of ischaemia on ECG or echocardiogram, or diabetics. Bisoprolol 5 mg daily should be commenced 2 weeks prior to surgery if possible.
- Preoperative ABPI measurements are vital for the later assessment of graft/vessel patency.
- Informed consent.
- Preoperative mapping of the long saphenous vein should be performed if it is being considered for use as a bypass conduit. Formal mapping using duplex imaging of the vein is useful as the size of the vein can be assessed, and the branches and main trunk marked.
- If the long saphenous vein is not suitable or has been stripped previously, the vein on the opposite leg should be mapped. If this is absent the cephalic or basilic veins of the arm should be mapped. It must be considered that this may be necessary when the patient is admitted and one arm spared the attentions of the phlebotomist.
- Prophylactic antibiotics should be given with the premedication or at the time of anaesthetic induction in theatre.
- Deep venous thrombosis prophylaxis using subcutaneous heparin should be used. Antiembolic compression stockings are contraindicated in patients with chronic ischaemia.
- A renal protective regime may be necessary, especially in patients undergoing endovascular procedures.

Endovascular techniques
ANGIOPLASTY

The treatment of patients with lower limb ischaemia has been revolutionized by the development of angioplasty. Using angiographic techniques a guide wire is passed across the lesion to be treated. A fine-bore catheter with a balloon at the tip is passed into the artery and positioned across the lesion. The balloon is inflated dilating the stricture.

STENT DEPLOYMENT

Re-stenosis may occur at the site of angioplasty. It is possible to place and expand a metal stent at the site of angioplasty to decrease this possibility. It is also possible to deploy a stent in an area of intimal flap dissection after angioplasty, thus preventing thrombosis.

STENT GRAFTING

A further advance is the use of a stent covered with prosthetic material (Dacron or polytetrafluorethylene [PTFE]) which is introduced into the artery using the same technique but when expanded forms an uninterrupted tube graft within the artery.

These techniques have limitations. Long-term success is greater in proximal vessels such as the iliac arteries. Stenoses greater than 10 cm long or occlusions greater than 5 cm have poor results. Distal vessel angioplasty has a lower success rate.

Procedure profile

Blood requirement	Group and save
Anaesthetic	LA
Operation time	30–120 minutes
Hospital stay	0
Return to normal activity	1 week

Operative techniques

There are a number of operative techniques available to help patients with chronic ischaemia:

ENDARTERECTOMY

The atheromatous lining of the narrowed artery is cored out. This procedure is particularly suitable for short stenoses in the larger vessels proximal to the superficial femoral artery and also for the removal of plaques in the internal carotid arteries in patients with cerebrovascular disease. It is usually associated with a patch closure which prevents narrowing of the artery.

BYPASS

Using this technique a conduit is anastomosed above and below the blockage. The conduit of choice is the patient's own long saphenous vein but because of its size, this is only suitable for bypass procedures below the inguinal ligament or for renal artery bypass. If a vein is not available, synthetic grafts are used but the results with these are not as good as they are prone to thrombosis. They are much more successful above the inguinal ligament as the vessels are larger and higher flow rates decrease the risk of thrombosis.

REPLACEMENT

The diseased artery is replaced by a prosthetic graft. The technique is used particularly in the replacement of aortic and other aneurysms.

Postoperative observations of pulse rate, blood pressure, respiratory rate, temperature and urinary output are required. Central venous pressure monitoring is valuable in patients with a history of cardiac failure. Low cardiac output or hypotension may precipitate thrombosis. The distal pulses should be recorded at the end of any arterial operation and should be checked regularly thereafter. If the pulses disappear, the surgeon should be informed immediately. If a bypass graft occludes in the postoperative period, it may be possible to unblock it if the situation is detected early.

All patients should be commenced on an antiplatelet agent, as this decreases the risk of graft occlusion in addition to reducing risk of cardiac and cerebrovascular events.

Patients should be entered in a graft surveillance programme using colour Doppler imaging. This may detect 'at-risk' grafts which can be modified to improve long-term patency.

Types of procedure

Each vascular operation is tailor-made for each patient using one or a combination of the techniques described above. The procedure may be named by the proximal and distal vessels to be dealt with, e.g. aortobifemoral bypass, femoroanterior tibial bypass, common femoral endarterectomy and patch angioplasty. Some of the commoner types of procedure are described below.

OPERATION: AORTOFEMORAL BYPASS
In this operation, disease of the aorta or iliac arteries which is
not amenable to angioplasty or stenting is bypassed. The aorta
is exposed transperitoneally or retroperitoneally. The femoral
arteries are exposed through groin incisions and a prosthetic
bypass graft is placed retroperitoneally and anastomosed to one
or both femoral arteries.

Procedure profile

Blood requirement	6 (and blood cell saver if available)
Anaesthetic	GA
Operation time	2–4 hours
Hospital stay	8–10 days
Return to normal activity	4–6 weeks

OPERATION: FEMOROPOPLITEAL
BYPASS/FEMORODISTAL BYPASS (Fig. 12.2.1)
 In this operation the femoral artery is exposed in the groin and
the popliteal artery or one of the distal leg vessels is exposed. The
long saphenous vein is excised along its length in the thigh and
calf, reversed so that the valves do not disrupt flow, and used to
bypass the blocked femoral artery. Sometimes the vein is left in
its bed ('in situ bypass') and the valves destroyed with a special
instrument called a valvulotome. If a vein is not available it is
possible to use prosthetic material usually a polytetrafleurethy-
lene (PTFE) graft.

Procedure profile

Blood requirement	4
Anaesthetic	GA/LA
Operation time	2–5 hours
Hospital stay	6–10 days
Return to normal activity	4–6 weeks

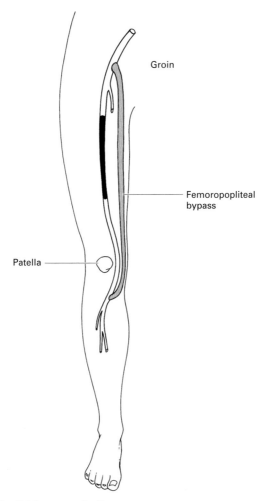

Fig. 12.2.1 Femoropopliteal bypass.

OPERATION: PROFUNDOPLASTY

This operation is performed if the origin of the profunda femoris artery is narrowed. It is sometimes combined with an endarterectomy. A vertical incision is made in the artery along the narrowed area and a patch of long saphenous vein or prosthetic material is inserted to widen the narrowed segment.

Procedure profile

Blood requirement	2
Anaesthetic	LA/GA
Operation time	1–2 hours
Hospital stay	7 days
Return to normal activity	3–6 weeks

OPERATION: AXILLOFEMORAL/AXILLOBIFEMORAL BYPASS

These operations are used to bring blood to ischaemic lower limbs in patients with an aortic occlusion who are not fit for an aortofemoral procedure. Also, it can be used in patients with an infected aortic graft. A long prosthetic graft is anastomosed to the axillary artery under the clavicle and tunnelled subcutaneously to the common femoral artery in the groin. If both legs are ischaemic an inverted Y graft may be used to bring blood to both femoral arteries.

Procedure profile

Blood requirement	4
Anaesthetic	GA
Operation time	1–3 hours
Hospital stay	7–10 days
Return to normal activity	4–6 weeks

OPERATION: ILEOFEMORAL/FEMOROFEMORAL
CROSS-OVER BYPASS
This is usually performed where there is an iliac blockage on one
side, which is not treatable by angioplasty or stenting and the
patient is not fit for a more major procedure. A prosthetic graft is
sutured from the normal iliac artery (using a retroperitoneal
approach) or the common femoral artery on the normal side and
tunnelled preperitoneally (from the iliac) or subcutaneously
(from the femoral artery) to the common femoral artery on the
diseased side.

Procedure profile

Blood requirement	4
Anaesthetic	GA/spinal
Operation time	2 hours
Hospital stay	7–10 days
Return to normal activity	4–6 weeks

Amputation
When all attempts to save an ischaemic limb have failed or the
patient presents with extensive gangrene, amputation may be
necessary to relieve the symptoms. The level of the amputation
will have to be high enough to ensure adequate healing of the
stump.

The option of amputation should be given to the patient against
the background of failure or unavailability of other options. It
should not be seen as a purely negative option as it gives excellent
pain relief and mobility is good with modern prosthetic limbs.
Always leave the final decision to the patient and their family.

OPERATION: ABOVE-KNEE AMPUTATION
The bone is divided approximately 40 cm from the greater
trochanter. Equal-sized anterior and posterior myocutaneous
flaps are formed 5 cm beyond this and closed over the cut end.
The wound is drained and the stump bandaged.

Procedure profile

Blood requirement	2
Anaesthetic	GA/spinal
Operation time	1 hour
Hospital stay	10–14 days
Return to normal activity	Variable

OPERATION: BELOW-KNEE AMPUTATION

This amputation is designed to use a long posterior flap of muscle and overlying skin to close the wound. The tibia is divided 10 cm below the tibial tuberosity, and the fibula 2.5 cm higher. The skin and muscle of the long posterior flap is folded forward over the divided bone and sutured to the skin anteriorly. This amputation has the advantage of preserving the knee joint, making rehabilitation easier.

Procedure profile

Blood requirement	2
Anaesthetic	GA/spinal
Operation time	1 hour
Hospital stay	10–14 days
Return to normal activity	Variable

OPERATION: RAY AMPUTATION

Where there is necrosis of a digit accompanied by necrosis or infection of the muscles of the foot especially in diabetics, a ray amputation of the toe and its metatarsal may be necessary. The incisions extend from the interdigital clefts at either side of the affected toe to the base of the relevant metatarsals. The wound is left open and dressed daily.

Procedure profile

Blood requirement	Group and save
Anaesthetic	GA/regional
Operation time	30–60 minutes
Hospital stay	10–14 days
Return to normal activity	Variable

OPERATION: TRANSMETATARSAL AMPUTATION

In this operation the forefoot is amputated. The sole of the forefoot is preserved as a flap which is sutured to the skin of the dorsum of the remaining foot.

Procedure profile

Blood requirement	Group and save
Anaesthetic	GA/spinal
Operation time	30–60 minutes
Hospital stay	2–3 weeks
Return to normal activity	Variable

OPERATION: AMPUTATION OF TOE

The toe is amputated with the head of the metatarsal, as exposed cartilage will impair healing. It is usually performed with a racquet-shaped incision, circumferential around the toe with the 'handle' extending onto the dorsum of the foot. The skin is closed with a number of loose sutures.

Procedure profile

Blood requirement	Group and save
Anaesthetic	GA/spinal
Operation time	30–60 minutes
Hospital stay	7–10 days
Return to normal activity	Variable

Postoperatively in the case of above-knee or below-knee amputation check that the bandages are not too tight after 8 h. Drains should be removed, without disturbing the dressings. Gentle physiotherapy should be commenced after 48 h to prevent development of contractures at the hip or knee joints. Liaise with limb fitting and rehabilitation services at an early stage. Patients with transmetatarsal and ray amputations may need orthotic shoe implants to aid them walking.

12.3 Aneurysms, acute ischaemia and arteriovenous fistulae

Arterial aneurysms

An aneurysm is an abnormal dilatation of a blood vessel, usually associated with atherosclerosis, which results in weakening of the arterial wall. The aneurysm occurs most commonly in the aorta, followed by the popliteal and femoral arteries, but may occur in any artery including the thoracic aorta.

Other causes include the following.

- Congenital. The best example is the berry aneurysm in the cerebral arteries.
- Traumatic. The arterial wall may be damaged during arteriography, surgery or by penetrating trauma with a sharp object or gunshot injury. These are usually referred to as false aneurysms.
- Inflammatory. Non-specific inflammatory aneurysms can occur, but mycotic aneurysms associated with specific bacterial infection can also occur. Syphilitic aneurysms are the best known but thankfully are now rare.
- Cystic medial necrosis is a degenerative condition of the arterial media and may occur as part of Marfan's syndrome.

Aortic aneurysm

Aortic aneurysms usually arise below the renal arteries and may extend into the iliac arteries. When small, aneurysms are usually asymptomatic. As they get progressively larger, the wall weakens.

Although an aneurysm may rupture at any size, it is unusual for this to occur if the maximum diameter is less than 5.5 cm. The risk of rupture is related to size and this is in the order of 20% per year for aneurysms greater than 5 cm. If the aneurysm ruptures, the likelihood is that the patient will die immediately. Even if they survive and undergo emergency surgery, the perioperative mortality is in the order of 50%. If the aneurysm is repaired as an elective procedure in a good centre, the mortality should be in the order of 5%. Therefore the aneurysm should be repaired before it ruptures. Aortic aneurysms may be lined with thrombus, some of which may break off and embolize to the smaller vessels of the legs causing acute ischaemia. Patients with aortic aneurysms may have aneurysms at other sites (e.g. iliac, femoral, popliteal).

Recognizing the pattern

The patient is usually over 50 years of age and males are more frequently affected than females. There may be associated atheromatous disease such as a history of myocardial infarction or angina or stroke.

Frequently the aneurysm is detected as an incidental finding at clinical assessment or during ultrasound examination. The patient sometimes notices an abdominal mass or pulsation. They may complain of back pain or epigastric discomfort as the aneurysm enlarges. There may be a sudden onset of pain and discoloration of the toes of one or both feet ('blue toe syndrome') which is caused by embolization of thrombus.

On examination, a pulsatile swelling is usually felt in the epigastrium and central abdomen. Palpation from side to side confirms that the pulsation is true and not transmitted. The essential characteristic however, is that this pulsatile mass is also expansile. When the examining index fingers are placed parallel to the lateral walls of the aneurysm, both fingers are pushed apart as the aneurysm expands during systole. In thin elderly patients with a prominent lordosis, the normal aorta is easily palpable and if somewhat tortuous may feel like an aneurysm. Careful bimanual palpation of its lateral and medial margins should demonstrate that it is not widened. It is important to examine for aneurysms at other locations especially in the femoral and popliteal arteries and also to assess distal pulses.

Proving the diagnosis

- A plain abdominal X-ray may show the characteristic curved line of calcification of the aneurysm wall.
- The best method of confirming the diagnosis is by using ultrasound.
- CT and MRI are the most accurate methods of measuring the size and extent of the aneurysm and determining whether it contains thrombus or not.
- Arteriography is not useful in the diagnosis of aortic aneurysm. However, it can give information with respect to the relationship of the renal vessels to the aneurysm and with newer methods of treatment, calibrated angiography to measure the exact length of the aneurysm and the angulation of its 'neck' is useful.

Management

The indications for repair are as follows.

- An aneurysm greater than 5.5 cm maximum diameter.
- An aneurysm giving rise to emboli.
- A rapidly expanding aneurysm.
- The onset of symptoms of abdominal or back pain as these may herald impending rupture.

If an aneurysm is less than 5 cm in diameter at presentation and is asymptomatic, its size should be observed every 3–6 months using ultrasound, to determine its rate of enlargement.

The patient and their relatives should be informed about the risks and benefits of surgery and the dangers of an untreated aneurysm. They should also be informed of the necessity of inserting a prosthetic graft to replace it. The patient's cardiac, respiratory and renal status should be assessed and optimized preoperatively. Perioperative β-blockade should be considered. Prophylactic antibiotics are given with the premedication or at induction of anaesthesia. Deep venous thrombosis prophylaxis using subcutaneous heparin should be used. The patient should have a urinary catheter inserted to measure urinary output during and after the procedure.

Endovascular repair of aortic aneurysm is undergoing clinical assessment at present. It requires a proximal and distal neck of suitable configuration to hold the stent graft. A tube graft or more usually a bifurcated graft may be inserted. A minority of aneurysms have a morphology suitable for this procedure.

OPERATION: CONVENTIONAL REPAIR OF AORTIC ANEURYSM

The aorta is exposed and the extent of the aneurysm confirmed. An aneurysm lying between the renal arteries and the aortic bifurcation may easily be replaced by a straight tube graft. If it extends into the iliac arteries it may be necessary to insert a bifurcated graft to the bifurcation of the iliac arteries or even to the femoral arteries in the groin. Once the aneurysm has been controlled proximally and distally, the lumbar vessels are suture ligated from within. The prosthesis is then sewn into the upper aorta and a similar anastomosis is made at the aortic bifurcation, iliac arteries or femoral arteries as indicated. The aneurysm wall is then wrapped around the graft.

Procedure profile

Blood requirement	6
Anaesthetic	GA/LA
Operation time	2–4 hours
Hospital stay	8–10 days
Return to normal activity	4–6 weeks

OPERATION: ENDOVASCULAR REPAIR OF AORTIC ANEURYSM

The femoral vessels are exposed and controlled through a groin incision. A guide wire is passed proximally into the aorta and a graft – previously prepared from the measurements obtained from calibrated angiography or CT – is passed over the wire through an incision in the femoral artery into the aorta. Bifurcated grafts with a main body consisting of one long limb and one short limb are inserted via one femoral and a second limb may be inserted into the short limb of the main body through the contralateral femoral artery excluding the aneurysm.

Procedure profile

Blood requirement	6
Anaesthetic	LA/GA
Operation time	2–4 hours
Hospital stay	2–5 days
Return to normal activity	4–6 weeks

Thrombus lining the aneurysm may become dislodged during the procedure. The presence of palpable pulses should be assessed before the patient leaves the procedure room. If previously palpable pulses are absent it is an indication for embolectomy. Haemodynamic monitoring is vital as hypotension, tachycardia and oliguria may indicate bleeding. A dopamine infusion to maintain renal output may be valuable especially in patients with impaired renal function, but must be used only when the patient is haemodynamically stable.

After open surgery the patient is mobilized on the third or fourth day postoperatively and may commence oral intake once the postoperative ileus has settled.

Follow-up of patients undergoing endovascular repair of aneurysms is vital as the long-term outlook is unknown. Patients undergoing standard operative repair need not be followed up beyond 6 weeks although there is the small possibility of developing graft infection or aortoenteric fistula where a loop of bowel becomes adherent and the graft fistulates into the bowel.

Ruptured aortic aneurysm

This is one of the most dramatic conditions which face the surgical team. The initial rupture is temporarily contained by the retroperitoneal tissues, in patients who survive long enough to be admitted to hospital. This gives a short time interval for the operation to be organized as the patient will die unless the aorta can be replaced before they exsanguinate. Rapid intervention is needed for the patient to survive.

Recognizing the pattern

The patient usually complains of sudden onset severe pain in the abdomen, back or flank, sometimes associated with collapse. The pain is more commonly on the left than the right. They may feel faint, cold and sweaty. Occasionally the presentation is less dramatic.

On examination the patient is pale and shocked with hypotension and tachycardia. The aneurysm is tender. Avoid palpating it more than is necessary. Note the presence or absence of distal pulses for future reference.

Proving the diagnosis

Time should not be wasted on investigations if the patient is shocked. A tender aneurysm in a shocked patient is an indication for surgery. If the situation is less acute, the diagnosis is in doubt and the patient is haemodynamically stable, a CT scan will confirm the presence of an aneurysm and demonstrate whether it is leaking.

Management

Warn the surgeon, anaesthetist and theatre as soon as possible that a patient with a leaking aneurysm has been admitted. Take blood for cross-matching (10 units) and baseline investigations (full blood count, urea and electrolytes and coagulation screen). Set up two large-bore intravenous lines and transfer the patient to theatre. If the patient is hypotensive, do not attempt to bring the blood pressure up at this stage as it may precipitate intraperitoneal rupture.

Prior to induction of anaesthesia pass a urinary catheter and give prophylactic antibiotics. Reassess the situation in the anaesthetic room if the patient is haemodynamically stable. Check how long it would be until the blood is available.

The patient will usually be induced on the operating table in theatre once the surgeon and the rest of the team are ready to start operating. The relaxation of the abdominal muscles associated with anaesthesia, reduces intra-abdominal pressure outside the vessel and so results in the loss of the tamponading effect. This frequently precipitates major blood loss.

*OPERATION: REPAIR OF RUPTURED AORTIC
ANEURYSM*

The abdomen is opened and a massive retroperitoneal haematoma is usually present. The aorta above the rupture and the iliac arteries below are controlled. Once this is done the haemorrhage is contained. The aneurysm is opened and a graft is sewn inside it as in an elective procedure.

Procedure profile

Blood requirement	10 (and cell saver if available)
Anaesthetic	GA
Operation time	2–5 hours
Hospital stay	8–21 days
Return to normal activity	Variable, 8–12 weeks

Postoperative care is as for an elective aneurysm repair. There is, however, a more prolonged period of intensive care as the patient has almost certainly been hypotensive for a period of time. Acute renal failure may occur in the postoperative period because of this. The patient will have a prolonged ileus because of the retroperitoneal haematoma and nutritional support may have to be considered. As the haematoma breaks down the patient may develop haemolytic jaundice which should resolve spontaneously.

Femoral aneurysms

These may present with acute thrombosis or embolization to the feet; they rarely rupture. They require resection or replacement with a graft if they are symptomatic or enlarge markedly.

Popliteal aneurysms

These frequently thrombose causing acute limb ischaemia. The presence of a large popliteal aneurysm is therefore an indication for surgery. The aneurysm may be tied off and a saphenous vein bypass graft inserted.

Acute arterial occlusion

This condition results in an acutely ischaemic limb, which has a high risk of limb loss unless intervention is swift. The causes are as follows.

- Acute arterial embolism. In this condition there is an acute blockage of an artery due to an embolus arising from thrombus formed proximally. Sources of emboli include the following:
  - atrial fibrillation
  - myocardial infarction with mural thrombus
  - subacute bacterial endocarditis
  - thrombus formation on an ulcerated atheromatous plaque
  - thrombus formation within an aneurysm.
- Acute thrombosis of chronic peripheral vascular disease. In this condition the patient has significant narrowing in an artery which thromboses when the flow through it decreases.
- Acute thrombosis of a popliteal artery aneurysm.
- Acute thrombosis of a previous bypass graft. In this condition the patient has had a previous bypass graft which occludes, usually as a result of stenosis within the graft or a progression of the atheromatous process above or below the graft.

Recognizing the pattern

Arterial emboli can occur in either sex and at any age but are more common in the elderly. Arterial thrombosis occurs in arteriopaths, typically middle-aged or elderly male smokers. Popliteal artery aneurysm thrombosis occurs in the elderly with a possible history of aortic aneurysm repair or surveillance. Graft occlusion can occur in anybody who has undergone a previous bypass graft.

Symptoms which occur in the affected limb are characterized by the following:

- pain
- pallor
- paralysis
- paraesthesia.

The history of embolism is characterized by sudden onset of these symptoms. If there is a previous history of intermittent claudication, the possibility of acute thrombosis should be considered. A history of previous vascular surgery is significant. The paraesthesia and paralysis are later symptoms and are due to ischaemia of the nerves. They are indicative that early intervention is indicated.

On examination the limb is pale, cold and immobile. Distal pulses are absent. There may be loss of pin-prick and light touch sensation in a stocking distribution over the distal leg. The pulse may be irregular and the patient may have other signs suggesting a source of embolus (e.g. a heart murmur, an aortic aneurysm or a localized arterial bruit). The contralateral limb should be assessed as peripheral vascular disease and popliteal artery aneurysms tend to be symmetrical.

Proving the diagnosis
Acute arterial embolism must be distinguished from thrombus on a previously existing atheromatous plaque or an occluded graft. The history and examination is a reliable guide. Arteriography is the definitive investigation.

Management
The treatment of acute ischaemia is urgent intervention to remove the blockage and restore the circulation. Blood is taken for group and cross-match and baseline haematological investigations (full blood count, urea and electrolytes and coagulation screen). Heparin infusion is commenced if there are no contraindications.

The treatments available to unblock the arteries include thrombolysis and surgery.

Thrombolysis is performed when there is limb-threatening acute arterial occlusion of short duration. It is contraindicated in patients with bleeding disorders, gastrointestinal bleeding, stroke, recent surgery or allergy to thrombolytic agents. It should not be considered in patients with paraesthesia and paralysis as the time taken to lyse the thrombus may result in irreversible ischaemia and limb loss. It is especially valuable in reopening occluded bypass grafts.

Surgery is indicated when thrombolysis is not possible or has failed.

OPERATION: INTRA-ARTERIAL CATHETER-DIRECTED THROMBOLYSIS

The radiologist should be aware that thrombolysis is being considered as the approach will probably be different if a diagnostic arteriogram is being performed. A catheter is placed in the artery percutaneously and an angiogram performed. The catheter is directed into the embolus or thrombus and a bolus of thrombolytic agent injected through the catheter directly into the clot. There are three thrombolytic agents in common usage, streptokinase, urokinase and tissue plasminogen activator. An infusion of thrombolytic agent is then commenced and the patient returned to the ward with the infusion running. A repeat arteriogram is performed at set intervals to assess clot dissolution. If the clot does not dissolve in 12 h, surgery should be considered.

If the procedure is successful, an angioplasty of the lesion causing thrombosis is indicated.

Procedure profile

Blood requirement	Group and save
Anaesthetic	LA
Operation time	2–12 hours
Hospital stay	2–5 days
Return to normal activity	2–4 weeks

OPERATION: CATHETER EMBOLECTOMY

The vessel where the embolus has lodged is isolated and controlled (commonly the femoral, occasionally the popliteal). An arteriotomy is made and visible clot extracted. The inflow of blood to the limb is checked. A Fogarty balloon catheter is passed down the arterial lumen. This is a thin catheter with a balloon at its tip. Once beyond the clot the balloon is dilated and gently pulled back towards the arteriotomy, extracting the clot. Once all the clot is extracted the arteriotomy is closed with a patch if necessary.

Procedure profile

Blood requirement	Group and save
Anaesthetic	LA/GA
Operation time	1–2 hours
Hospital stay	3–10 days
Return to normal activity	Variable

The postoperative care is similar to that following other arterial operations. The possibility of compartment syndrome, due to swelling of revascularized ischaemic muscles, must be considered if the patient develops pain or swelling of the leg after successful treatment. This is an emergency and the patient may require fasciotomies.

Arteriovenous fistulae

An arteriovenous fistula is a condition in which there is an abnormal connection between the arterial and the venous circulations. The common causes are as follows.

- Congenital – often associated with haemangioma or hamartoma formation.
- Post-traumatic – arteriovenous fistulae may follow penetrating injury or damage done to vessels during operation.
- Iatrogenic – arteriovenous shunts are created, usually in the forearm, as a route of access to the circulation for those on dialysis.

  The high pressure and increased flow causes the vein to dilate and become tortuous. There may be an increased cardiac output and a high pulse pressure if the shunt is large.

Recognizing the pattern
Arteriovenous fistulae are rare but can occur at any age from birth onwards.

The patient may have noticed prominent pulsatile veins, the mass of a haemangioma or the appearance of a 'throbbing' swelling at the site of previous trauma. Occasionally they complain of 'buzzing' associated with the flow disturbance. Rarely they present with high output cardiac failure.

Superficial fistulae are usually associated with dilated pulsatile veins. Subcutaneous fistulae present as a swelling beneath the skin, possibly associated with a scar suggestive of an old wound. On palpation there is an expansile pulsation. The characteristic sign is that of an audible 'machinery murmur' over the lesion present in both systole and diastole. It may be abolished by proximal arterial compression. There may be a palpable 'thrill'. Limb enlargement may be associated with congenital arteriovenous malformations.

Proving the diagnosis
Colour Doppler imaging will prove the diagnosis. Arteriography is required in planning appropriate therapy.

Management
Small arteriovenous fistulae may not require treatment. If there are dilated veins associated with the fistula, a graduated compression stocking or sleeve may be beneficial. Larger arteriovenous fistulae may be treated by embolization or surgery.

EMBOLIZATION
The radiologist performs an angiogram to identify the vessels forming the fistula. These are selectively cannulated and a thrombogenic substance is injected via the catheter, blocking the vessels and occluding the fistula.

OPERATION FOR ARTERIOVENOUS FISTULA
The feeding vessels (defined by preoperative arteriography) are dissected out and tied off and the fistula excised. There may be multiple feeding vessels especially in congenital arteriovenous fistulae and blood loss may be high. For this reason embolization is the preferred treatment.

Procedure profile

Blood requirement	4–6
Anaesthetic	GA
Operation time	2–5 hours
Hospital stay	7–14 days
Return to normal activity	4–6 weeks

12.4 Other arterial conditions

Carotid artery disease

The brain is supplied by four major arteries, the two internal carotid arteries and the two vertebral arteries. These communicate within the cranial cavity through the circle of Willis.

An atheromatous plaque in the carotid artery may affect the blood supply to the brain. Plaques are commonly formed at the bifurcation of the carotid arteries or at the origin of the internal carotid artery. Although reduction in cerebral blood flow is unusual because of the excellent collateral circulation through the circle of Willis, the plaque may undergo ulceration, thrombus formation and distal embolization resulting in a transient ischaemic attack or a stroke. A transient ischaemic attack is a focal neurological deficit lasting less than 24 h (usually lasting only a few minutes) with complete recovery. The symptoms depend upon the region supplied by the vessel in which the embolus lodges. Approximately one-third of patients who suffer from a transient ischaemic attack will have no further symptoms, another third will have further transient ischaemic attacks and the final third will progress to stroke. Acute, total occlusion of a carotid artery may cause a stroke resulting in a complete hemiparesis. This is often, but not always, preceded by transient ischaemic attacks.

The ophthalmic artery is the first branch of the internal carotid artery after it enters the skull. An embolus to this artery may lodge in the retinal artery, giving rise to transient mono-ocular blindness or amaurosis fugax. The embolus usually breaks up with full restoration of vision. If this does not occur the patient will suffer a retinal infarct in the area supplied by that branch of the retinal artery.

The unpredictability of the situation has made choosing which patients benefit from intervention difficult, but the indications for surgery are becoming clearer.

Recognizing the pattern

The patient is usually an arteriopath, middle aged or elderly, a smoker and hypertensive. They may have had previous peripheral or coronary arterial problems.

There may be a history of a single or multiple transient ischaemic attacks or an established stroke. These will affect the cerebral cortex on the same side as the carotid lesion and will result in a weakness or paraesthesia of the arm and leg on the opposite side of the body and possibly a speech disturbance. Amaurosis fugax will present as a transient blindness on the same side as the carotid lesion, which the patient may describe as a shutter coming down over the eye involved.

There may be nothing to find on examination but a localized bruit over the lateral side of the neck, which may arise from a narrowed carotid artery. The neurological and eye signs may be transient. Examination of the visual fields may reveal defects and fundoscopy may reveal evidence of previous emboli.

Proving the diagnosis

To confirm carotid artery disease, bilateral colour Doppler ultrasound imaging (Duplex) of the carotid arteries should be performed. This is a very accurate method of diagnosing carotid artery stenosis. On the basis of recognized blood velocity criteria, the degree of narrowing can be assessed as < 20%, 20–49%, 50–69% and 70–99%. Its limitation is in the differentiation of a very tight stenosis and an occlusion of the artery where operation is contraindicated. In this situation arteriography is helpful.

MRI angiography is non-invasive but at present its availability is limited to certain centres. It can confirm blood flow in the carotid arteries and simultaneously give information about the brain.

Conventional arteriography and intra-arterial digital subtraction arteriography give better images of the arteries, but there is a risk of causing a stroke when they are performed.

CT of the brain is useful to rule out other pathology (if an MRI study has not been performed).

Patients with suspected carotid artery disease should have the same risk factor assessment as those presenting with peripheral vascular disease.

Management

All patients should undergo risk factor modification to decrease the risk of disease progression. There are two approaches to treatment.

- The use of antiplatelet medication, such as aspirin, dipyridamole or clopidogril, and/or anticoagulants such as warfarin.
- Surgical endarterectomy to remove the plaque.

The decision over which treatment to use depends upon the symptomatic status of the patient and the degree of narrowing of the carotid arteries.

Management of asymptomatic bruit

Where a bruit is found in the neck but the patient has no symptoms, a Doppler imaging study should be requested. If there is a less than 70% narrowing of the carotid artery the patient should be commenced on low-dose aspirin (75 mg daily) to reduce the risk of stroke. If there is a 70–99% stenosis, most clinicians would treat the patient conservatively although there are ongoing clinical trials to determine whether surgery would be beneficial.

Management of transient ischaemic attacks

If a patient presents with transient ischaemic attacks and carotid Doppler studies show a narrowing of < 69%, treatment should be with aspirin or some other antiplatelet agent. Warfarin should be considered in patients with atrial fibrillation. If there is a stenosis of 70–99% surgery is indicated and is of definite benefit in preventing a stroke. If the carotid artery is occluded, surgery is not indicated.

Preoperatively the patient should be fully informed of the nature of the operation and of the risks of developing a stroke if surgery is not performed. They should be warned about the possibility of developing a stroke during or immediately after the operation. Such occurrences are thankfully rare and usually transient. The neck should be shaved on the relevant side. Medications should be reviewed preoperatively and the surgeon should be asked about continuing anticoagulants and antiplatelet agents preoperatively. Duplex scanning immediately preoperatively should be considered to rule out occlusion of the artery in the period between presentation and operation.

OPERATION: CAROTID ENDARTERECTOMY

The common, internal and external carotid arteries are exposed and controlled through an incision along the anterior border of the sternomastoid muscle. The patient is heparinized and the arteries clamped. A longitudinal incision is made in the common carotid artery extending into the internal carotid artery. The surgeon may decide to use a shunt. This is a tube placed in the common and internal carotid arteries to carry blood to the brain during the procedure. The localized plaque is removed by endarterectomy. The artery is closed and a vein or a prosthetic patch may be used to prevent narrowing.

Procedure profile

Blood requirement	2
Anaesthetic	GA/LA
Operation time	2 hours
Hospital stay	3–7 days
Return to normal activity	4–6 weeks

Postoperatively patients should undergo neurological observation in addition to the routine haemodynamic observations. Maintaining the blood pressure between 100 and 180 mmHg systolic is important. With hypertension there is a risk of bleeding from the arterial suture line and possibly a haemorrhagic stroke. Hypotension may result in thrombosis of the endarterectomy site resulting in stroke. Any neurological deficit should be reported to the surgeon immediately. Tongue deviation to the side of operation on protrusion indicates a hypoglossal nerve lesion, the majority of which recover. The patient may complain of headache, which is due to cerebral reperfusion. The patient should be reassured and given adequate analgesia. It usually settles within days but the patient should be observed until it does so.

Antiplatelet therapy should be prescribed postoperatively in all patients.

Raynaud's phenomenon

This is a clinical condition characterized by a sequence of colour changes in the digits on exposure to cold or emotional stress. The colour changes result from intense vasospasm of the digital vessels which cause the fingers (or toes) to go white initially, then cyanosed as the spasm relaxes in the arterioles but not in the venules and then red with reactive hyperaemia as there is complete relaxation of the spasm. The spasm may be due to a normal vasoconstrictive response to cold in diseased arteries or an excessive response to cold in normal vessels. The latter occurs more frequently and is called Raynaud's disease. It is a disease of unknown aetiology.

Secondary Raynaud's phenomenon usually occurs in diseased vessels and is seen in scleroderma, systemic lupus erythematosus and other connective tissue diseases. Other conditions which can cause stenoses in the arteries include cervical rib, atherosclerosis, Buerger's disease, cryoglobinaemia and certain drugs (e.g. the contraceptive pill). Certain occupational hazards such as working with vibrating tools, exposure to vinyl chloride and heavy metals may also cause it.

Recognizing the pattern
The patient is usually a woman in her late twenties or early thirties.

There is a history of colour changes following exposure to cold as described above. In Raynaud's disease the changes usually occur in all the fingers or toes and are symmetrical. In secondary Raynaud's phenomenon, the changes may be asymmetrical. There is usually numbness or pain associated with the attacks.

During an attack the characteristic sequence of colour changes are evident. Between attacks, the hands may appear normal. The skin of the fingers may be dry and fissured or there may be ulceration and gangrene at the tips of the fingers in extreme cases. Peripheral pulses are usually normal. It is important to rule out a cervical rib.

Proving the diagnosis

The diagnosis of Raynaud's disease is based on the history and exclusion of underlying causes. Delayed or abnormal hand rewarming after cold provocation can be measured using thermography. This will confirm a vasospastic tendency. Upper limb and digital pressure measurements will rule out occlusive disease in the arteries of the upper limb. Haematological investigations should be performed to rule out other underlying causes. These should include full blood count, plasma viscosity, liver function tests, thyroid function tests (TFTs), rheumatoid factor, antinuclear antibodies and cryoglobulins.

Management

Conservative measures are the mainstay of treatment, and are based on keeping the extremities warm (gloves and socks) and the avoidance of sudden exposure to cold. Battery-heated gloves are available for patients with frequent attacks. Skin care with moisturizing creams should be advised. It is important to maintain the central body core temperature and not just concentrate on the hands. Ulcers or infection should be treated with antibiotics as indicated. Patients should be advised to stop smoking as nicotine is a powerful vasoconstrictor.

Medications used include the calcium-channel blockers nifedipine and nicardipine, and the α-adrenergic blockers prazosin and thymoxamine. Response to medication is variable.

If symptoms are severe or trophic changes are present cervical sympathectomy may be indicated. This is effective in only 50–75% of cases and the benefit may be short-lived.

OPERATION: CERVICAL SYMPATHECTOMY

The anaesthetist must be informed whether the procedure is unilateral (which side) or bilateral.

This operation is best performed thoracoscopically (see p. 575). In the open operation the sympathetic chain may be approached using a supraclavicular incision or by an axillary incision, where access to the chest is gained by resecting a portion of the third rib. The second and third cervical ganglia are exposed and resected or destroyed. Chest drains may be used if a bilateral procedure is performed.

Procedure profile

Blood requirement	Group and save
Anaesthetic	GA
Operation time	1–2 hours
Hospital stay	2–7 days
Return to normal activity	1–2 weeks

Postoperatively a chest X-ray is performed in the recovery room to rule out pneumothorax. As well as routine haemodynamic observations, oxygen saturation should be assessed by oximetry. Atelectasis and chest infection are recognized complications of a thoracotomy. Horner's syndrome may occur, especially after supraclavicular cervical sympathectomy and is usually transient.

12.5 Venous disorders

Varicose veins

Varicose veins are elongated, dilated and tortuous veins, which usually occur in the skin of the lower limb. The veins in the leg may be divided into the skin (superficial) veins and the deep veins. They are connected by 'perforator' veins, which cross the deep fascia of the leg and drain blood from the superficial veins into the deep veins. The deep veins tend to lie within the muscle mass of the calf and thigh. When these muscles contract they act as an auxiliary pump to aid venous return. Valves in the perforating

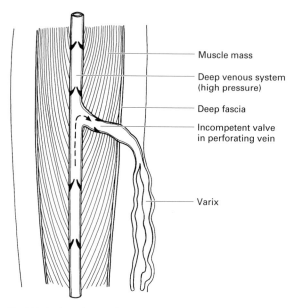

Fig. 12.5.1 The mechanism of varicose vein production.

veins prevent blood flowing into the skin veins under normal circumstances. During muscle relaxation, reverse flow of blood is prevented within the deep veins by valves.

If the valves in the connecting veins become incompetent, pressure will be transmitted from the deep veins into the skin veins resulting in the formation of varicose veins (Fig. 12.5.1).

Common sites for incompetent valves to occur are as follows.

· Where the long saphenous vein joins the femoral vein in the groin.
· Where the short saphenous vein joins the popliteal vein in the popliteal fossa.
· Where there are perforator veins in the medial aspect of the midthigh.
· Where calf perforators connect the deep veins and the skin veins behind the medial border of the tibia.

Recognizing the pattern

The clinician's task is to determine if the patient's symptoms are due to the varicosities and to determine the site of reflux from the deep to the superficial system.

Patients are usually female in their twenties or thirties but may be either sex or any age.

A history of previous deep venous thrombosis should be sought. Symptoms, which may be associated with varicose veins, include the following.

- Cosmetic. The patient is upset about the appearance.
- Pain. Varicose veins characteristically give rise to ache in the leg especially after prolonged standing. It is relieved by leg elevation and support stockings.
- Itching. This often occurs over the varicosities, is worse in warm weather or after a hot bath and may occur in the presence of eczema.
- Other symptoms due to the complication of varicose veins. These include oedema or leg swelling (worse at the end of the day), pigmentation and thickening of the skin in the region of the medial malleolus, eczema and even ulceration.

On examination the site of reflux through an incompetent perforator or perforators should be sought. On inspection and palpation the presence of varicosities is self-evident and different patterns of visible varicosities are outlined in Fig. 12.5.2. A dilated saphenofemoral junction presenting as a 'lump in the groin' is a saphena varix. The presence of complications of varicose veins should be sought. Peripheral pulses should be palpated.

Proving the diagnosis

It is possible to confirm the presence of reflux using a hand-held Doppler. With the patient standing, the saphenofemoral junction is identified (medial to the femoral artery) and the probe placed over it. The patient's calf is squeezed and an augmentation of blood flow is heard. On release of the calf normally nothing is audible, but in patients with saphenofemoral junction incompetence, sustained reverse flow is heard. The saphenopopliteal junction can be assessed in a similar manner.

The results of treatment depend on the accuracy of the diagnosis of the site of valvular incompetence. Colour Doppler

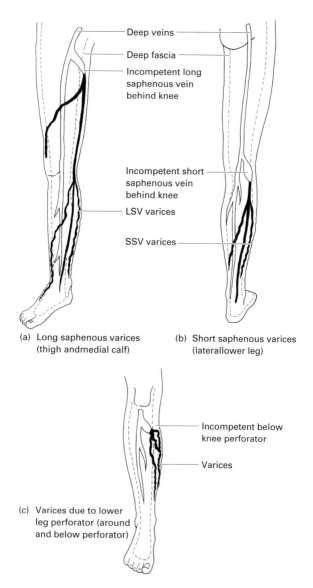

Deep veins

Deep fascia

Incompetent long
saphenous vein
behind knee

Incompetent short
saphenous vein
behind knee

LSV varices

SSV varices

(a) Long saphenous varices
(thigh andmedial calf)

(b) Short saphenous varices
(laterallower leg)

Incompetent below
knee perforator

Varices

(c) Varices due to lower
leg perforator (around
and below perforator)

imaging of the veins may be helpful in the accurate localization of sites of reflux as the veins can be visualized and the direction of flow can be assessed simultaneously.

Ascending phlebography may occasionally be useful in localizing calf perforator incompetence but only in selected cases.

Management

Conservative treatment is advised if the varices are not very severe or if intervention is contraindicated. Loosing weight, skin care and graduated compression hosiery are the mainstay of conservative treatment. Hosiery should be renewed every 4–6 months as it tends to lose its elasticity. The indications for intervention are severe disfiguring varices, aching or pain, the presence of skin changes or ulceration. Intervention may be contraindicated if there is any evidence of deep venous occlusion (usually after previous deep venous thrombosis). Active treatments are foam or sclerosant injection with ultrasound guidance, or surgery.

INJECTION SCLEROTHERAPY

This is suitable treatment for patients with isolated, residual (after surgery) or recurrent varicose veins where there is no reflux of blood from the deep to the superficial system.

It is performed in the outpatient department. A sclerosant is injected into the superficial veins and compression bandaging immediately applied and maintained for 6 weeks. The patient is advised to walk frequently to decrease the risk of deep venous thrombosis.

OPERATION: FOR VARICOSE VEINS

Operation is the treatment of choice in patients with reflux of blood from the deep to the superficial system, especially into the long saphenous and short saphenous veins. Increasingly, varicose vein surgery is being carried out as a day-case procedure. If this is the case it may be better to operate on one leg at a time to encourage postoperative mobility.

Fig. 12.5.2 (*Opposite*) The three examples of varicose veins due to incompetent perforating veins. (a) Long saphenous varices (thigh and medial calf); (b) short saphenous varices (lateral lower leg); (c) varices due to lower leg perforator (around and below perforator). LSV, long saphenous vein; SSV, short saphenous vein.

Preoperatively the patient is measured for a full-length graduated compression stocking. With the patient standing, the veins are marked as they are difficult to localize when the patient is supine. This should be performed by the operating surgeon. If saphenopopliteal junction reflux is present, the saphenopopliteal junction may be marked preoperatively using colour Doppler imaging as there is anatomical variation in the level of the saphenopopliteal junction. Deep venous thrombosis prophylaxis is given.

There are a number of operations performed for varicose veins surgery. The technique involves ligating the site of reflux from the deep to the superficial venous systems and removing the varicose veins.

OPERATION: HIGH TIE OF THE LONG SAPHENOUS VEIN (SYN: FLUSH LIGATION)

The long saphenous vein is ligated at its origin flush with the saphenofemoral junction. This is synonymous with flush ligation. All its branches in the groin should be ligated.

OPERATION: STRIPPING

The long saphenous vein may be removed by passing a wire with a metal 'olive' attached at one end, down through its lumen. The vein is tied around the wire and the 'olive' strips the vein when the wire is pulled. This procedure is done to disconnect the vein from its branches and from midthigh perforators. The long saphenous vein used to be stripped to the ankle but a high incidence of saphenous nerve damage was associated so now the vein is only stripped to knee level. It has been shown to decrease the risk of recurrence.

OPERATION: MULTIPLE AVULSIONS

The actual varicosities are avulsed through small incisions over the vein.

OPERATION: SAPHENOPOPLITEAL JUNCTION LIGATION

The short saphenous vein is ligated at its junction with the popliteal vein behind the knee. The short saphenous vein is rarely stripped because of the risk of damage to the sural nerve which is intimately related to it.

Procedure profile

Blood requirement	0
Anaesthetic	GA
Operation time	1–2 hours
Hospital stay	Day case or overnight stay
Return to normal activity	1–2 weeks

Postoperatively the leg is bandaged in theatre and the patient is discharged later that day on appropriate analgesics. Patients are encouraged to mobilize the following day. After a week the bandages are removed and the graduate compression stocking which has been fitted preoperatively is worn for a further 5 weeks. At that stage the patient is reviewed in the outpatients and discharged if all is well, or scheduled for surgery on the other leg if this is indicated.

Venous ulceration

Chronic venous hypertension leads to damaged capillaries, oedema and induration. Red cells leaking out of the capillaries are broken down in the interstitial tissue resulting in haemosiderin deposition and brownish discoloration of the leg. The nutrition to the skin is impaired which leads to eczema and ulceration.

Venous ulceration is ultimately a complication of chronic venous hypertension following valvular damage in the deep system after deep venous thrombosis or in the superficial system following chronic varicose veins. It is important to recognize that there may be an arterial component to the ulceration in up to 15% of patients.

Recognizing the pattern
Women are more commonly affected and usually present over the age of 40 years.

There is chronic painful reddening or discoloration of the skin above the medial malleolus. The ulcer is commonly precipitated by minor trauma. The ulcer is frequently painless but any discomfort is exacerbated when the leg is dependent. There may be a history of previous deep venous thrombosis.

The typical site for a venous ulcer is the lower third of the calf on the medial aspect. There may be slough on the ulcer surface or a seropurulent discharge. The base is covered with granulation tissue and never penetrates the deep fascia. There is usually an irregular shelving edge which is usually a dark blue colour. The surrounding skin is usually pigmented, dry and flaky but there may be cellulitis present. Varicose veins are invariably present and the sites of valvular incompetence should be sought. Peripheral pulses should be sought and documented and the ABPI (see p. 493) should be measured prior to treatment.

Proving the diagnosis

The ABPI will confirm or rule out the presence of peripheral vascular disease. In cases where the diagnosis is uncertain, full blood count and plasma viscosity (PV), culture of the ulcer, TPHA and Mantoux tests may be indicated. If an ulcer is chronic, biopsy of the edge is indicated to rule out malignant change (Marjolin's ulcer). The underlying sites of venous reflux can be confirmed using colour Doppler imaging or phlebography.

Management

There are three aspects to the management of venous ulceration.
- The prevention of ulceration in patients with the preulcerative changes associated with venous hypertensive disease.
- Healing an established ulcer.
- Prevention of recurrent ulceration in patients who have a healed ulcer.

PREVENTION OF ULCERATION

Skin care. Patients who have thickened dry skin benefit from having an emollient in their bath water and in applying unperfumed oil to their skin after bathing. Patients with eczema may benefit from local application of a steroid ointment. Cellulitis should be treated with systemic antibiotics; locally applied antibiotics are of no benefit and may induce sensitivity.

Compression. Graduated compression hosiery (class II, pressure 18–24 mmHg or class III, pressure 25–35 mmHg), below knee, above knee or tights should be prescribed. Two pairs should be prescribed at a time as the patient should always wear one set when the other is being washed. These should be replaced every 4–6 months as they tend to lose their elasticity over time. It is important that the patient is satisfied as compliance is vital.

Surgery. Surgical correction of underlying sites of valvular incompetence must be performed if possible to prevent ulceration:

TREATMENT OF ESTABLISHED ULCERATION
Patients with venous ulceration need to have an ABPI measurement prior to treatment. If the ABPI measurement is less than 0.8, an arterial assessment should be performed, as improvement in arterial blood flow may be required to heal the ulcer. A culture swab should be taken from the ulcer if it is infected and the skin care measures outlined above should be commenced.

If ABPI is above 0.8, four-layer compression bandaging should be applied. The ulcer is cleaned with saline and a non-adhesive dressing applied. A layer of padding bandage is applied from the level of the metatarsal heads to the tibial tuberosity. A light crêpe bandage is then applied to smooth the contour of the limb. A light compression bandage is then applied and finally an elasticated cohesive bandage. The dressing is changed weekly in patients with clean ulcers or twice weekly in those with sloughy ulcers. Using this technique it is possible to heal 75% of venous ulcers in 12 weeks.

If the deep venous system is normal, then surgical correction of the underlying venous disorder may accelerate healing and prevent recurrence. If the deep system is not functioning correctly, patients need to wear support stockings for the rest of their life to prevent ulcer recurrence.

PROPHYLAXIS
Anyone who develops a deep venous thrombosis should wear 'blue line' elastic bandages until the tendency to swelling is controlled. They should then be encouraged to wear good supportive stockings until all tendency to oedema formation has disappeared. If the tissues are adequately supported in this way (for 3–6 months) induration can be prevented and risk of ulceration decreased. Tubigrip elastic supports are not adequate (see p. 529).

12.6 Lymphoedema

Fluid and a small quantity of protein normally leaks out of the capillaries into the interstitial space to form interstitial fluid. Most of the fluid is resorbed at the venous end of the capillaries but some, together with the protein is collected in the lymphatic channels and returned to the circulation after being filtered through the lymph nodes. Obstruction to the flow of lymph produces chronic oedema. Causes may be grouped as follows.

- Primary. This is a rare condition affecting 1 in 33 000 of the population. It is due to absent, hypoplastic or hyperplastic (dilated) lymphatics with absent valves.
- Secondary. The lymphatics are blocked due to external causes such as:
  ◦ fibrosis, e.g. following infection or radiotherapy
  ◦ infestation, e.g. filariasis
  ◦ infiltration by neoplasm, e.g. malignant melanoma
  ◦ trauma, e.g. following block dissection of the groin or axilla.

Recognizing the pattern
Primary lymphoedema frequently affects females. It may present at birth (when it may be called Milroy's disease if associated with a family history of leg swelling) but usually presents in the teens or at any time up to middle age. Secondary lymphoedema can occur at any age.

The patient notices painless swelling of one or both limbs which is worse at the end of the day. Primary lymphoedema always presents in the legs, secondary lymphoedema may occur in the arms or legs, depending on the underlying cause. Occasionally, the patient presents with cellulitis in which case the limb will be painful.

On examination in early cases, the oedema is of the pitting type, however, in chronic cases the oedema is brawny and non-pitting. The quality of the skin should be noted and the size of the limb measured (circumferential measurements at recorded points from bony landmarks) and recorded.

Proving the diagnosis
It is necessary to exclude other causes of limb oedema such as cardiac failure, renal failure, hypoproteinaemia, hepatic

impairment, and hypothyroidism (usually bilateral) or venous hypertensive disease (usually unilateral).

A positive diagnosis of lymphoedema can be obtained by a lymphoscintogram. Technetium^{99m}-labelled sulphur colloid is injected into a web space of the foot and its clearance is monitored by a gamma camera. Lymphoscintograms may also demonstrate hypoplastic or hyperplastic lymphatics or abnormalities in the proximal lymphatics.

Management

The management is conservative and surgery is rarely indicated.

CONSERVATIVE TREATMENT

Initial therapy. The aim of initial therapy is to treat any infections, heal any ulcers and reduce the size of the limb. Cellulitis occurring in patients with lymphoedema is a serious-condition and needs admission and treatment with intravenous antibiotics. Skin care with moisturizing creams or lotions is important to improve the quality of the skin and decrease the risk of infection. Limb volume reduction methods include, elevation, manual lymphatic drainage (a physiotherapy technique), external elastic compression bandaging, and external pneumatic compression. These treatments can be provided on an out-patient basis.

Maintenance therapy. Once the limb volume has been reduced, continued skin care is required. The patient should be fitted with fully supported graduated compression hosiery as for chronic venous insufficiency. Tubigrip is contraindicated as it applies constant pressure through out its length and impedes lymphatic drainage from the foot. If the patient suffers from recurrent cellulitis, long-term, low-dose penicillin may be required. Diuretics are rarely of value.

OPERATIVE TREATMENT

Most surgical treatments for lymphoedema have not been subject to rigorous evaluation. The patient should be informed that there are no effective methods of restoring lost lymphatic channels. Two operations have been performed in the past but are rarely performed now. The operations are performed under tourniquet control to reduce blood loss and the leg is elevated

and supported during the operation using a Kirschner wire
through the calcaneum.

HOMANS' OPERATION
An area of skin with a wider area of subcutaneous tissue is
excised from the medial aspect of the lower leg, reducing its bulk.
A similar procedure may be carried out on the lateral aspect, usually at a later date.

CHARLES' OPERATION
A circumferential excision of all the skin and subcutaneous tissue
from the knee to the ankle is excised and skin grafts applied to the
defect.

13 Skin surgery

13.1 Benign lesions of the skin

Much differing pathology presents as lumps in the skin. Skin 'lumps and bumps' are therefore popular in examinations. Your examination technique for these should include determination of the following 11 points.

- Shape – rounded, irregular, elliptical, etc.
- Size – in centimetres, including depth, width and length.
- Surface – smooth, nodular, irregular, ill defined.
- Consistency – hard, soft, fluctuant.
- Colour.
- Edge – well defined, ill defined.
- Fixation – to superficial layers of skin or deep to the muscle or fascia.
- Transillumination?
- Pulsation?
- Bruit?
- Relationship to surroundings – where are the regional nodes and are they enlarged?

  Make a habit of running through each of these headings each time that you encounter a lump in the skin.

Papilloma (skin tag, fibroepithelial polyp)

This is a benign overgrowth of normal skin. It consists of a core of connective tissue and blood vessels covered by epidermis. Intradermal naevi and neurofibromas can produce a similar appearance.

Surgery: Diagnosis and Management, 4th edition. Edited by N. Rawlinson and D. Alderson. © 2009 Blackwell Publishing, ISBN: 978-1-4051-2921-3

Recognizing the pattern

Papillomas occur at any age but are more common in the elderly.
Patients request removal for cosmetic reasons or because they
catch on clothing or have been traumatized.

Papillomas occur at any site and occur in all shapes and sizes.
They are either soft and compressible, or solid, smooth pedun-
culated nodules. There may be surface ulceration due to trauma.
Multiple tiny tags are common around the neck and axilla.

OPERATION: REMOVAL OF SKIN PAPILLOMA

Small tags (1–5 mm diameter) can be snipped off with scissors
without using anaesthetic, but it is painful (Fig. 13.1.1). Bleeding will stop spontaneously. When larger tags are snipped off
anaesthetic is required mainly to enable cautery to be used for
haemostasis. In both instances the wound will heal spontaneously providing it is kept clean. Alternatively, the papilloma
pedicle can be removed using an elliptical excision. The ellipse
direction should follow the skin crease lines. The wound is closed
with monofilament nylon sutures. All papillomas should be sent
for histology.

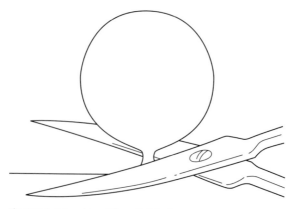

Fig. 13.1.1 Snip excision of fibroepithelial polyp.

Procedure profile

Blood requirement	0
Anaesthetic	LA
Operation time	15 minutes
Hospital stay	Outpatient
Return to normal activity	Less than 24 hours

Seborrhoeic keratosis (seborrhoeic wart, basal cell papilloma)

This is a benign overgrowth of the basal cells of the epidermis.

Recognizing the pattern

The patient is usually elderly and concerned because the lesion is unsightly, itchy or slowly getting bigger.

On examination it is a flattened well-defined, greasy, tan or dark brown warty plaque that appears to be 'stuck onto' the skin rather than an integral part of it. Any site can be affected. Multiple warts are commonly present on the trunk, head and neck.

Management

Reassurance is usually sufficient. Seborrhoeic warts can be removed by curettage (Fig. 13.1.2) or destroyed by cryotherapy. Lesions that do not curette off easily may be warty pigment naevi and these have to be excised. In general elliptical excision of seborrhoeic warts is unnecessary and produces an inferior cosmetic result. Any seborrhoeic wart removed should be sent for histology.

Infective warts

Common warts are the result of a human papilloma virus infection. They are thus contagious and common on children's hands. Immunity to the virus is conferred by previous infection

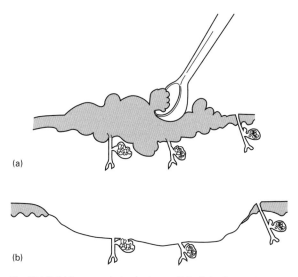

Fig. 13.1.2 (a) Curettage of seborrhoeic wart. (b) Eroded surface remaining with retained hair follicles and sweat ducts after curettage.

so that viral warts are uncommon in older immunocompetent people. On the sole of the foot, pressure pushes the wart into the skin producing the characteristic verruca.

Recognizing the pattern

A wart is a slow-growing nodular lesion of the skin which eventually regresses spontaneously. Many warts last for more than 2 years. Warts may bleed on trauma, become painful particularly if infected, but are principally social embarrassments.

Without repeated injury, e.g. on the face, a wart will develop multiple frond-like surface growths. At sites exposed to regular minor trauma, e.g. fingers and feet, these frond-like growths are worn away leaving a hard keratinized papule with a warty or irregular surface. This is characteristically surrounded by an acorn-cup like rim of normal skin (Fig. 13.1.3).

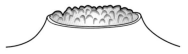

Fig. 13.1.3 Viral wart with typical 'acorn cup' appearance.

Management

Treatment is not necessary. Reassurance that warts regress spontaneously is usually sufficient. Regression can be hastened by topical keratolytics (salicylic acid and lactic acid), curettage or cryotherapy. Because warts are infectious none of these treatments are definitively curative.

Keloid

In a keloid the overgrowth of fibrous tissue spreads beyond the original scar boundaries and never resolves spontaneously. By contrast in a hypertrophic scar the thickening remains localized to the original scar and eventually softens and flattens (Fig. 13.1.4).

Recognizing the pattern

Keloids are common in Afro-Caribbeans, Asians and young people. The lump is slow growing, tender or itchy. There is usually a

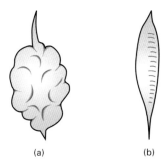

(a)   (b)

Fig. 13.1.4 Comparison of (a) a keloid and (b) a hypertrophic scar.

history of previous trauma or surgery although keloids may form after minimal trauma (e.g. acne scarring).

On examination red-brown or purple firm scar tissue is heaped up above the level of the skin and it may even become pedunculated. Keloids can occur anywhere but are commonest at keloid-prone sites (central chest, upper back and shoulders). The whole or part of the scar may be involved.

Management

Keloids are difficult to manage. No treatment is uniquely effective. The surgeon should avoid the temptation to excise a keloid as it is almost certain to recur. Repeated injection of steroids into the keloid (triamcinolone 10–40 mg/mL) will reduce scar thickness. Silicone gel sheeting is useful for large hypertrophic scars. Radiotherapy should be avoided because of the risk of inducing tumour formation. Excision of keloids that are easy to excise (e.g. ear lobe) is advocated with intraoperative and postoperative intralesional steroid injection and pressure therapy.

Hypertrophic scars, by contrast, will improve spontaneously. Intralesional steroids will hasten this outcome but, as with keloids, there is the risk of perilesional steroid atrophy.

Lipoma

This is a benign tumour composed of fat cells divided into large lobules by loose fibrous septa. Lipomas are frequently multiple. Painful lipomas are actually angiolipomas.

Recognizing the pattern

The patient is usually an adult. The lesion is rare in children. The lump takes several years to reach the size of a walnut. Advice is usually sought when the lump becomes unsightly. There may be a family history of similar lesions.

Lipomas occur anywhere there is adipose tissue but are commoner on the upper limb and trunk. They may be of any size from a few millimetres to several centimetres in diameter. Occasionally a lipoma arises in the muscle or close to the deep fascia, in which case it appears to be attached to the muscle. The tumour has a smooth, lobulated surface with a well-defined edge. It is usually soft although small lipomas may be quite firm. It often lies in the subcutis, and the skin can then be moved over it.

Management
If the lipoma is causing trouble it should be removed.

OPERATION: REMOVAL OF LIPOMA

An incision is made over the lipoma in the direction of the skin creases and deepened until the lipoma is reached. The lipoma is then gently freed from the surrounding skin. Soft lipomas can be squeezed out through the incision. If a large lipoma has been removed the cavity may be need to be drained.

Procedure profile

Blood requirement	0
Anaesthetic	LA or GA depending on size
Operation time	10–30 minutes
Hospital stay	Outpatient or 24 hours
Return to normal activity	1–2 days

Epidermoid cyst, implantation dermoids and pilar cysts (sebaceous cysts, steatoma, epithelial cyst)

The term epidermoid cyst causes great confusion. Epidermoid cysts are lined with stratified squamous epithelium which produces keratin; this slowly accumulates to form a foul smelling cheesy material. Epidermoid cysts are not derived from sebaceous glands. Most cysts arise spontaneously. When they appear on the face and back some are the result of old acne scarring blocking a hair follicle. Epidermoid cysts characteristically have a punctum through which the contents can be expressed and via which infections sometimes enter.

An implantation dermoid is an acquired condition due to implantation of epidermis into the subcutaneous tissue. The epidermis continues to grow and forms a cyst that is lined with stratified squamous epithelium. The patient may be a gardener or manual worker likely to suffer hand injuries.

Pilar cysts (sebaceous cyst, trichilemmal cyst) are very similar except that they mainly occur on the scalp, do not have punctum, are lined by a non-stratified epithelium and are much thinner walled and thus burst more easily during removal. They contain more watery contents than an epidermoid cyst. Both types of cyst can be treated in the same way. Rarely a pilar cyst can develop into a proliferating pilar (trichilemmal) cyst which may be confused with a squamous cell carcinoma of the scalp.

Recognizing the pattern

Epidermoid cysts occur at any age but are rare in children. They may be multiple. The patient presents because they are unsightly, infected or discharging. On examination the lump is a spherical, smooth, well-defined swelling of variable size, which may be visible as a white cyst through the overlying stretched skin. A punctum is frequently visible. Epidermoid cysts are common on the scalp, face and upper back.

Management

An infected epidermoid cyst must first be drained and excised later. Inflamed epidermoid cysts are not invariably infected. If the cyst wall bursts, usually because of injudicious squeezing by the patient, the keratin leaks out into the surrounding tissues and provokes a brisk foreign-body reaction. Inflamed or infected cysts are best left to settle with antibiotics before removal is attempted because the tissues are friable and excision is difficult. A non-infected cyst can be removed under a local anaesthetic.

OPERATION: EXCISION OF EPIDERMOID CYST

On a hair-bearing site adjacent hair should be shaved off. Lignocaine 1% with adrenaline (1 : 200 000) should be infiltrated around and immediately above the cyst so as to partly separate the skin and the cyst wall. The punctum should be excised with the cyst using an ellipse centred on the punctum (Fig. 13.1.5). Alternatively, large cysts can be incised, the contents expressed and the cyst lining grasped with artery forceps and enucleated.

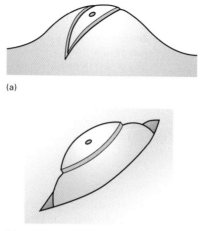

(a)

(b)

Fig. 13.1.5 Excision of an epidermoid cyst. (a) The ellipse should be centred on the punctum. (b) The cyst can be removed intact using the ellipse to manoeuvre the cyst.

Removal of the intact cyst is a surer way of guaranteeing complete removal because retained wall fragments may cause recurrence. Pressure should be applied to occlude the remaining dead space and the skin closed with a monofilament nylon suture. If the cyst has previously ruptured or been infected, the cyst plus the surrounding fibrotic tissue should be removed.

Procedure profile

Blood requirement	0
Anaesthetic	LA
Operation time	15–30 minutes
Hospital stay	Outpatient
Return to normal activity	1–2 hours

Dermoid cysts

Dermoid cysts are different. These are rare developmental abnormalities developing at embryological lines of skin fusion when a piece of epidermis comes to lie beneath the skin's surface. Seventy per cent present in children as soft nodules on the midline of the head and neck, or outer third of the eyebrow (external angle dermoid). Surgery is potentially complicated because a proportion have deeper attachments to bone or periosteum. Preoperative CT scanning may therefore be required.

Ganglion

The cause of ganglia is not established. Ganglia may arise from the leakage of synovial fluid secondary to myxomatous degeneration occurring in fibrous tissue close to a joint capsule or tendon sheath. The cystic lesion contains 'glairy', sticky, clear fluid. On the finger a similar lesion, called a myxoid cyst, results from leakage of synovial fluid from the distal interphalangeal joint into the posterior nailfold.

Recognizing the pattern
The patient is usually an adult who presents with a disfiguring, painful or movement-restricting lump.

The lump is commonly around the hand or wrist or on the foot, close to the joints. The swelling is lobulated with a smooth surface and a well-defined edge. It may be of any size and consistency. It often becomes more tense when the joint is flexed or extended. It is attached deeply but not to the skin.

Management
A ganglion can sometimes be dispersed by pressure (being 'hit with the family bible') or by aspiration with a needle, but tends to recur. The favoured method of treatment is excision.

OPERATION: REMOVAL OF A GANGLION
It is usually possible to remove the ganglion under a local anaesthetic but, at difficult sites or in a young patient, a general

anaesthetic is preferred. An exsanguinating tourniquet is used where possible. Ganglia are often intimately related to tendons, arteries and nerves and must be dissected out with great care.

Procedure profile

Blood requirement	0
Anaesthetic	LA or GA
Operation time	30 minutes
Hospital stay	Outpatient
Return to normal activity	Depends on occupation

Neurofibroma

These are benign tumours arising from both the nerve sheath and neural tissue. In neurofibroma the whole nerve is therefore involved and complete removal inevitably results in removal of the nerve. Neurofibromas may arise from unnamed small nerve radicals, larger nerve branches, individual major nerves and dorsal nerve roots in the paraspinal region.

Neurilemmomas (schwannoma) by contrast arise from the myelin-producing Schwann's cells only and have a true capsule. Whilst they may press on the nerve axon they do not involve it. A neurilemmoma can therefore be carefully dissected out without damage to the nerve function (Fig. 13.1.6).

Multiple neurofibromatosis (Von Recklinghausen's disease, neurofibromatosis type 1 or NF1, peripheral neurofibromatosis) is caused by an autosomal dominant gene on chromosome 17. Patients have multiple neurofibromas, café-au-lait patches, axillary freckling, Lisch nodules (brown specks) in the iris, optic gliomas, and skeletal and endocrine abnormalities including phaeochromocytoma. Neurofibromatosis type 2 (NF2) patients (syn: central neurofibromatosis) also have multiple neurofibroma but in association with bilateral acoustic neuromas and other neural tumours but none of the other skin or skeletal changes and

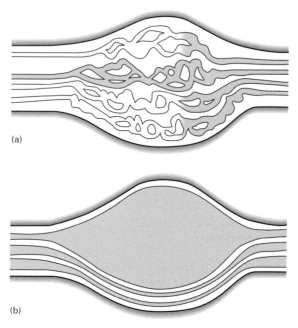

Fig. 13.1.6 Comparison of (a) a neurofibroma in which both neural tissue and nerve sheath are involved with (b) a neurilemmoma in which just the neural sheath is affected.

different eye abnormalities. The abnormal autosomal dominant gene is on chromosome 22.

Recognizing the pattern

The patient may present at any age but is usually adult. When taking a history ask about other affected family members. A neurofibroma is often asymptomatic but is occasionally painful. It may be disfiguring or rarely cause paraesthesiae or motor weakness in the distribution of the nerve involved. Rapid size increase and pain may be caused by haemorrhage into the neurofibroma or malignant transformation.

On examination three types of neurofibromas are recognized.

- Discrete cutaneous neurofibromas that move when the skin is moved. These are soft, lilac or flesh coloured, pedunculated or sessile, cutaneous or subcutaneous tumours.

- Subcutaneous neurofibromas that are not attached to the skin and appear as a firm, possibly tender, subcutaneous oval swelling. These may be attached to a large nerve and consequently are relatively fixed in the direction of the nerve but mobile at right angles to the nerve trunk. Pressure on it may cause tingling in the nerve distribution.

- Plexiform neurofibromas, which arise from larger nerves and may be very large and infiltrate into adjacent structures. All types may undergo sarcomatous change although this is more likely in plexiform neurofibromas.

Management

Neurofibromas need only be removed if they interfere with normal function, or are disfiguring, excessively big or painful. Complete removal may be difficult because some cutaneous neurofibromas are diffuse and difficult to excise. Large, proximally based, neurofibromas may be associated with potentially serious loss of function due to nerve damage during removal. If this is suspected thorough investigation of the potential for sensory or motor loss should be carried out before surgery and the patient warned. Sarcoma formation occurs in approximately 5% of multiple neurofibromatosis patients and is characterized by increasing pain and size of the neurofibroma. The diagnosis should be confirmed by incisional biopsy and excision thereafter. Plexiform neurofibromas may bleed significantly during excision.

OPERATION: EXCISION OF A NEUROFIBROMA

An attempt should be made to excise the neurofibroma fully. The nerve ends may need to be resutured if the function supplied is vital. The risk of sarcomatous change is not increased by incomplete excision.

Procedure profile

Blood requirement	0
Anaesthetic	LA or GA
Operation time	30 minutes
Hospital stay	Inpatient/outpatient
Return to normal activity	Variable – 24 hours for a small lesion

Postoperatively the patient may occasionally need admitting and the limb immobilizing to protect a nerve anastomosis.

Keratoacanthoma (molluscum sebaceum)

This is a self-healing tumour of keratinocytes that arises on sun-damaged sites. It is easily confused, both clinically and histologically, with squamous cell carcinoma and if there is doubt about the diagnosis it should be treated as a squamous cell carcinoma.

Recognizing the pattern
The patient is usually elderly and complains of a rapidly expanding lesion with a dark central core. The nodule should reach its maximum size by 3 months and begin to regress in size thereafter.

Keratoacanthomas arise on chronically sun-exposed skin as a round symmetrical nodule with a smooth shoulder of stretched skin. The central keratin horn (Fig. 13.1.7) becomes necrotic in older lesions.

Management
A clinical diagnosis of keratoacanthoma should only be made if there is a history of a rapidly growing lesion that starts to spontaneously decrease in size after 3 months. The lesion should be symmetrical with an edge of normal skin rather than tumour. If a confident clinical diagnosis is made the lesion can be allowed to resolve spontaneously leaving a small crateriform scar. If

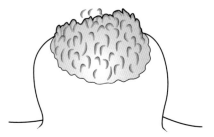

Fig. 13.1.7 Characteristic appearance of a keratoacanthoma with a symmetrical shape and shoulder of normal skin expanded by the enclosed tumour.

removal is required this can be done by excision, curettage or radiotherapy. If there is doubt about the diagnosis the lesion should be managed as a squamous cell carcinoma by wide local excision.

13.2 Pigmented naevi and malignant skin conditions

Moles (pigmented naevi)

Moles commonly appear in the first two decades of life. An average adult in their late twenties will have 20–30 naevi. There are several normal variants of benign naevi. Moles evolve and therefore change in appearance with time.

Benign naevi evolve through three stages (Fig. 13.2.1) and these changes are characteristically best seen on facial naevi. Initially they appear as flat brown moles. Histologically these are junctional naevi with clumps of melanocytes centred around the junction between the epidermis and dermis. This evolves into a compound naevus when some melanocytes move deeper into the dermis whilst others remain at the junction. These appear as raised brown moles. Finally all the naevus cells move into the

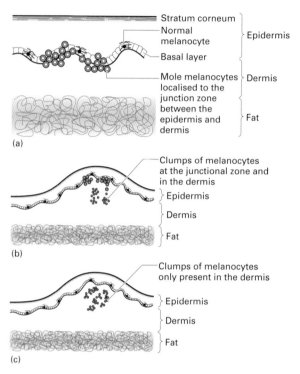

Fig. 13.2.1 Stages in the development of a normal mole. These start as (a) a flat brown junctional naevus, then become (b) raised brown compound naevi and finally (c) raised flesh-coloured intradermal naevi.

dermis to create a papular, flesh-coloured, often hairy intradermal naevus.

Normal variants of benign naevi include the following.

- Congenital naevi are moles present at birth or that appear in the first few months of life. Giant congenital naevi have greater risk of melanoma transformation. There is debate about whether the commoner small congenital naevus have similar higher frequency of malignant transformation.

- A blue naevus is slatey grey or blue in colour. The striking colour is produced by melanin deposited by melanocytes that remain deep in the dermis.
- Spitz naevus (juvenile melanoma). These appear as red facial papules in children and brownish red papules on limbs in adults. They are clinically and histologically distinct from malignant melanoma.
- Halo naevus. Some naevi disappear spontaneously. The first indication of this is a white halo appearing around the pigmented papule.
- Dysplastic naevus. Clinically they may have features suggestive of a melanoma (pigment and edge irregularity) but histologically they are benign. Patients with multiple dysplastic naevi or a family history of melanoma have a greater risk of developing melanoma.

Benign naevus

A benign mole has uniform colour (i.e. all brown, all tan, and so on) and a regular margin, and is usually symmetrical about one axis and sometimes hairy. Moles on the scrotum, palms and soles are no more likely to turn malignant than moles elsewhere. Moles in the nail fold manifest as a pigmented streak in the nail and should be biopsied.

Management

A benign naevus that is causing no symptoms can be left alone. The lesion is usually excised either because it is cosmetically unattractive, or because it is showing some features suggestive of malignant change.

OPERATION: SHAVE EXCISION OF BENIGN PAPULAR NAEVI

Removal of benign papular pink naevi for cosmetic reasons is usually best done by shave excision because this simple procedure produces a good cosmetic result. Pigment and hair will remain in 25% of brown or hairy naevi. If this is unacceptable an elliptical excision is appropriate.

Anaesthetic is injected into the mole to stiffen the tissue and make is easier to shave off. The protruding part of the mole is

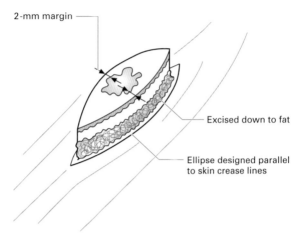

Fig. 13.2.2 Excision of a suspect mole or staging excision of a malignant melanoma.

shaved off flush with the skin. Bleeding is stopped using cautery and the wound allowed to heal spontaneously.

OPERATION: REMOVAL OF A SUSPICIOUS NAEVUS
Removal of suspect moles should be done under a local anaesthetic using an elliptical incision, parallel to skin crease lines, down to fat, taking a 2 mm margin on either side of the edge of the mole (Fig. 13.2.2). The wound should be sutured using absorbable and nylon surface sutures. The specimen should always be sent for histology. If this shows evidence of malignant change, the scar will need to be re-excised.

Malignant melanoma

Appproximately 50% of malignant melanomas arise in an existing naevus. The remainder develop spontaneously. Five clinico-pathological types are recognized. In all these types the best guide to prognosis is the depth (Breslow thickness) to which malignant melanocytes have penetrated at the time of excision (Fig. 13.2.3).

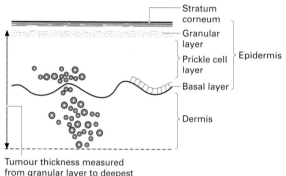

Fig. 13.2.3 Measurement of melanoma thickness by the Breslow method.

- Lentigo maligna (Hutchinson's melanotic freckle). This is a completely flat brown or black macule usually on the face. Malignant melanocytes are only present in the basal layer of the epidermis. Solid melanomas (lentigo maligna melanoma) develop in approximately 25% of cases.
- Superficial spreading melanoma. The malignant melanocytes grow laterally through the epidermis for some time before clumping together and growing downwards into the dermis. This type occurs at any site as a just-palpable irregularly pigmented lesion.
- Nodular melanoma. The malignant melanocytes invade deeply into the dermis from the start. These appear as raised pigmented nodules at any site.
- Amelanotic melanoma. These melanomas do not produce sufficient pigment to make them change colour. They are usually misdiagnosed as squamous cell carcinomas or pyogenic granulomata. Because of the potential delay in diagnosis amelanotic melanomas may present late. They are, however, no more likely to metastasize than a pigmented melanoma of similar thickness.
- Acral lentiginous melanoma. This type develops around nails and on the feet. They present with nail destruction, pigment

streaks or solitary nail dystrophy. They are commonly mis-diagnosed as ingrown toenail, fungal infections, etc.

TUMOUR STAGING

The stage of a melanoma refers to its extent of spread and gives some indication of prognosis. There are three clinical stages.

- Stage l: confined to the primary lesion (including satellite lesions within a radius of 5 cm). The prognosis depends on tumour thickness (Fig. 13.2.3).
- Stage 2: involvement of the first single group of regional lymph nodes and cutaneous secondaries in this course.
- Stage 3: involvement of two or more groups of lymph nodes with visceral metastases particularly to the liver, lungs and brain.

Recognizing the pattern

Malignant melanoma usually occurs after adolescence. Melanomas in prepubertal children that have not developed from giant congenital naevi are extremely rare. Melanoma is commoner in white-skinned people exposed to the sun. It occurs in approximately 10 : 100 000 individuals in Europe (a male to female ratio of 1 : 2) and 40 : 100 000 in Australia.

There may be a positive family history. The patient usually presents because the mole has changed or a new pigmented lesion has appeared.

The malignant lesion can occur anywhere but is more common on the limbs, head and neck. Signs suggestive of malignant change are as follows.

- Colour change. Melanomas have pigments of different hues in the same lesion, e.g. red and black, grey and brown.
- Change in shape. Melanomas are asymmetrical. Extensions or margin irregularities (notching) are characteristic.
- Increasing size. Most melanomas are greater than 7 mm. Bleeding and itching are not specific. Ulceration is a late feature. Benign moles may be traumatized accidentally or because they are itchy.

Examine the adjacent skin for satellite nodules around the melanoma and examine draining lymph nodes. Systemic symptoms of weight loss or metastasis to other organs may be present.

Management

OPERATION: EXCISION OF MALIGNANT MELANOMA

A staging excisional biopsy down to fat with a 2-mm margin of normal skin is done to confirm the diagnosis and establish the tumour thickness. Pretreatment liver function tests and a chest X-ray are commonly done to exclude distant metastasis in thicker melanoma.

Tumours less than 1 mm thick require a 10-mm margin of excision. Tumours 1–2 mm thick can be excised with a 10–20-mm margin and tumours thicker than 3 mm are normally excised with a 30-mm margin. In all cases excision should be carried down to, but not including, the deep fascia. The defect can be closed directly, or using a skin graft. Split skin graft should be taken from the opposite limb to avoid transferring a metastasis in situ.

Procedure profile

Blood requirement	0
Anaesthetic	GA/LA
Operation time	1–2 hours depending on site
Hospital stay	Day case or 5–7 days
Return to normal activity	3–4 weeks

OPERATION: BLOCK DISSECTION OF THE GROIN

There is no established role for elective node dissection in melanoma. However, if there is evidence of spread to the regional nodes, a block dissection may be performed.

A fine-needle aspiration or an excision biopsy of the enlarged node is taken. If tumour is present, all the groin nodes are excised. The long saphenous vein is tied lower down the thigh and a block of tissue removed from the front of the femoral vein and artery. The upper end of the saphenous vein is again divided as it enters the femoral vein. The block may be continued up under the inguinal ligament to remove nodes in the iliac region. Drains must be used postoperatively as seroma is a common complication and there is a significant risk of wound breakdown.

Procedure profile

Blood requirement	Group and save
Anaesthetic	GA
Operation time	2–3 hours
Hospital stay	7–10 days
Return to normal activity	4–6 weeks

Postoperatively the leg is likely to swell due to lymphoedema. It is important to keep it elevated and to apply heavy-duty elastic bandages before the patient is mobilized. The patient should continue to have the foot of the bed raised for 2 or 3 months after the procedure until the tendency to oedema has subsided. The oedema may be permanent.

PALLIATIVE AND ADJUVANT THERAPY

Melanomas tend to be chemo- and radioresistant but patients with thick (> 1.5 mm) melanomas may benefit from inclusion in ongoing trials. All melanomas should be referred to your local skin cancer multidisciplinary team. Other treatments include the following.

- Radiotherapy. This is useful for the treatment of bone pain or cerebral metastases.
- Chemotherapy. This can occasionally be helpful in advanced disease. The effective agents are the following:
  - melphalan – especially when used for isolated cytotoxic hyperthermic limb perfusion
  - combination chemotherapy – various combinations are undergoing trials, e.g. VBM (vindesine, bleomycin, methotrexate) or BOLD (bleomycin, vincristine, 1-(2-chloroethyl)-3-cyclohexyl-1-nitrosourea, 5-(3, 3-dimethyl-1-triazino)imidazole-4-carboxamide). Toxicity of these regimes is significant.
- Interferon-α2b has been shown to reduce the risk of metastasis in high-risk patients with thick tumours.

Other malignant skin conditions
Squamous cell carcinoma in situ (Bowen's disease)

This is carcinoma of the skin limited to the epidermis. Approximately 5% of cases develop into an invasive squamous cell carcinoma.

Recognizing the pattern

Bowen's disease occurs on sun-exposed sites, particularly the lower legs in elderly women. Previous arsenic ingestion, in the form of 'tonics', predisposes to Bowen's disease.

The lesion is painless, slowly enlarging and patients complain of the appearance. It can be distinguished from psoriasis because lesions are solitary, crusted rather than scaly and have an irregular edge. Biopsy will confirm the diagnosis.

Management

Lesions can be treated by topical 5-fluorouracil application, curettage, cryotherapy, excision or radiotherapy.

Squamous cell carcinoma

This is a malignant keratinizing tumour of stratified squamous epithelium. It is locally invasive and also metastasizes via the lymphatics and the bloodstream.

Recognizing the pattern

Squamous cell carcinoma occurs on chronically sun-exposed sites particularly in elderly men. Characteristic sites include the lower lip, top of the ear, back of the hand and other head and neck sites. The tumour can arise in immunosuppressed younger patients, particularly following organ transplantation.

Most patients give a history of previous regular excess exposure to sunlight. Other carcinogenic factors include coal tar exposure (road workers) and tobacco (lip tumours). The lesion enlarges slowly and has usually been present for several months before presentation. Squamous cell carcinomas are sometimes painful.

The nodule is hard, irregular in outline, and usually has a keratin and crust-covered surface or a central necrotic ulcer and everted edge. There may be evidence of local or distant metastases. It is important to examine draining lymph nodes.

Management
The lesion can either be excised or treated with radiotherapy.

Basal cell carcinoma (BCC, basal cell epithelioma, rodent ulcer)
This is a locally malignant condition arising from basal epidermal cells. BCCs grow into surrounding tissues and can cause extensive local destruction but only exceptionally metastasize.

Recognizing the pattern
The patient is usually elderly but BCC also occurs in the 20+ age group. The condition is more common in white-skinned people with a history of repeated sun exposure.

The tumour is painless and slow growing. Patients sometimes notice the enlarging nodule or an ulcer that does not heal, occasionally bleeds, scabs over and then re-ulcerates.

An early nodular BCC is a smooth pearly papule. As the tumour enlarges the centre becomes necrotic, ulcerates and crusted. At this stage only the edge is raised (rolled) and pearly white in colour; this feature is best seen if the skin is stretched. The lack of keratin formation and the presence of the characteristic pearly-coloured edge distinguish BCC from squamous cell carcinoma. BCCs may also be scarring (morphoeic), superficial (plaque-like patch on the trunk) or pigmented.

Management
BCCs can be treated by cryotherapy, curettage, radiotherapy or excision.

OPERATION: EXCISION OF BASAL CELL CARCINOMA
The excision margin depends on the tumour characteristics. Small (< 2 cm), well-defined tumours can be excised with a 3–4-mm margin. Large (> 2 cm), recurrent or ill-defined tumours are more likely to recur using this excision margin. These tumours can be treated by wide (10-mm) local excision using histological control to confirm the adequacy of excision. The defect is closed either directly, using local flaps or with a skin graft.

Procedure profile

Blood requirement	0
Anaesthetic	LA or occasionally GA
Operation time	Depends on size and need to graft; 30–90 minutes
Hospital stay	Day case or 24–48 hours
Return to normal activity	1 day or more depending on size of lesion

Skin metastases

Metastases from visceral carcinoma can present as a swelling or ulceration in the skin. They are particularly common on the scalp. The treatment consists of chemotherapy or radiotherapy appropriate to the original primary tumour. The diagnosis is made by biopsy to help identify the primary malignancy.

13.3 Skin infections and hyperhidrosis

Skin infections

Skin abscess

This is the result of a *Staphylococcus aureus* infection producing a collection of pus surrounded by granulation tissue in the subcutaneous tissues or dermis.

Recognizing the pattern

There is a painful swelling. The pain is throbbing and characteristically worse at night or if the affected part is dependent. It may have discharged pus.

On examination there is a localized swelling which is warm, red and tender. It is initially firm but as suppuration occurs it becomes softer, spherical and fluctuant. It may later discharge. The patient is usually pyrexial and the regional lymph nodes become enlarged and tender.

Management

The abscess must be drained unless it ruptures spontaneously. A swab should be sent for culture and sensitivity.

OPERATION: INCISION AND DRAINAGE OF ABSCESS

An incision is made over the most fluctuant area. A closed haemostat is inserted into the cavity and then opened. A drain is inserted.

Procedure profile

Blood requirement	0
Anaesthetic	LA
Operation time	15 minutes
Hospital stay	Outpatient
Return to normal activity	1–2 days

Postoperatively any predisposing cause (e.g. diabetes) should be treated. Antibiotics are only appropriate if there is associated cellulitis or constitutional disturbance.

Hidradenitis suppurativa

This is a troublesome recurrent infection of apocrine sweat glands and characteristically affects the axillae, groins and perineum. Mild cases respond to antibiotics according to sensitivities. Oral estrogens or antiandrogens can also be used in females. Surgery may be the only effective treatment in resistant cases. Sinus tracts may need to be laid open and allowed to granulate as described for pilonidal sinus. Eventually areas of recurrent sepsis may need to be fully excised.

Pilonidal sinus

In this condition broken-off hairs come to lie in a subcutaneous sinus. Lesions characteristically occur over the sacrum in the gluteal cleft. It can also occur in the hands, axillae or umbilicus.

The lesion in the sacral area probably starts as a preformed congenital pit. Hairs break off the head and back and tend to gravitate towards the cleft. It seems likely that the barbed surface of the hair results in it working its way under the skin once its tip has become lodged in the pit. Several hairs follow down the sinus, which then becomes infected. The patient complains of recurrent abscesses in this area. The abscess usually points to the skin at the side of the midline.

Recognizing the pattern

The patient is typically male with thick black hair. The condition is more common between the ages of 15 and 40 years. There are recurrent episodes of pain and sepsis, often with several months between each episode. As the sinus becomes larger, the episodes become more frequent. Pilonidal sinus can occur in barbers and in this case the sinus lies between the fingers. The hairs are derived from the customer rather than the sufferer.

On careful inspection the pit is seen in the midline. There may be several such pits. The abscess is visible and palpable laterally.

Management

A small sinus may settle with antibiotic treatment but once the condition has become recurrent surgery is required. An acutely inflamed abscess will need to be drained.

Three operative procedures are described. The sinus may be incised and laid open, it may be completely excised or it may be curetted and injected with phenol.

OPERATION: FOR PILONIDAL SINUS

When the lesion is laid open, a probe is passed along the track and an incision is made onto it from above. Granulation tissue in the base of the sinus and the hairs and debris are removed. Any lateral extensions into an abscess cavity are also laid open.

If the sinus is excised, the skin is closed directly over the wound.

Procedure profile

Blood requirement	0
Anaesthetic	GA or LA, depending on size
Operation time	30–45 minutes
Hospital stay	3–7 days depending on size
Return to normal activity	3 weeks, depending on occupation

If the sinus has been excised, and if the wound heals by primary intention, the postoperative care is uncomplicated. If the wound breaks down due to tension or infection it can be allowed to heal by secondary intention.

If the sinus has been laid open, it is dressed daily by inserting a plug of silicone dressing or silastic foam. As the wound granulates and the epithelium grows in from the edges, the bulk of the dressing is reduced. It is important to make certain that no 'bridging' of the skin edges occurs as this will lead to renewed pit formation and a recurrent sinus. Similarly, the hairs around the wound must be shaved regularly to prevent them sticking into the granulation tissue and reforming a sinus. Laser hair removal may be helpful in preventing recurrence.

OPERATION: PHENOL INJECTION OF PILONIDAL SINUS
The surrounding skin is carefully protected using petroleum jelly. Phenol (80%) is injected and left in the sinus for 1 min. This is repeated three times. The sinus is then gently curetted and the hairs removed. A small drain may be inserted.

Procedure profile

Blood requirement	0
Anaesthetic	GA
Operation time	10 minutes
Hospital stay	24 hours
Return to normal activity	48 hours

After phenol injection the area remains painless as the phenol destroys local nerves. Occasionally a sterile abscess develops, which requires drainage. The recurrence rate is about 17% if the sinus has fewer than three openings.

Boil (furuncle) and carbuncle

A boil is a small abscess developing in an infected hair follicle. A carbuncle is an infection of a group of adjacent follicles. In both instances *Staphylococcus aureus* is the infecting organism. Necrosis of the skin between the follicles is a common associated feature. This results in the formation of a large ulcer, which slowly heals to leave a substantial scar. Infections are more common in diabetics, the malnourished and patients on long-term steroid therapy.

Recognizing the pattern

The presentation is initially similar to a skin abscess. There is a spreading, very painful lesion of the skin with constitutional disturbances.

The neck is the most common site affected. The lesion is diffuse, hard and reddened with a central area of slough surrounded by multiple sinuses extruding pus.

Management

Release any pus by lancing.

The initial management is conservative with regular cleaning and dressing. Culture the pus and prescribe antibiotics to control the infection. The necrotic central area of skin may need to be excised. Check for predisposing causes such as diabetes.

Conditions of the nails

Ingrowing toenail

Ingrowing toenails are caused by:
- incorrectly cutting the toenails
- poorly fitting shoes
- trauma
- congenital nail abnormalities.

Toenails should be cut transversely so that the corners of the free nail edge protrude beyond the lateral nailfolds. If the nail

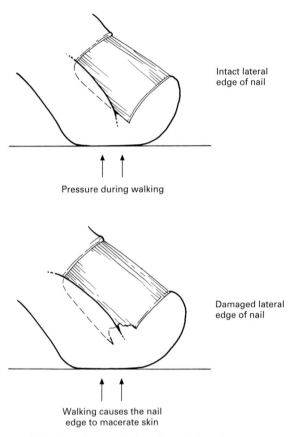

Intact lateral
edge of nail

Pressure during walking

Damaged lateral
edge of nail

Walking causes the nail
edge to macerate skin

Fig. 13.3.1 One mechanism producing an 'ingrowing' toenail.

corners are trimmed further back the cut may not quite reach the
lateral edge of the nail leaving a spicule of nail. This grows into
and finally penetrates the lateral nailfold (Fig. 13.3.1). The resulting foreign-body reaction and secondary infection produce the
symptoms.

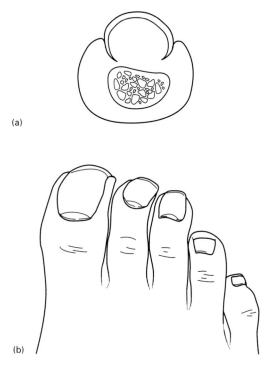

(a)

(b)

Fig. 13.3.2 Congenital malformations of the toenails producing (a) a pincer toe and (b) congenital malalignment of the great toe.

Footwear should allow the toes to spread adequately. High heels that cause the toes to be forced into a narrow pointed shoe may also force the lateral nail margin into the nailfold. Trauma may split the side of the nail and the sharp edge may grow into the nailfold.

Congenital abnormalities that predispose to ingrowing toenails should be distinguished (Fig. 13.3.2). These include overcurvature of the nail (pincer nails) and malalignment of the big toenails. All the toenails are affected although symptoms are most frequent in the great toe. In pincer nails the deformed nailplate grips the nailbed like a claw and the lateral and medial nail borders need to be removed. Malaligned nails should be realigned rather than destroyed.

Recognizing the pattern

The patient may present at any age though the condition is unusual before the age of 5 years.

The usual complaint is of a painful big toe, which is swollen, red and intermittently discharges pus. Attempt to establish the likely cause in acquired disease.

On examination the nailfolds are affected to a variable extent on one or both sides of the nail. Identify congenital abnormalities that predispose to ingrowing toenail.

Management

Conservative management of acquired ingrowing toenail is as follows.

- Prevent secondary infection and reduce pain by keeping the feet dry, using oral antibiotics if required and avoiding tight shoes or socks.
- Reduce granulation tissue formation. Potent topical steroid (clobetasol proprionate) application or cryotherapy will reduce inflammation and granulation tissue.
- Redirection of nail growth. Pack cotton wool pledglets moistened with surgical spirit or tincture of iodine under the corner of the nail so that the free edge of the nail grows out without puncturing the lateral nailfold.
- Prevent recurrence. Teach the patient how to cut their nails correctly (Fig. 13.3.3). Advise on the need for correct size and shape of shoe. Minimize the consequences of excessive foot sweating. Generally improve foot hygiene.

OPERATION: AVULSION OF THE BIG TOENAIL

The toe is anaesthetized by digital nerve block. If a tourniquet is applied this should be as wide as possible to prevent digital nerve damage and left on for no longer than 20 min. The nail is halved with strong scissors ensuring that the proximal edge under the skin fold is divided. A strong haemostat is passed under one cut edge of the nail, the nail grasped and twisted off. Ensure that the

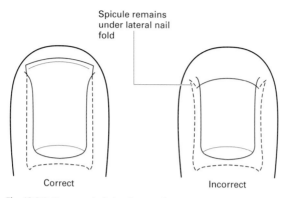

Spicule remains
under lateral nail
fold

Correct   Incorrect

Fig. 13.3.3 Correct method of cutting toenails.

lateral proximal corner is included. The procedure is repeated with the other half. The toe is dressed with paraffin gauze, a gauze pad and then a bandage. The foot should be kept elevated overnight and the toe redressed within 48 h.

Simple avulsion of the nail removes the source of infection and pain. It may be all that is needed on first presentation. Recurrence after such conservative treatment can be managed by excision (Zadik's operation) or destruction (phenol matricectomy) of the whole nail matrix and hence the entire nail. Alternatively, only one side of the matrix and hence nail can be excised (wedge excision) or destroyed (lateral nailfold phenol matricectomy).

OPERATION: ZADIK'S OPERATION (NAIL MATRIX EXCISION)

The nail is removed and the skin is incised diagonally from the corners of the posterior nailfold and folded back. The exposed nail matrix is then excised down to bone taking care to include the lateral horns of the matrix (Fig. 13.3.4). The skin edges are then stitched loosely together and a dressing applied and changed at 24 h. Avoid operating if there is active infection because of the risk of osteomyelitis in the distal phalanx.

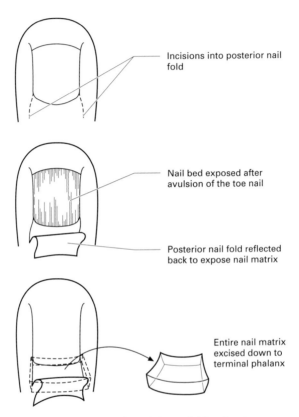

Fig. 13.3.4 Zadik's procedure for surgical removal of the nail matrix.

Procedure profile

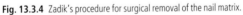

Blood requirement	0
Anaesthetic	LA
Operation time	30 minutes
Hospital stay	Outpatient
Return to normal activity	2–5 days

OPERATION: WEDGE EXCISION

This is similar to the Zadik's procedure except that only the side of the nail matrix is removed. It is performed for re-current ingrowing toenail where only one nailfold is involved. The resulting nail is narrow but patients may prefer this outcome for functional and cosmetic reasons.

Phenol can be used to destroy part, or the entire, nail matrix. This procedure is simpler, results in less pain postoperatively and in skilled hands produces better functional and cosmetic results than surgical matricectomy.

OPERATION: PHENOL MATRICECTOMY OF INGROWN TOENAIL

An exsanguinating tourniquet is applied because phenol is neutralized by blood and bleeding will reduce its effectiveness. If the complete nail matrix is to be destroyed the entire nail is avulsed. A cotton wool bud dipped in phenol (40% in water) is placed beneath the proximal nailfold and rolled from side to side and into the lateral horns of the matrix.

Three 1-min phenol applications are required. There is little postoperative pain. The patient should change dressings daily for the first week.

Only one side of the nail matrix can be destroyed if required. The side of the nail is separated from the nailbed and lateral nailfold using a nail elevator. A piece of nail approximately 4–5 mm wide is then trimmed off down to the base of the nail using nail splitters. The phenol-tipped applicator is then inserted into the gap created under the posterior nailfold and into the lateral nail matrix horn (Fig. 13.3.5). Two 1-min phenol applications are required.

Acute paronychia

Paronychia is a soft tissue infection of the lateral and posterior nailfolds. Acute paronychia is usually caused by *Staphylococcus aureus* and may require surgery. Herpes simplex infections around the nail, or herpetic whitlow (particularly common in nurses and doctors), should be distinguished and treated medically. Chronic paronychia (usually due to *Candida albicans*) occurs in persons whose hands are regularly in water, rarely follows acute paronychia and is relatively painless. Surgical removal

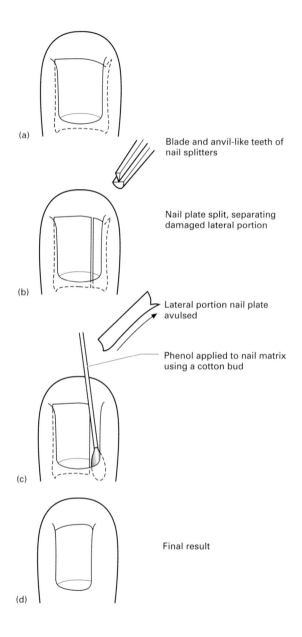

(a)

Blade and anvil-like teeth of nail splitters

(b)

Nail plate split, separating damaged lateral portion

Lateral portion nail plate avulsed

Phenol applied to nail matrix using a cotton bud

(c)

(d)

Final result

of part of the posterior nailfold is occasionally used in recalcitrant chronic paronychia.

Recognizing the pattern

Acute paronychia is very painful and there is erythema, swelling, tenderness and possibly visible pus in the nailfold. If pus has spread under the nail, pressure over the nail will be painful. Advanced infection may spread to the pulp space.

Management

In the first 48 h the infection may resolve with antibiotic therapy. Splinting the finger and elevation of the limb will reduce pain. Once pus has formed it must be drained.

OPERATION: INCISION AND DRAINAGE OF A
PARONYCHIA

Under digital nerve block and with a tourniquet applied, the skin is incised at one or both proximal corners of the nailfold and a flap raised to release the pus. The entire slough must be excised. If pus is trapped beneath the nail, that part of the nail must also be removed. The finger is dressed with paraffin gauze. Inadequate primary treatment may result in nail dystrophy or destruction.

Procedure profile

Blood requirement	0
Anaesthetic	LA
Operation time	10 minutes
Hospital stay	Outpatient
Return to normal activity	1–2 days

Fig. 13.3.5 (*Opposite*) Phenol wedge matricectomy for unilateral ingrown toenail. (a) The problem; (b) the sliver of nail snipped off; and (c) a phenol-tipped cotton bud inserted into the space under the posterior nailfold and into the lateral horn of the matrix. (d) Final result.

Postoperatively the dressing is changed daily until the finger heals.

Subungual haematoma
This is a collection of blood beneath the nail following a crushing injury to the fingertip. It is painful because the rigid nailplate prevents the inflamed tissue from expanding.

Recognizing the pattern
The patient presents following trauma with a very painful finger and a collection of blood beneath the nail.

Management
The digit must be X-rayed to exclude fracture of the phalanx. The blood is released by burning a hole in the nail over the clot with the end of a red-hot paper clip (trephining the nail). This procedure is surprisingly painless.

A fracture of the phalanx beneath does not usually require manipulation and the nail provides sufficient splintage. However, a finger splint and elevation of the arm in a sling for 24–48 h will help to ease the pain. The patient needs antibiotics (penicillin and flucloxacillin) because trephining makes the fracture compound.

Hyperhidrosis
Excessive sweating usually affects the axillae, hands and feet. This causes social embarrassment and the sweat may damage paper, shoes and clothing.

Management
Medical management is not very effective; 20% aluminium chloride applied at night helps axillary hyperhidrosis, 1% formaldehyde soaks can be used on the feet and iontophoresis tried at any site. Botulism toxin is effective in treating axillary hyperhidrosis.

When conservative measures fail, hyperhidrosis of the hands can be treated by transthoracic cervical sympathectomy. Lumbar sympathectomy may help foot sweating but is a radical procedure for a relatively minor problem. Quadrilateral sympathectomy is not advisable as it produces postural hypertension.

Preoperatively check there is no history of chest trauma or infection as these may be associated with pleural adhesions. Warn the patient of the possibility of Horner's syndrome, compensatory sweating and the very slight chance of the need for a thoracotomy or a persistent chest drain. Horner's syndrome is due to inadvertent damage to the sympathetic supply to the eye resulting in a small pupil and drooping eyelid (ptosis) on the side of the lesion. It is rare with transthoracic sympathectomy. Look for and note any pre-existing ptosis. Compensatory sweating is a postoperative increase in sweating from other areas of the body. Usually it is not a problem with unilateral sympathectomy but is more pronounced after bilateral or extensive sympathectomies.

OPERATION: TRANSTHORACIC ENDOSCOPIC CERVICAL SYMPATHECTOMY

Two axillary ports may be required, one for the telescope (5 or 10 mm) and one for a diathermy hook (5 mm). An excellent view of the sympathetic chain is obtained. The lung is deflated either by using a double-lumen endotracheal tube and blocking off one bronchus, or by insufflating the chest with a low pressure of CO_2. The chain is destroyed from the lower edge of the stellate ganglion to the third thoracic ganglion to denervate the hand. Progressing distally may denervate the axilla. The pleura is emptied of any gas by inserting a drain at the end of the procedure.

Axillary hyperhidrosis is best treated by local excision of the sweat glands. The disadvantage of this approach is the large scar produced and general poor healing due to wound tension. Alternatively, only part of the axillary skin is excised and the sweat glands in the remainder are damaged or removed by curettage, extensive undermining (Hurley–Shelley procedure) or liposuction.

OPERATION: EXCISION OF AXILLARY SWEAT GLANDS

The day before operation the sweat gland area is mapped out using either a starch iodine reaction or quinizarin, both of which change colour when moist. Alternatively, just the hair-bearing portion of the axilla can be excised and the wound closed with suction drainage to the subcutaneous space.

Procedure profile

Blood requirement	0
Anaesthetic	LA/GA
Operation time	1 hour
Hospital stay	Day case or 3–5 days
Return to normal activity	2 weeks

After the wound has healed active shoulder exercises with or without physiotherapy may be required to restore full arm movements.

14 Surgery of children

14.1 Surgical conditions of neonates

Abdominal wall defects

Developmental defects present on the anterior abdominal wall. Gastroschisis is a defect in the anterior abdominal wall lateral to the umbilicus which permits partial evisceration in utero. The bowel is thickened and distorted by exposure to amniotic fluid. Exomphalos is a wide open umbilical ring permitting herniation of abdominal contents into the base of the umbilicus. In severe cases there is associated pulmonary hypoplasia. Malrotation is an associated feature. Chromosomal defects and major congenital anomalies are common.

Recognizing the pattern
Usually diagnosed antenatally. The diagnosis is self-evident at birth.

Proving the diagnosis
Chromosome studies as well as echocardiography are necessary in exomphalos. A contrast meal will exclude malrotation.

Management
The torso is wrapped in clingfilm to reduce heat and fluid loss. Care is taken to avoid mechanical trauma. Rehydration is essential.

OPERATION FOR GASTROSCHISIS/EXOMPHALOS
Reduction of the abdominal contents and closure of the abdominal wall defect is attempted in the first few hours of life. If primary closure cannot be achieved a silo is sutured to the margin of

Surgery: Diagnosis and Management, 4th edition. Edited by N. Rawlinson and D. Alderson. © 2009 Blackwell Publishing, ISBN: 978-1-4051-2921-3

the defect and gradual reduction achieved at the bedside over 5–7 days.

Procedure profile

Blood requirement	1 (rarely needed)
Anaesthetic	GA
Operation time	1 hour
Hospital stay	4–6 weeks
Return to normal activity	Not applicable

Following surgery inpatient stay is 4–6 weeks to allow functional recovery.

Diaphragmatic hernia

This is a posterolateral defect in the (left) diaphragm associated with herniation of abdominal contents into the chest and pulmonary hypoplasia.

Recognizing the pattern
If the diagnosis has been missed antenatally the baby may present with respiratory collapse at birth or within the first few hours of life.

Proving the diagnosis
A chest X-ray confirms the diagnosis.

Management
Early intubation and mechanical ventilation is undertaken to allow stabilization of the baby. There is a 50% mortality that is not reduced by early surgery.

OPERATION: REPAIR OF DIAPHRAGMATIC HERNIA
Reduction of abdominal contents back into the abdomen and primary closure of the diaphragmatic defect is attempted. A patch may be required.

Procedure profile

Blood requirement	1 (rarely needed)
Anaesthetic	GA
Operation time	2.5 hours
Hospital stay	1–3 weeks
Return to normal activity	Not applicable

Oesophageal atresia

Failure of separation of the dorsal foregut (oesophagus) from the ventral trachea at 26 days' gestation may result in formation of a tracheo-oesophageal fistula. In 85% of cases the proximal oesophagus ends as a blind pouch, with the distal oesophagus arising from the trachea (Fig. 14.1.1).

Recognizing the pattern
The baby is unable to swallow saliva (bubbly baby) and if fed coughs and becomes cyanosed as milk spills into the lungs.

Proving the diagnosis
Gentle attempts to pass a nasogastric tube reveal the blockage, the level being apparent on chest X-ray. Abdominal X-ray shows bowel gas only if there is a tracheo-oesophageal fistula.

Management
Place a tube in the oesophageal pouch and aspirate secretions.

OPERATION: REPAIR OF OESOPHAGEAL ATRESIA
A right thoracotomy gives good access. The tracheo-oesophageal fistula is ligated and divided and primary anastomosis usually achieved. With a long gap it may be necessary to raise a feeding gastrostomy and bridge the gap at a later date with a stomach, colon or small bowel interposition graft.

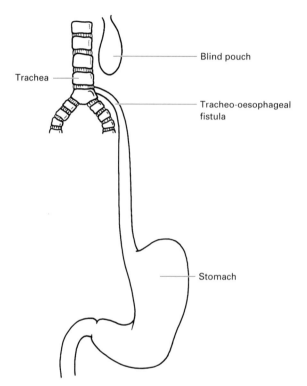

Fig. 14.1.1 The most common form of oesophageal atresia.

Procedure profile

Blood requirement	1 (rarely needed)
Anaesthetic	GA
Operation time	2.5 hours
Hospital stay	1–3 weeks
Return to normal activity	Not applicable

Neonatal intestinal obstruction

Bile-stained or persistent vomiting in the newborn may indicate a life threatening problem and should be investigated promptly.

Mechanical obstruction may be:

- intrinsic; atresia, stenosis or web
- secondary to external compression by bands, malrotation/ volvulus or an incarcerated inguinal hernia
- secondary to lumen obstruction by inspissated meconium as in cystic fibrosis
- functional as in Hirschsprung's disease
- secondary to sepsis at any site leading to ileus.

Recognizing the pattern

Antenatal ultrasound may predict intestinal obstruction in the presence of polyhydramnios or echogenic bowel. Postnatally the presenting features are vomiting, abdominal distension and delayed passage of meconium, the contribution of each depending on the level of obstruction.

Proving the diagnosis

A plain abdominal X-ray will show dilated bowel loops and may reveal the level of obstruction, but contrast studies from above or below are often required.

Management

The baby must be rehydrated. A nasogastric tube is mandatory. Definitive treatment depends on the underlying pathology.

Small bowel atresia

An atresia is a missing segment of bowel, occasionally with a fibrous cord joining the two ends. Obstruction is complete, resulting in gross dilatation proximally and distal atrophy. Related problems include stenosis (a narrowing where obstruction may be only partial) and luminal web (a mucosal barrier which may be complete or perforated).

Recognizing the pattern

The patient presents with bile-stained vomiting. Abdominal distension is greater if obstruction is distal.

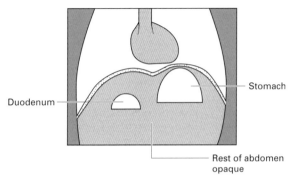

Fig. 14.1.2 The double bubble seen on erect X-ray.

Proving the diagnosis

Abdominal X-ray shows dilated proximal bowel. In duodenal atresia a typical 'double bubble' is seen in the upper abdomen (Fig. 14.1.2). A contrast enema shows a hypoplastic microcolon as a result of disuse.

Management

OPERATION FOR SMALL BOWEL ATRESIA

A laparotomy is performed via a transverse incision. The affected segment is resected and an end-to-end anastomosis performed. Resection is avoided in duodenal atresia and a side to side bypass duodenoduodenostomy performed.

Procedure profile

Blood requirement	1 (rarely needed)
Anaesthetic	GA
Operation time	1.5 hours
Hospital stay	Varies with site of atresia. 3 weeks–months
Return to normal activity	Not applicable

It can take days or even weeks for the dilated upstream segment and disused distal segment to achieve coordinated function and during this period intravenous feeding is required.

Malrotation

During early development the gut is a midline structure. As it elongates it herniates through the abdominal wall (Fig. 14.1.3). At 10 weeks in utero it returns to the abdominal cavity, rotating 270° anticlockwise about the axis of the superior mesenteric artery. This places the caecum in the right iliac fossa. If the process is not fully completed the caecum may lie in the right hypochondrium, where its peritoneal attachments ('Ladd's bands') cross the duodenum. There is an increased risk of midgut volvulus, as the close proximity of caecum and duodenojejunal flexure results in a short-based mesentery.

Lateral view

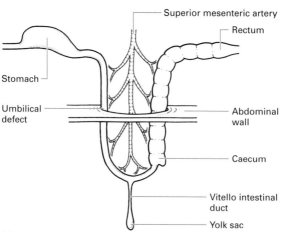

(a)

Fig. 14.1.3 (a) Normal development of the gut: ventral view. The midgut is originally a midline structure protruding through the umbilical defect.

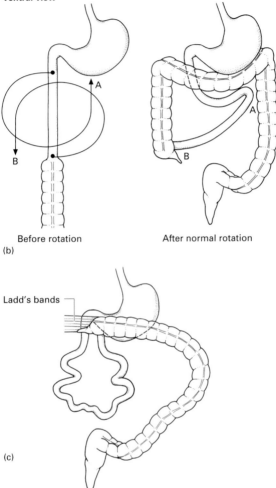

Ventral view

Before rotation

After normal rotation

(b)

Ladd's bands

(c)

Fig. 14.1.3 (*Continued*) (b) Normal development of the gut: ventral view, before and after normal rotation. Points A and B rotate 300° anticlockwise to achieve the adult position of the gut. The colon comes to lie over the proximal gut. (c) Malrotation: the caecum lies over the duodenum. The duodenojejeunal junction is close to the ileocaecal valve.

Recognizing the pattern

Presentation is with bilious vomiting at any age, with 50% occurring during the first week. Failure to make the diagnosis will result in rapid deterioration and death.

Proving the diagnosis

Emergency contrast meal is diagnostic showing the duodeno-jejunal (DJ) flexure lying to the right of the midline. Barium enema confirms the abnormal position of the caecum.

Management

Immediate emergency laparotomy.

OPERATION FOR MALROTATION

If there is a volvulus present, this is untwisted. Ladd's bands are divided and the duodenum mobilized to broaden the base of the mesentery. The bowel is returned to the abdomen in a position of non-rotation placing the large bowel on the left and the small bowel on the right to reduce the risk of future volvulus. Delayed diagnosis leads to loss of the entire midgut and an open and close procedure.

Procedure profile

Blood requirement	1 (rarely needed)
Anaesthetic	GA
Operation time	1 hour
Hospital stay	7–10 days
Return to normal activity	Not applicable

Meconium ileus

Deficient pancreatic function results in inspissated meconium, causing complete obstruction. This occurs in 15% of patients with cystic fibrosis (mucoviscidosis), a familial condition with a recessive inheritance.

Recognizing the pattern
The baby vomits bile and may have a distended abdomen with palpable loops of bowel.

Proving the diagnosis
Abdominal X-ray shows dense meconium pellets resembling ground glass. If antenatal perforation occurs it results in widespread peritoneal calcification. A sweat test will confirm cystic fibrosis.

Management
A gastrografin enema will confirm the diagnosis and may liquefy the inspisated meconium. Scrupulous attention must be paid to hydration as hypovolaemia can be precipitated by this procedure.

OPERATION FOR OBSTRUCTION DUE TO MECONIUM ILEUS
Where gastrografin enemas are unsuccessful laparotomy, enterotomy and removal of inspisated meconium is necessary. Stoma formation is rarely necessary.

Procedure profile

Blood requirement	1 (rarely needed)
Anaesthetic	GA
Operation time	1 hour
Hospital stay	7–10 days
Return to normal activity	Not applicable

Postoperatively respiratory complications are common, requiring treatment with oxygen, physiotherapy and antibiotics. Long-term care is a specialist area. Pancreatic enzyme supplements will be required.

Hirschsprung's disease

Absence of intramural ganglia in the distal bowel results in a functional obstruction due to lack of peristalsis and tonic contraction of smooth muscle. The rectum is involved in all cases. In 70% the lower sigmoid is involved as well, and in 15% the whole colon. The bowel proximal to the affected segment is grossly dilated (megacolon).

Recognizing the pattern

It classically presents with delayed passage of meconium (> 48 h) and abdominal distension. There is a significant risk of fulminating enterocolitis. Late diagnosis occurs in a small number of cases.

Proving the diagnosis

Barium enema may show a dilated proximal bowel and narrowed distal segment. Suction biopsy with acetylcholinesterase staining confirms the absence of ganglia, but requires an experienced pathologist.

Management

Traditionally staged surgery was performed with a defunctioning colostomy in distal ganglionic bowel (frozen sections mandatory). The aganglionic segment is resected and the ganglionic bowel anastomosed to the anus by one of several alternative techniques, e.g. Duhamel or Soave. More recently primary pull-through has gained popularity.

Anorectal malformations

On inspection of the neonate the anus is found to be absent or ectopic. With low lesions a rectocutaneous fistula is present. With higher lesions a rectourethral (boys) or rectovulvar fistula (girls) is present. Other congenital malformations are frequently present.

Recognizing the pattern

The absent anus is usually noted at birth. Untreated the baby will become increasingly distended. An abdominal X-ray taken with the baby in the knee chest position (invertogram) or ultrasound may used to assess distance between distended rectum and anal dimple (> 1 cm in a term infant = high lesion). Absence of a cutaneous fistula strongly favours a high lesion.

Management
Low anorectal malformations: a VY anoplasty is commonly undertaken. Constipation is a long-term problem.

High anorectal malformations: a colostomy is formed in the first few days of life. Between 3 and 6 months a posterior sagittal approach is used to close the fistula and bring the lower rectum down through the sphincter mechanism to the perineum. Colostomy closure is delayed until adequate dilatation is achieved (2–3 months). Results are often disappointing, with poor continence. A permanent stoma may be necessary in 10% of cases.

Necrotizing enterocolitis (NEC)
This is most common in premature infants, or babies asphyxiated during birth. The aetiology is unknown but NEC is very rare in babies who have not yet been fed.

Recognizing the pattern
Bloody or mucous stools are passed. The baby is ill, hypothermic and distended. Abdominal X-ray may show gas in the bowel wall. Free air may be seen if there is perforation.

Management
Feeds are withheld and intravenous fluids are given. Broad-spectrum antibiotics are given, including cover for anaerobes. Daily abdominal X-rays are taken to assess progress. In the event of perforation or development of an intra-abdominal mass, laparotomy is required to resect the affected segment with stoma formation or primary anastomosis. Second-look operations may be required. Those babies managed conservatively may develop strictures which need resection later.

Paralytic ileus
Infections are a common cause; the baby is characteristically floppy and may be hypothermic although external signs of infection may be minimal.

Proving the diagnosis
A full septic screen is required, including an active search for:

- line infections
- pneumonia
- urinary tract infection
- meningitis
- umbilical stump infection.

Management
Infections are treated with appropriate antibiotics and careful fluid balance. Idiopathic functional obstruction usually resolves on conservative management.

14.2 Surgical conditions of children

Congenital hypertrophic pyloric stenosis

There is obstruction of the outlet of the stomach by hyperplasia of the circular muscle of the pylorus. The aetiology is not known. There is a male predominance and a family history is common.

Recognizing the pattern
Presentation is typically between the ages of 3 and 6 weeks. There is projectile vomiting of non-bile-stained vomit, following which the baby is eager for further feed. The baby fails to gain weight and is often dehydrated. After a test feed, an olive-like 'tumour' may be palpable in the right hypochondrium.

Proving the diagnosis
A test feed is usually diagnostic. Where doubt remains an ultrasound scan in skilled hands is invaluable showing the thickened, lengthened pylorus.

Management
Vomiting results in dehydration and potassium depletion with a hypochloraemic alkalosis. Preoperative correction is essential and may take 48 h.

OPERATION: RAMSTEDT'S PYLOROMYOTOMY
The 'tumour' is delivered through a transverse right upper
quadrant incision and the muscle layer split until the mucosa
pouts through. Care is taken to avoid perforating the mucosa.
An umbilical approach is becoming increasingly popular.

Procedure profile

Blood requirement	0
Anaesthetic	GA
Operation time	30–60 minutes
Hospital stay	2 days
Return to normal activity	Not applicable

Full-strength feeds are rapidly reintroduced if a clear feed is
tolerated at 12 h. Persistent vomiting may be controlled by
antireflux medication.

Intussusception

A segment of proximal bowel is passed distally along the lumen
as a result of peristalsis (Fig. 14.2.1). Five per cent of cases result
from a lead point such as a polyp or Meckel's diverticulum.

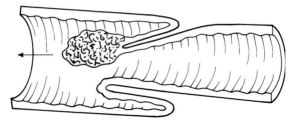

Fig. 14.2.1 The production of an intussusception. Peristalsis propels an
enlarged Peyer's patch or polyp through the bowel.

Idiopathic cases may follow mild upper respiratory infections, perhaps as a result of enlargement of Peyer's patches. The commonest site is ileocaecal.

Recognizing the pattern

Idiopathic intussusception classically presents between 2 months and 2 years with a peak at around 10 months. Outside this age range a pathological lead point should be sought. There is a classic triad of symptoms.

- Pain. A healthy child suffers recurrent spasms of pain, with pallor, screaming and drawing up of the legs. Between spasms the child is normal.
- Vomiting. Initial vomiting is due to pain. This settles, but recurs as obstruction becomes established.
- Bleeding per rectum. Bloodstained mucus resembling redcurrant jelly is passed. Obstruction occurs later.

On examination a tender, sausage-like mass may be felt in the right hypochondrium. The right iliac fossa feels 'empty'. Rarely the apex of the intussusceptum may be felt (or even seen) per rectum.

Proving the diagnosis

Diagnosis is now made on ultrasound scan with a visible target sign.

Management

Ressuscitation and analgesia are usually necessary before reduction. A sick child may require paediatric intensive care and there are deaths each year from inadequate management. These children should be transferred to a tertiary centre preoperatively.

RADIOLOGICAL REDUCTION OF INTUSSUSCEPTION BY AIR ENEMA

The use of barium is no longer recommended. Air enema is now the method of choice, using pressures of up to 100 mmHg. There is a 10% recurrence rate.

OPERATION: REDUCTION OF INTUSSUSCEPTION

A transverse incision is used and the intussusception reduced by 'milking' (not by traction). Any gangrenous bowel or causative lesion is resected. About 3% of cases recur even after bowel resection.

Procedure profile

Blood requirement	Group and save
Anaesthetic	GA
Operation time	1 hour – longer if resection required
Hospital stay	3–5 days
Return to normal activity	Not applicable

Inguinal hernia and hydrocoele

Inguinal hernia is the commonest paediatric surgical referral and is much more common in boys. It results from failure of closure of the processus vaginalis, a peritoneal pouch related to the testis during its descent into the scrotum (Fig. 14.2.2a,b). Hydrocoeles arise from the same structure (Fig. 14.2.2c).

Recognizing the pattern
Most childhood hernias occur in the first year of life. The incidence in boys is 1 in 50 and in girls is 1 in 500. They are more common in premature babies where there is a high risk of small bowel strangulation. The history is of an intermittent swelling in the groin, especially on crying or straining. Incarceration is not uncommon, resulting in emergency presentation. On examination the swelling may or may not be visible. In girls a sliding hernia containing an ovary results in a firm 1-cm lump in the inguinal canal.

Hydrocoeles present as a swelling of the testis. Occasionally a swelling proximal to the testis may result from an encysted hydrocoele of the cord.

Proving the diagnosis
The diagnosis is proved by feeling the swelling. If no swelling is present, the characteristic history of intermittent groin swelling is virtually diagnostic.

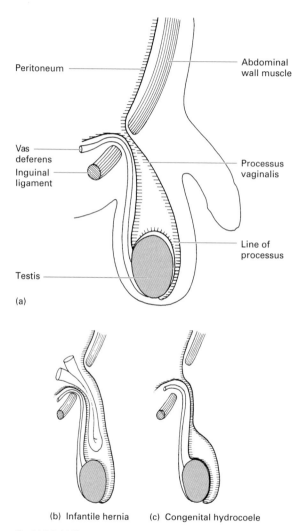

Fig. 14.2.2 (a) The processus vaginalis; (b) infantile hernia; (c) congenital hydrocoele.

Management
Operation is required. All babies less than 6 months or children who have had an episode of incarceration should have their operation on the next available list. The presence of both testes in the scrotum should be checked.

OPERATION: HERNIOTOMY IN CHILDREN
The spermatic cord is exposed through a transverse groin incision. The hernial sac is separated from the cord structures, to which it is closely related, and ligated at the level of the internal ring. At the end of the operation the testis must be at the base of the scrotum, since, if it is in the groin, it may become fixed there by postoperative fibrosis.

Procedure profile

Blood requirement	0
Anaesthetic	GA
Operation time	15–40 minutes
Hospital stay	Day case or 24 hours
Return to normal activity	1–2 days

Umbilical hernia

Umbilical hernias in children are of two types.
- True. This results from failure of closure of the umbilical ring. Closure usually occurs spontaneously in the first few years of life.
- Paraumbilical. This is a true defect in the linea alba close to the umbilicus. This type of hernia does not close spontaneously.

Recognizing the pattern
There is a bulge in the region of the umbilicus. Strangulation almost never occurs in true hernias and is rare in paraumbilical hernias in children.

Management

A true umbilical hernia may be followed up to ensure that it closes. If it does not do so operative closure may be offered before school age. Paraumbilical hernias should be repaired at the same age.

OPERATION: REPAIR OF UMBILICAL HERNIA

The defect is closed through a small semilunar incision.

Procedure profile

Blood requirement	0
Anaesthetic	GA
Operation time	30 minutes
Hospital stay	Day case
Return to normal activity	1–2 days

Umbilical discharge

A granuloma may develop following separation of the umbilical cord and result in a mucous discharge A swab should be taken but antibiotics are rarely required. Cauterization with a silver nitrate stick or the use of topical Sofradex or Terra Cortril will speed resolution. A more profuse, persistent discharge may indicate a congenital fistula or sinus. These are extremely rare.

Rectal bleeding in children

Most cases are mild and result from straining. The stool should be examined, as worms may be responsible. Piles are rare in children. Stool softeners are used to ease passage of motions and the child is prevented from staying on the potty for long, as this may cause venous congestion.

An anal fissure causes pain and bleeding. Constipation results, as the child is frightened to pass motions, which compounds the problem. Stool softeners are given together with dietary advice. An examination under anaesthetic may be necessary if there is no improvement after 3 months.

Intermittent passage of blood and mucus may be due to a benign rectal polyp. A polyp can be ligated at its base and will slough off painlessly a few days later.

Massive haemorrhage is most often due to a Meckel's diverticulum. Peptic ulcer, intussusception, blood dyscrasias, intestinal duplications and angiomas are rarer causes.

The incidence of inflammatory bowel disease in children is increasing and should be remembered in a child with cramping pains and passage of bloody mucus.

Rectal prolapse in children

Rectal prolapse in children is associated with potty training and is prompted by the squatting position which is adopted. A true full-thickness prolapse or a partial (mucosal) prolapse may occur.

Recognizing the pattern
The child is usually 2–3 years old when the alarming symptom of something protruding from the anus is noted during defaecation. There may be a history of excessive staining or constipation by the child. The prolapse usually reduces spontaneously.

Proving the diagnosis
The diagnosis is usually made on the mother's history.

Management
Reassurance and the use of stool softeners is routine. Raising the potty off the floor by several inches to allow the child to sit with 90° hip and knee flexion may be useful. All children with full thickness rectal prolapse should undergo a sweat test because of the association with cystic fibrosis. In most cases the condition resolves spontaneously. If mucosal prolapse persists, sclerosant injections (oily phenol) may be required.

Constipation in children

This is the infrequent passage of stools. The passage of hard stools, sometimes referred to as constipation, is usually the result of a low-residue diet and is treated with high fibre and high fluid intake. Transient constipation may result from dietary changes.

Chronic constipation may have an organic cause such as neurological deficits or anal stenosis but the majority of cases are functional, often precipitated by pain associated with an acute anal fissure. It can result in acquired megarectum due to incomplete emptying, and the consequent impaction of faeces causes spurious diarrhoea and soiling.

Management
Management is difficult and often prolonged, requiring specialized nursing. Toilet training and dietary manipulation are aided by the judicious use of laxatives, suppositories and enemas. Occasionally manual evacuation under GA is necessary.

Urinary tract infection in children

Urinary tract infection in children must be taken seriously as long-term complications are likely unless properly treated.

Recognizing the pattern
Infants may present with abdominal pain, vomiting, pyrexia or failure to thrive. Older children may present with wetting by day, having previously been fully continent. Only a minority present with loin pain, rigors and dysuria.

Making the diagnosis
'Clean catch' midstream urine specimens are required in older children. In infants suprapubic bladder aspiration may be necessary. Confirmed infections require ultrasound, to assess the kidneys and ureters as congenital anomalies are commonly found. A micturating cystourethrogram is required, since vesicoureteric reflux is commonly responsible. Nuclear isotope scans (MAG3,

DTPA, DMSA) are used where appropriate to assess renal function and structure.

Management
Initial infections are treated with antibiotics. All cases require investigation to seek associated anomalies.

14.3 General management of the paediatric patient environment

Infants have a high surface area to volume ratio and are therefore prone to heat loss. This is maximal in newborn and premature infants whose thermoregulatory system is also immature.

Nursing
The gag reflex is poor, so there is increased risk of aspiration, and regular aspiration of nasogastric tubes is essential to reduce the risk of vomiting.

Fluids
Fluid overload is a significant risk, especially in neonates. A 1-day-old baby should be given no more than 60 mL/kg/24 h intravenously gradually increased over several days to a standard 120 mL/kg/24 h. For oral fluid intake the standard is 150 mL/kg/24 h. Postoperative fluid requirements are reduced because of high levels of antidiuretic hormone. For older children, maintenance fluid requirements can be calculated from the following formula.

- Give 100 mL/kg/24 h for each of the first 10 kg = 4 mL/kg/h.
- Give 50 mL/kg/24 h for each of the next 10 kg = 2 mL/kg/h.
- Give 10 mL/kg/24 h for each kilogram above 20 kg = 1 mL/kg/h.

For example, a 22-kg child requires 1.54 L/24 h (64 mL/h) for ordinary maintenance.

Dextrose saline (0.45% sodium chloride, 5% dextrose) is suitable. Additional fluid losses e.g. from nasogastric tube or stoma must be replaced mL/mL with i.v. fluid. A urine output of 1–2 mL/kg/h is expected in a healthy child. A child that is peripherally shut down and has a low urine output should receive a fluid bolus of 20 mL/kg of either colloid or normal saline.

Weight can be calculated from the formula (age in years + 4) × 2.

Electrolytes

As with adults, hypokalaemia can result from diarrhoea or vomiting and must be considered in any intravenous fluid regime.

Hypocalcaemia can cause collapse or fits. Initial treatment is with intravenous calcium gluconate 10%. If this fails to raise the calcium level, check for low magnesium levels.

The poor glycogen reserves of the neonate result in a risk of rapid onset hypoglycaemia. BM-stix testing is routinely done 6-hourly postoperatively, and corrective action taken if the level falls below 3 mmol/L.

15 The management of trauma

15.1 Dealing with a major accident

The principles of management of the trauma victim are taught on the Advanced Trauma Life Support (ATLS) course. This is essential for all doctors who, following their foundation years, will be involved in the management of trauma.

When a major trauma victim arrives in hospital, there may be many people involved in the initial assessment and resuscitation. There is often great danger for the patient and urgent decisions need to be made. Good organization is imperative, and action, however rapid, has to be methodical and thoughtful. Priorities must be decided and one doctor (the team leader) should assume overall control of the progress of resuscitation without being too embroiled in the action.

Accurate notes are always important, particularly for victims of assault, road accidents or industrial injuries. Legal action may be taken many months after the injury when the actual details have been forgotten.

How do you cope when the victim of a major accident suddenly comes under your care? The following plan is helpful. There are six stages.

- Primary survey to assess vital functions.
- Resuscitation.
- Secondary survey – a full history and examination.
- X-ray and special investigations.
- Priorities for management.
- Treatment.

Surgery: Diagnosis and Management, 4th edition. Edited by N. Rawlinson and D. Alderson. © 2009 Blackwell Publishing, ISBN: 978-1-4051-2921-3

Primary survey and resuscitation

The primary survey and resuscitation are considered together because in practice they are combined. The principle of care is 'treat as you find'. A problem with the airway must be sorted before moving on to assess breathing. Do not go on, until the step you are doing is complete. When there are two or three doctors working together, steps can be done simultaneously.

The primary survey assesses A (airway), B (breathing), C (circulation), D (disability) and E (exposure). Resuscitation manages life-threatening injuries to A, B and C.

Airway
- Beware cervical spine injury. Immobilize the neck until this is excluded (see p. 640). Never do a chin-lift or head tilt.
- Open the airway. Is it clear? 'Look' with a sucker.
- Clear potential obstruction, including broken teeth, debris, vomit, etc.
- The airway may need frequent aspiration.
- Perform a jaw thrust, and then use an oropharyngeal (Guedel) airway to hold the tongue forward and keep the airway open. Beware using a nasopharyngeal airway in head injury with risk of base of skull fracture.
- If the patient is still not breathing adequately and remains cyanosed, consider intubation and ventilation. Severe head injury, coma or maxillofacial injuries are also indications for intubation.
- Rarely the patient may need an emergency cricothyroidotomy (e.g. for facial burns).
- Give the patient high-flow oxygen.

Breathing
- Is the patient breathing? Is mechanical ventilation effective?
- Look, feel and listen. What is the respiratory rate? Is there a trend? Is the trachea central? Listen for breath sounds. Compare the two sides.
- Is there adequate gaseous exchange, i.e. is the patient cyanosed or adequately oxygenated?
- Check whether there is any injury to the chest that may embarrass respiration.

- Does the patient have a tension pneumothorax or haemo-thorax? Crepitus in the skin indicating surgical emphysema is a sign of tension pneumothorax.
- Treat any life-threatening injury of the chest immediately, e.g. tension pneumothorax or haemothorax (see pp. 626–27).

Circulation

- Check the pulse, capillary re-fill and blood pressure.
- Stop any external bleeding with direct pressure.
- Beware of bleeding into 'hidden body cavities'. These are the chest, abdomen, pelvis and retroperitoneum.
- Insert two large-bore intravenous cannulae. The antecubital fossa is the best site unless injured.
- Take blood for investigations and cross matching. Request 8 units. Warn the labs if more is likely.
- Treat any hypovolaemia with crystalloid or blood. O-negative blood can be used if blood is needed before the cross-match is completed. The longer the delay in instituting such therapy, the more collapsed are the veins and therefore the more difficult intravenous cannulation will be.
- Expect hypotension where there is multifocal injury.

Disability

- Check the basic level of consciousness. Is the patient *a*lert, or responding to *v*oice, *p*ain, or *u*nresponsive (AVPU)? Record the Glasgow Coma Scale.
- Look at the pupils and limbs for lateralizing signs (see p. 618).

Exposure

- Ensure the patient is completely undressed.
- Do a log roll and rectal examination. Examine the spine.
- Insert a urinary catheter (see p. 453) and nasogastric tube unless contraindicated. Test the urine for blood.
- Order a portable series of X-rays (lateral cervical spine, chest and pelvis) in the resuscitation room.
- Monitor the patient's response to your resuscitation.
- If deterioration occurs then re-assess from the beginning. The consequences of trauma may develop during this primary survey – e.g. a tension pneumothorax.

At the end of the primary survey and resuscitation the immediate life threat should be averted, there should be adequate cerebral perfusion of oxygenated blood, and a fuller assessment of all the injuries can begin.

Secondary survey

A full history and examination are then undertaken together with documentation of the injuries. Monitor vital functions during this time.

The exact order in which this is done will be governed by events. However, it must be thorough and, if urgent treatment interrupts it, it must be completed at the earliest opportunity. Patients have, for instance, had a fractured finger left untreated because in the excitement of the initial effort to save life, no one has had time to examine the digits.

The history

Try to determine exactly what happened and how long ago. Obtain a detailed account of the mechanism and direction of injury. This may be obtained from the patient, bystanders, ambulance personnel or police. A description of the patient's condition when first found is essential and should be recorded. Try and picture it. A clear and 'vivid' history informs the examination. Form some idea of the degree of force; for example 'How high was the fall?', 'On what did he land?', or 'How fast was the car travelling?'.

If the patient is conscious, find out about any areas of particular pain. If there is deterioration, this information may be valuable later.

Remember to find out the patient's normal medical condition including any allergies, any current medication such as insulin or steroids, past medical history (e.g. diabetes, myocardial ischaemia or previous chest injury), and the time of their last meal.

On examination

The examination must be a thorough assessment and include all systems. The findings should be accurately recorded, ideally at the time the examination is being carried out. Examine the patient methodically, starting with the head, neck and trunk and working down both arms and both legs, looking for possible injuries. This is especially important in an unconscious patient.

Use what is known of the mechanism of the accident to predict sites of injury. For example a person hit by a car bumper while standing may have ligament injuries to the knee. A passenger in a car hit on the left side may have a ruptured spleen or kidney.

Start with the head, looking for lacerations, bruising, haematoma or deformity. Check the pupil reaction and size. Measure the conscious level using the GCS (see p. 611). Examine the ear drums and fundi.

Logroll the patient (if not done earlier) and examine the neck, including a careful palpation of the cervical spine for localized tenderness or deformity. Then feel the thoracic and lumbar spine for any possible fracture. If there is any likelihood of an unstable spinal fracture, this must be stabilized before the patient is moved (see p. 640). The neck needs immobilizing until cervical spine injury is excluded. This is achieved by demonstrating:

- no bony tenderness
- normal X-rays – three views
- no neurological signs in arms or legs
- no distracting injury.

This may not be possible in the emergency department.

Examine the upper limbs next, including the clavicles, joints, bones and soft tissues down to the individual fingers. Re-examine the chest for rib, lung or mediastinal injury. Surgical emphysema is often a sign of tension pneumothorax. Then feel the abdomen. Palpate methodically around the various organs observing the patient's reaction for any sign of a localized site of tenderness.

Finally, examine the pelvis and the lower limbs down to the toes.

X-ray

- The following are routine in all cases of major trauma:
  - cervical spine – three views. Some practitioners do the lateral C-spine in the resuscitation room. If it does not show C7/T1, this can be scanned at the same time as other scans are done (a CT is often done before other plain imaging)
  - chest

  ◦ pelvis.
- Include the following, depending on injuries observed:
  ◦ thoracic spine
  ◦ lumbar spine
  ◦ limbs
  ◦ facial views.
- Specialist imaging, such as CT, ultrasound or contrast radiology.

Special investigations
- Send off blood to the laboratory for haemoglobin, cross-matching 8 units, urea and electrolytes, blood sugar, amylase.
- Test the patient's urine for blood.
- All women of child-bearing age must have a pregnancy test.

Decide on priorities for management
Decide on the priorities for management. This can be started whilst the patient is being X-rayed. It may well be difficult. The order should be as follows.
- Conditions threatening life – usually treated during the primary survey.
- Conditions which are at present stable but could threaten life if they deteriorate.
- Major injury, no threat to life.
- Minor injury.

Management
Management will be considered under the following headings.
- Head injuries   Section 15.2
- Chest and abdominal injury   Section 15.3 (p. 622)
- Spinal and pelvic injuries   Section 15.4 (p. 640)
- Trauma to the skin and limbs   Section 15.5 (p. 647)

15.2 Head injuries

Patients present with either:
- major head injuries, where the patient's injury is obvious and their conscious level may be reduced

- minor head injuries where there is a history of head injury but the patient 'appears' unaffected
- a deteriorating head injury, particularly one that was 'minor' and then becomes 'major'. Prompt recognition and rapid management saves life and brain function.

Brain survival depends on adequate perfusion with oxygenated blood. This is governed by the intracranial pressure (ICP), the mean blood pressure and respiratory function. The brain compartment in the skull is of constant volume (once the bones have fused at about 18 months of age), containing brain, blood and CSF. There is limited room for expansion either by brain swelling or haematoma (Fig. 15.2.1a). As additional volume is added, cerebrospinal fluid (CSF) shifts into the spinal compartment, the venous sinuses are compressed and there may be some vasoconstriction. There is thus little initial change in ICP. Once this leeway is taken up, the ICP starts to rise, until eventually a small increase in volume causes a dramatic rise in pressure (Fig. 15.2.1b).

The brain perfusion pressure (BPP) is the sum of the mean blood pressure (MAP) minus the ICP. A minimum of 60 mmHg is required for adequate brain function. Less than this causes first electrical and then structural damage. In a major injury with head involvement the ICP may rise and the MAP may fall, both resulting in inadequate brain perfusion (Fig. 15.2.1c). In addition cerebral autoregulation of blood flow is impaired. The priority is to restore the blood pressure before correcting ICP.

Remember that it is not possible to lose enough blood into a head injury to cause hypovolaemia. Therefore if hypovolaemic shock is present look for extracranial injury. If this is not visible assume bleeding into the chest, abdomen, pelvic space or retroperitoneum.

Pathology of brain injury

Brain injury is divided into primary damage sustained at the moment of injury, and secondary damage occurring in the minutes/hours following the impact (Fig. 15.2.2).

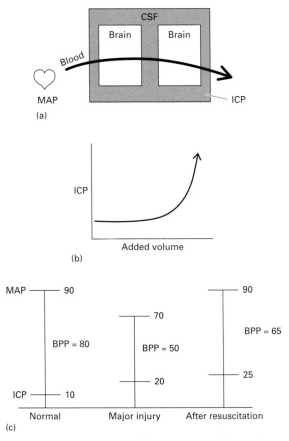

Fig 15.2.1 The physiology of brain perfusion and intracranial pressure changes with trauma and space-occupying lesions.

Primary brain damage

Primary brain damage occurs by distortion and sudden movement within the dura and skull. Damage may be focal (e.g. after assault injury), the rest of the brain being relatively normal, or

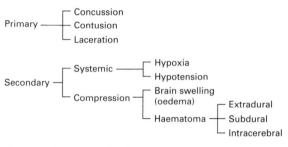

Fig. 15.2.2 The pathology of head injury.

may be a combination of focal and diffuse injury typical of a high-momentum impact. There are three categories of primary injury.

- Concussion. This is a generalized injury resulting in diffuse loss of nerve function. It is an 'electrical injury' which is reversible.
- Contusion. This is more localized and consists of bruising of the cortex.
- Laceration of the cerebral cortex. This is often associated with bleeding into the subdural space. This is primary structural damage, and is irreversible. Diffuse axonal injury is included in this category and is seen after high-momentum rotational injuries (e.g. pedestrian being hit by a bus).

Secondary brain damage
Secondary brain damage is caused by the following.
- Systemic factors, including:
  ∘ hypoxia
  ∘ hypotension.
- Compression (raised intracranial pressure), caused by:
  ∘ brain swelling
  ∘ haematoma:
    ▪ extradural
    ▪ subdural
    ▪ intracerebral.

If brain compression is asymmetrical, focal shift occurs between the various brain compartments. The most important of these are as follows.

- The medial temporal lobe herniates beneath the falx and presses on the third cranial nerve causing dilatation of the ipsilateral pupil.
- The temporal lobe herniates through the tentorial hiatus and compresses the midbrain causing decorticate posture.
- The cerebellar tonsils herniate through the foramen magnum ('coning') and cause major cardiorespiratory disturbance/arrest.

The assessment and management of head injury is governed by the need to prevent, detect and treat this secondary injury. Systemic and local factors responsible for secondary brain damage are correctable. The prevention of hypoxia and hypotension is crucial to the outcome of brain damage and is most important in the first few hours after head injury.

Major head injury

Recognizing the pattern
The initial assessment is combined with resuscitation. The following steps are performed.
- Is the airway patent? If not an airway must be inserted or the patient intubated. All patients in coma need intubation.
- Cervical spine. A patient with a major head injury must be assumed to have a cervical spine injury until this is excluded. Until then the head is immobilized in hard collar, sandbags and tape. All airway care is mindful of this. Use a jaw thrust, and not chin lift or head tilt.
- Is the patient breathing effectively? There may be active breathing movements but inadequate air flow due to a flail chest.
- Is ventilation adequate? Central cyanosis indicates inadequate gaseous exchange, which may be due to pulmonary contusion. Blood gases should be performed as soon as possible. Hypercapnia is a potent cause of cerebral vasodilatation and therefore increased ICP.
- Pulse and blood pressure. Is there a pulse and is it strong? Is there evidence of any external bleeding? If so, this must be controlled. Remember that isolated head injury does not cause hypotension so look elsewhere for blood loss.
- Carotid perfusion. Are there carotid pulses?

- Chest X-ray. An early chest X-ray is mandatory to exclude pneumothorax or haemothorax.

Emergency management aims to achieve cardiorespiratory stability. This may include blood transfusion, insertion of a chest drain for a tension pneumothorax or haemothorax or even laparotomy (e.g. for ruptured spleen). At the end of this assessment and resuscitation, the mean blood pressure should be restored such that cerebral perfusion is improved even though the ICP may still be elevated.

Once the primary survey and resuscitation is complete the secondary survey can begin. Start a monitoring record of Glasgow Coma Scale (GCS), pulse rate, blood pressure, respiratory rate and body temperature to detect any deterioration. If this occurs, go back and repeat the primary survey.

THE HISTORY
Establish full details of the injury, especially from the ambulance personnel. Include the position in which the patient was lying (an unconscious patient lying on their back may have aspirated), the time of the injury, any changes in conscious level, any history of fitting and whether the patient was ever cyanosed or unable to breathe.

Find out about any allergies, medications and medical illnesses.

NEUROLOGICAL EXAMINATION
Assess the conscious level. Make a note of eye opening, verbal response and motor response. The GCS is the standard method of recording the level of consciousness and facilitates comparisons later on (Table 15.2.1). It is dynamic, and a series of measurements showing the trend of change is more valuable than a single reading. A falling GCS suggests systemic disorder (hypoxia or hypotension) or rising ICP.

Examine the head for scalp lacerations or bruising. Localized tenderness and a boggy swelling due to haematoma may be felt over a fracture site. You may feel a depression in the outline of the skull if the fracture is depressed. Look in the nose and ears for blood or CSF leakage, which may indicate a base of skull fracture in the floor of the anterior (nose) or middle (ear) cranial fossa.

Table 15.2.1 Glasgow Coma Scale. (From Jennett B, Teasdale G. (1977) Aspects of coma after severe head injury. *Lancet* i 878–81.)

Function	Type of response	Points
Eyes	Open:	
	spontaneously	4
	to verbal command	3
	to pain	2
	Closed	1
Best verbal response*	Orientated and converses	5
	Disorientated and converses in sentences	4
	Inappropriate words	3
	Incomprehensible sounds	2
	No response	1
Best motor response	To verbal command:	
	obeys	6
	To painful stimulus:†	
	localizes pain	5
	flexion – withdrawal from pain‡	4
	flexion – abnormal (decorticate rigidity)	3
	extension (decerebrate rigidity)	2
	No response	1
Total		3–15

* Arouse patient with painful stimulus if necessary.
† Apply the thumb to the underside of the supraorbital ridge, find the notch and press up, observing the arms. To localize pain a hand must come above the chin.
‡ Elicit pain by squeezing a finger-nail bed.

Anterior fossa fractures, as well as causing traumatic rhinorrhoea, cause bilateral black eyes ('panda eyes'). Bleeding may extend into the orbit and cause an effusion of blood, leading to unilateral exophthalmos, disturbance of eye movements and subconjunctival haemorrhage. The posterior border of this haemorrhage cannot be seen. The cranial nerves may also be affected. Bruising behind the ear (Battle's sign), with or without facial nerve palsy, and/or CSF otorrhoea indicate a fracture through the petrous temporal bone, the floor of the middle crania fossa.

Examine the eyes noting the pupil size, equality and reaction to light. Try to assess eye movement.

Examine the limb movements, noting the tone and testing the reflexes.

Management

Early management is governed by the stability or otherwise of the patient's conscious level. If the unconscious patient is stable, investigations can proceed in an orderly fashion. These should include the following.

- Repeat blood gases to check respiratory function.
- Haemoglobin.
- Urea and electrolytes.
- Blood sugar.
- Liver function tests.
- CT scanning. The indications for CT scanning include the following:
  - a patient who is in coma (GCS 8 or less) after resuscitation
  - GCS less than 13 at any time
  - GCS 13–14 (confusion) at 2 h after injury
  - any patient with an open skull fracture
  - depressed skull fracture or clinical evidence of skull base fracture
  - neurological signs
  - post-traumatic seizure
  - a history of penetrating injury such as stabbing or gun shot.
  - age over 65
  - coagulopathy, including warfarin therapy
  - dangerous mechanism (e.g. fall of 1 metre, ejection from car).

The presence of deterioration adds urgency. The faster the drop in GCS the quicker the scan is done (once ABC are stable).

- Skull X-ray. There is now very little place for skull X-rays in head injury except:
  - in the assessment of non-accidental injury in children
  - in conjunction with close observation where CT resources are limited.

These patients should be discussed with the regional neuro-surgical centre.

GENERAL CARE OF THE UNCONSCIOUS PATIENT
The priorities are to minimize brain swelling, maintain oxygenation and blood pressure and monitor regularly for evidence of deteriorating conscious level.

Nurse the patient with the head elevated 30°. In some centres ICP monitoring is performed. There is no place for steroids in acute head injury.

RESPIRATION
If respiration is not adequate, the patient will need to be ventilated. This enables better control of blood gases. Hyperventilation to lower the P_aCO_2 (partial pressure of carbon dioxide) below the lower limit of normal is not now routine, since the vasoconstriction can cause brain ischaemia. Sedation and analgesia are necessary during this period if the patient is restless or in pain.

If ventilation is required for longer than 7 days, a tracheostomy may be required.

The daily assessment of the chest should include:
· examination
· chest X-ray
· blood gases.

Chest physiotherapy should be carried out regularly and if possible coincide with turning the patient. Tracheobronchial suction or bronchoscopy may be required.

CARDIOVASCULAR SYSTEM
Aim to ensure cerebral perfusion and avoid hypertension. If the blood pressure increases, exclude raised ICP, pain, hypoxia or a distended bladder and then treat as indicated.

NUTRITION
This may be given either through a nasogastric tube or by an intravenous route. If the nasogastric route is used, it is important to watch for regurgitation. Also remember that patients with multiple injuries may have an ileus.

BLADDER
This should be catheterized. Retention of urine is a common cause of restlessness.

BOWELS
They should be controlled by enemas.

FLUID BALANCE
A strict watch should be kept on the patient's fluid balance together with measurements of urea and electrolytes and blood sugar, particularly if mannitol has been given. If anything, a slight fluid deficit should be maintained to prevent cerebral oedema.

GENERAL BODY CARE
The pressure points on the skin should be looked after by regular turning and putting the patient on a sheepskin and/or a ripple mattress. The eyes should be cleaned and kept closed to prevent corneal ulceration. The mouth should be regularly cleansed and kept moist to prevent parotitis or stomatitis. Regular limb physiotherapy is needed to prevent contractures developing.

EPILEPSY
Fits following head injury are common, particularly after conditions such as depressed skull fracture with dural penetration and brain damage. Epilepsy requires treatment with anticonvulsants, such as phenytoin or carbamazepine. In an emergency intravenous diazepam is a safe drug to use. There is no indication for prophylactic anticonvulsants.

DETERIORATION IN CONSCIOUS LEVEL
Deterioration may be seen in the emergency department or after a period of observation in hospital. The faster the deterioration occurs, the faster must be the response if one is to save the patient's brain. Deterioration is due to secondary brain damage, often caused by a developing haematoma.

The signs of deterioration are as follows:
- a decreasing level of consciousness
- bradycardia
- hypertension
- deep breathing.

Changes in the pupillary reactions and focal neurological signs such as arm or leg weakness indicate the probable side of such a lesion (lateralising signs). Pupil dilatation occurs on the side of the lesion, and weakness on the opposite side.

Exclude new problems with the airway, breathing and circulation, and then carry out a CT scan. This differentiates between generalized brain swelling, brain contusions and haematoma.

Contact the neurosurgical centre. Transfer of the patient may be indicated. This is potentially dangerous. Ensure the patient is intubated, ventilated and stable prior to moving off. Active measures can be taken to reduce cerebral oedema. Mannitol (20% 250–500 mL (1 gm/kg) i.v. over 20–30 min) or frusemide may be given. Discuss with the neurosurgeon.

HAEMATOMA

A haematoma causing cerebral compression and midline shift must be removed. This may be done at the referring hospital, or by at the neurosurgical centre. Usually transfer is advised, following the resuscitation described above. The management of haematoma is described further on p. 617.

Minor head injury

This is defined as a head injury where there has been no loss, or only transient loss, of consciousness, with or without loss of memory. The patient is conscious when seen. In other words 'the patient has had a minor injury to the head but appears OK'. The primary decision is to identify those patients who are at risk of secondary deterioration and therefore need imaging and/admission for observation.

Recognizing the pattern

A careful enquiry as to the nature of the injuries is undertaken. Establish whether the patient remembers the whole event clearly or if there is any retrograde or post-traumatic amnesia. Are there any disturbances of smell or hearing which may indicate a fracture causing damage to the olfactory or auditory nerves? Are there disturbances of vision, photophobia, nausea, vomiting or headache? Has the patient had a fit?

On examination the examination is performed as for a major head injury, but in this case with the cooperation of the patient.

Proving the diagnosis

The indications for CT scan include the following.
- Loss of consciousness or amnesia at any time.
- GCS 13–14 (confusion) at 2 h after injury.
- An open skull fracture.
- Neurological signs.
- Post-traumatic seizure.
- Depressed skull fracture or clinical evidence of skull base fracture.
- A history of penetrating injury such as stabbing or gun shot.
- Age over 65.
- Coagulopathy, including warfarin therapy.
- Dangerous mechanism (e.g. fall of 1 metre, ejection from car).

There is now very little place for skull X-rays in head injury except:
- in the assessment of non-accidental injury in children
- in conjunction with close observation where CT resources are limited.

Management

The main decision is whether the patient needs admission to hospital or can be sent home. The indications for admission to hospital are as follows.
- A history of loss of consciousness more than 5 min (i.e. significant).
- Confusion or other impairment of conscious level at the time of examination.
- Evidence of a skull fracture.
- Vomiting or increasing headache.
- Neurological symptoms or signs.
- No witness to the accident, and no history.
- An unreliable history (usually due to alcohol or drugs).
- Lack of adequate supervision at home.

A normal CT scan does not avoid admission if other symptoms are present. Sometimes the CT scan is done too early.

If the patient can go home, then an instruction sheet should be given to the patient's carer which includes the address and telephone number of the hospital, the date, and advice that the patient should return to hospital immediately if he or she develops symptoms of nausea, vomiting, headache, drowsiness, photophobia or weakness.

Patients who are admitted should have the following observations quarter- or half-hourly (in order to look for signs of raised ICP).

- Conscious level, which should be described using the Glasgow Coma Scale (p. 611).
- Pulse, blood pressure, respiratory rate and body temperature.
- Pupil size, equality and reaction.
- Limb tone and movement.

Observations should ideally be continued for 24 h, after which the a stable asymptomatic patient can be discharged. Children may stay longer because this age group can develop raised ICP from brain swelling within the first 48 h.

Intracranial haematoma

Haematomas may be extradural, subdural or intracerebral (Fig. 15.2.3).

- Extradural haematoma occurs between the bone and the dura and is classically due to rupture of the middle meningeal artery following a fractured overlying temporal bone.
- Subdural haematoma occurs between the dura and brain, and is usually associated with severe head injury causing cerebral laceration. It is typically less brisk than an extradural haemorrhage.
- Intracerebral haematoma is a collection of blood within the substance of the brain and is associated with major brain damage. Occasionally intracerebral haemorrhage due to aneurysm or hypertension is the primary event which caused the head injury.

Recognizing the pattern

A head-injured patient develops signs of secondary deterioration and rising ICP, as described above. The other presentation of

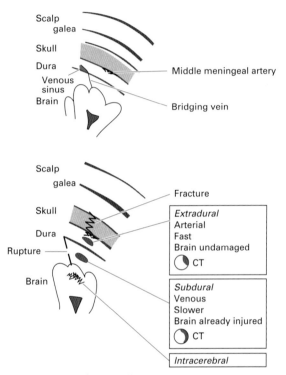

Fig. 15.2.3 The sites of intracranial haematoma.

intracranial haemorrhage is of a patient who is unconscious and begins to show signs of rising pressure.

On examination focal lateralizing signs may indicate the side of the compression.

- Pupillary size. There is contraction followed by dilatation of the pupil on the side of the haemorrhage (Hutchinson's pupil). As the pressure further increases, the opposite pupil shows similar signs. Bilateral fixed and dilated pupils may be a sign of brain-stem death, seen as the terminal evidence of coning. Remember, though, the effects of drugs, including alcohol, and of fits.

- Hemiplegia. This is usually contralateral to the side of the first dilated pupil.

Proving the diagnosis

The diagnosis is made on a CT scan. If the patient is deteriorating rapidly emergency intubation and ventilation are indicated. They should still be scanned, if possible, even if this is one or two slices simply to confirm the diagnosis. Occasionally a patient deteriorates so quickly that even this is not possible.

Management

The management is surgical evacuation provided that the patient's clinical condition warrants it. A patient found to have a haematoma but who is clinically improving can be managed conservatively.

An acute extradural or subdural intracranial haematoma is solid and therefore has to be removed by craniotomy, usually by a neurosurgeon. Skilled anaesthesia is mandatory. Mannitol is given while theatre is being prepared, and during patient transfer to the neurosurgical centre.

Burr holes are very occasionally indicated in the receiving emergency department/hospital. Sometimes a CT has confirmed the diagnosis of an extradural haematoma in a patient who has quickly deteriorated, and when the journey time to the neurosurgeon is too long. A burr hole is done to let the compressing haematoma out, and then the patient transferred. A rarer event is a patient being taken to theatre on clinical grounds only (clinical extradural, no CT available and a surgeon trained in this procedure). In determining which side burr holes should be done without CT guidance, the site of a skull fracture and the side of the first dilated pupil are of more significance than localization by observed limb weakness.

OPERATION: CRANIAL BURR HOLES

The burr hole is situated either next to the fracture or at a point 5 cm up from the midpoint of a line drawn between the external auditory meatus and lateral angle of the eye. This lies over the middle meningeal artery. A linear incision is made in a direction that can be converted into a scalp flap if a craniotomy is to be performed. The temporalis muscle/fascia is divided and a burr hole drilled. If a haematoma is found, it is evacuated. An acute extradural haematoma has the consistency of 'redcurrant jelly'. If necessary the burr hole may be enlarged (craniectomy) to find and control the bleeding vessel. This is usually beneath the fracture. It is then acceptable to place a swab in the wound and transfer the patient to the local neurosurgical centre.

Procedure profile

Blood requirement	2
Anaesthetic	GA
Operation time	1 hour
Hospital stay	Variable
Return to normal activity	Variable

The long-term management of head injuries is multidisciplinary. Complications such as epilepsy, chronic subdural haematoma, external hydrocephalus and infection may occur.

Skull fracture

A skull vault fracture can be closed (simple) or open (compound). An open fracture is one where there is an associated scalp injury, rendering the fracture site open to the atmosphere, with the secondary risk of meningitis or abscess formation. Fractures that run into the nose or middle ear (base of skull) with CSF leakage are also regarded as open.

A vault fracture may be undisplaced (a linear or fissured fracture) or depressed. A depressed fracture will cause local injury and loss of function depending on its site. The site, depth and the presence of dural penetration determine the treatment required.

Recognizing the pattern
Skull fracture is caused by focal injury. Blunt injury (e.g. hammer) that breaks the skin has more force than an incision injury

and so is more likely to cause fracture. There is bony tenderness away from the impact site. If there is a scalp wound a fracture may be seen in its base, or felt with a gloved finger. A depressed fracture is sometimes cosmetically visible. Brain or CSF coming for the wound indicates a fracture with dural penetration.

Signs of a base of skull fracture include 'panda eyes', CSF rhinorrhoea, haemotympanum, Battles's sign (bruised mastoid) and CSF otorrhoea.

Proving the diagnosis

This is made on CT scan. Underlying brain injury and air in the head are also detected.

Skull X-ray is rarely indicated. The appearances can be difficult to interpret. A linear fracture is characteristically thinner and darker and has a more angular course than the vascular markings. It is straighter and more defined than the cranial suture lines.

Management

A closed linear fracture requires no additional management, other than that already described for head injuries. The patient is admitted and regular observations are carried out.

An open linear fracture requires surgical treatment. The wound must be thoroughly cleaned and the fracture inspected. If hair is present, it must be removed, if necessary by craniectomy. Broad-spectrum antibiotics are given (e.g. cefuroxime 1.5 g i.v.). If there is CSF leakage, the patient remains in hospital until it stops. If the leak persists more then 1 week, surgical repair of the defect may be necessary.

A closed depressed fracture is managed conservatively unless there is evidence of dural penetration or the fracture is overlying an important area of function, e.g. the speech or motor cortex. In this case surgery is indicated. The depressed fracture is elevated and any fragments of bone or damaged brain removed.

An open depressed fracture requires urgent operation to clean the area and remove any dirty bone, fragmented dura or damaged brain. The wound can be closed and skull reconstruction may be carried out at a later date. Antibiotics are required as above.

15.3 Chest and abdominal injury

Chest trauma

With any chest injury there is a danger that respiration may be compromised. You should also consider whether there has been associated injury to the underlying pleura, lungs or mediastinal structures including the heart.

Injuries to the chest involve one or more of the following.
- Chest wall:
  - fractured ribs
  - flail chest
  - fractured sternum.
- Pleura:
  - pneumothorax
  - tension pneumothorax
  - traumatic haemothorax.
- Lung:
  - pulmonary contusion
  - pulmonary laceration.
- Mediastinal structures:
  - closed chest injury
    - ruptured thoracic aorta
    - ruptured bronchus
    - ruptured diaphragm
    - ruptured oesophagus
  - blunt injury to the heart
  - haemopericardium.
- Penetrating injuries: bullet and stab wounds to the chest.

Fractured ribs

Ribs are usually fractured as a result of a direct blow to the chest or a crushing injury. The fractures may be single or multiple and simple or compound. Pneumothorax may occur, either due to perforation of the underlying lung by the fractured rib, or a compound fracture with air entering through the wound (open pneumothorax). A traumatic pneumothorax is at higher risk of developing tension and so must be excluded by X-ray.

Recognizing the pattern

The patient complains of severe, localized, pleuritic pain and difficulty in breathing. The latter may either be due to inability to take a deep breath because of pain, or secondary to a pneumothorax.

On examination the characteristic sign is of extreme tenderness at one point along the rib. There may also be bruising or laceration at the site of the injury. Remember to look for signs of an associated pneumothorax, particularly if there is an open wound. An obvious sucking noise when the patient inspires is diagnostic and requires immediate attention.

Proving the diagnosis

The diagnosis of rib fracture is clinical. The fracture may not be seen on a chest X-ray. If the patient is seen within 24 h of injury a chest X-ray is done to exclude a pneumothorax.

Management

For patients with a sucking chest wound, a large square occlusive gauze pad should be taped over the wound on three sides leaving the inferior border free. This will allow egress of air on expiration but limits entry through the chest wall wound on inspiration. This immediate measure is followed by placement of a chest drain and temporary complete occlusion of the wound. A decision to close or explore the wound depends upon the circumstances of the injury. See penetrating injuries below.

ANALGESIA

Analgesia must be adequate to allow effective respiration. This is especially important in the elderly and debilitated who are likely to develop an underlying hypostatic pneumonia. Intercostal bupivacaine nerve blocks are very useful but need to be repeated every 6 h or so. Non-steroidal anti-inflammatory agents such as diclofenac are particularly useful, as they do not cause respiratory depression.

BREATHING

The patient is given breathing exercises and physiotherapy.

STRAPPING

Opinions differ about the value of strapping. Strapping relieves pain but restricts normal chest expansion. It is rarely used now.

Flail chest

A flail chest develops when the chest wall has lost its mechanical rigidity due to multiple fractures. One segment of the rib cage becomes separated from its surroundings and can move paradoxically (i.e. inwards on inspiration, outwards on expiration). This results in inadequate ventilation of the lung and retention of pulmonary secretions. There is associated pulmonary contusion. A dangerous vicious circle ensues in which the lung becomes increasingly oedematous, the patient more and more anoxic and respiratory movements increasingly active. This further exacerbates the paradoxical movement, and progressive anoxia ensues.

Recognizing the pattern

The patient has signs of fractured ribs. Initially respiration may be satisfactory but after 24–48 h there is increasing dyspnoea and the patient becomes more and more distressed. On inspection the flail segment will be seen to move paradoxically.

Proving the diagnosis

The diagnosis is confirmed on chest X-ray. Blood gas estimations are of value and show a low PO_2, (partial pressure of oxygen) and an elevated PCO_2. CT scanning shows underlying damage.

Management

The patient should be sat up and given oxygen. As a temporary measure the flail segment may be supported with strapping. Strong analgesia will be required in all cases and is best given either as intercostal blocks or as a thoracic epidural anaesthetic. The patient is observed carefully and, if the respiratory rate begins to climb, further action may be required. Serial blood gas estimations are also used to monitor progress. In severe cases intermittent positive pressure ventilation is needed. A tracheostomy reduces the dead space and facilitates good tracheobronchial toilet. If the flail segment is depressed (stove-in chest), it will require elevation.

Fractured sternum

This is a rare injury. It commonly follows road traffic accidents where there is a forceful impact against the seat belt, steering wheel or dashboard.

Recognizing the pattern

The patient complains of pain over the sternum and is usually breathless. The pattern of bruising from the seat belt may be seen. On examination the sternum is very tender and there may be a palpable step or deformity. Pulmonary complications are rare, but there may be associated damage to the trachea, great vessels or heart.

Proving the diagnosis

- Chest X-ray.
- X-ray sternum.
- ECG.
- Cardiac enzymes.

Management

The patient is admitted and treated with strong analgesia (e.g. pethidine) to allow chest expansion. If there is severe displacement with a reduction in the anteroposterior diameter of the chest, the depressed segment is pulled forward at open operation and fixed with wires. Cardiac monitoring is vital.

Traumatic pneumothorax

Air may get into the pleural space either following damage to the lung after a penetrating wound or rib fracture, or through a deep wound. There is a risk of developing tension.

Recognizing the pattern

Apart from the pain of the original injury, the patient complains of breathlessness and pleuritic pain. On examination the affected hemithorax is hyper-resonant. The breath sounds are decreased on that side.

Proving the diagnosis

This is confirmed on chest X-ray. The absence of lung markings in the periphery of the pleural space is noted, as is the edge of the lung.

Management

Because of the risk of tension, a traumatic pneumothorax must be drained with a large intercostal drain attached to an underwater seal. The insertion and management of a chest drain is described on p. 248.

Tension pneumothorax

A tension pneumothorax develops when there is a 'one-way valve' leaking air from the lungs into the pleural cavity. Air accumulates, compressing the lung, and urgent treatment is required. Severe respiratory embarrassment develops and vascular compromise can ensue due to kinking of the great veins secondary to mediastinal displacement. This eventually obstructs venous return to the heart and death occurs due to cardiac arrest.

Recognizing the pattern

Deterioration is a vital clue to diagnosis. A breathless patient with the clinical features of a pneumothorax becomes progressively worse with increasing dyspnoea and evidence of increasing mediastinal shift.

The patient is distressed with a hyperexpanded immobile hemithorax, 'drum' hyper-resonance and absent breath sounds. Tracheal displacement only occurs when a tension is developing. There may be associated surgical emphysema of the chest wall, neck and face (which feels like crackling in the skin). Impaired venous return causes a tachycardia and hypotension. The final deterioration can occur very rapidly.

Proving the diagnosis and management

The presence of a tension pneumothorax is a clinical diagnosis, and is confirmed by inserting a chest drain. No time should be wasted doing an X-ray. If this is a possibility, a chest drain should be inserted urgently. A needle thoracocentesis will buy time as you set up for the chest drain. The rush of air under pressure confirms the diagnosis. Once the tension has been released, normal chest drainage connected to an underwater seal can be established (see p. 250). The presence of a pneumothorax and the position of the drain are confirmed by urgent chest X-ray.

OPERATION: NEEDLE THORACOCENTESIS

After cleaning the skin a large venflon is inserted in the second intercostal space in the midclavicular line. Feel the sternal angle and then identify the second rib. Follow it out laterally. Feel the midpoint of the clavicle and drop an imaginary line down. This avoids hitting the internal mammary artery that runs behind the costochondral junction. Insert the venflon onto the rib and walk up and into the pleural space (see Fig. 6.1.1).

Traumatic haemothorax

An accumulation of blood in the pleural cavity can occur from injury to the lung, heart, great vessels or chest wall. There may be an associated pneumothorax, which can tension (see above).

Recognizing the pattern

The presence of blood is irritant and causes pleuritic pain and breathlessness. The patient may be shocked. On examination there are signs of a pleural effusion with lack of breath sounds and a dull percussion note at the lung base.

Proving the diagnosis

The blood in the pleural cavity is seen on chest X-ray and confirmed on tapping the chest.

Management

Unlike a tension pneumothorax which can be released immediately it is found, a haemothorax can tamponade itself, and will start bleeding again once it is released. So set up i.v. lines and give fluid first. After this resuscitation, with cross-matched (or O-negative) blood available, immediate drainage is required. An underwater seal is used and the level of the water in the bottle is marked so that the blood loss can be measured. Further management is usually conservative until the bleeding stops. However, if more than 1500 mL is removed, or if the rate of bleeding is more than 200 mL/h, a thoracotomy may be required.

Pulmonary contusion or laceration

This is bruising, and oedema of the lung beneath chest wall trauma. There may or may not be an associated rib fracture. The injury to the lung has a severe effect on respiration. There may also be an associated pulmonary laceration with blood or air in the pleural cavity.

Recognizing the pattern

The patient is breathless, apprehensive and cyanosed, and coughing produces sputum tinged with blood.

Proving the diagnosis
A chest X-ray shows a progression from a patchy diffuse opacity in the lung fields (12–24 h after injury) to a complete 'white out'. Blood gases show hypoxia and hypercapnia.

Management
It is important to keep the patient relatively dehydrated and diuretics may be helpful. Intravenous fluid therapy must be carefully regulated to avoid overtransfusion. Oxygen, adequate analgesia and physiotherapy will help, but the patient may eventually need ventilating. Monitoring on a high-dependency unit is helpful.

Closed chest injury
Closed chest injuries are often caused by shearing forces generated during extreme deceleration. The following will be considered.
- Rupture of the thoracic aorta.
- Rupture of the bronchi.
- Rupture of the diaphragm.

Rupture of the thoracic aorta
Rupture of the ascending thoracic aorta is usually fatal. Rupture of the descending aorta usually involves the intima and media only, resulting in a large periaortic haematoma.

Recognizing the pattern
The patient complains of severe central chest pain. The diagnosis is made by noting widening of the mediastinum on a chest X-ray and it is important to be aware of this potentially lethal condition. Where there is doubt a repeat chest X-ray may show progressive change.

Management
After control of blood pressure, urgent operation is required. Under cardiopulmonary bypass repair or replacement of the aorta by a Dacron graft is undertaken.

Ruptured bronchus
This commonly occurs distal to the carina as the bronchus leaves the support of the mediastinum. There is a large escape of air

causing bilateral pneumothoraces and mediastinal emphysema. There may be haemoptysis.

Recognizing the pattern
The patient is acutely dyspnoeic and shocked, and surgical emphysema may be felt in the neck.

Proving the diagnosis
This is confirmed on chest X-ray and on bronchoscopy.

Management
Immediate operative repair is required to restore lung function. Any significant delay will result in infection around the bronchial wound and later stricture formation.

Rupture of the diaphragm
This occurs after a crush injury to the abdomen. The diaphragm usually tears on the dome from front to back adjacent to the pericardium. There may be herniation of the stomach or other organs through the rent. The stomach may distend, collapsing the lung and shifting the mediastinum. Occasionally it becomes strangulated. Small tears may be asymptomatic and without visceral herniation. This occurs later, perhaps related to events that raise intra-abdominal pressure. A history of significant prior trauma can often be elicited from adults with late symptoms related to a diaphragmatic hernia.

Recognizing the pattern
The patient presents with increasing respiratory difficulty following an abdominal injury.

Proving the diagnosis
The chest X-ray may show a raised hemidiaphragm and, if the left side is involved, a stomach bubble may be visible in the chest. If a nasogastric tube has been passed, it will be seen to lie in the chest. A decubitus film will also show a horizontal fluid level in the chest. A barium swallow is useful.

Management
Following resuscitation and passage of a nasogastric tube, surgical repair is required urgently. If there is no other thoracic

injury requiring operation, the diaphragm may be exposed from below through the abdomen. This decreases the incidence of pulmonary complications postoperatively and allows the surgeon to check that the spleen is not damaged.

Ruptured oesophagus

This is an extremely rare injury in isolation, and is usually encountered in association with other major thoracic injuries. Air in the mediastinum may become apparent as subcutaneous emphysema in the neck. CT scan reveals air in the mediastinum and/or pleural space. Emergency thoracotomy is required. The approach is determined by the range of injuries thought to be present.

Blunt injury to the heart

Blunt injury to the heart may cause contusion of the myocardium with necrosis of muscle fibres. Dysrhythmia or heart failure may follow. Occasionally there may be rupture of the papillary muscles or interventricular septum. The thin walls of the atria and right ventricle may burst, causing cardiac tamponade (see below). Cardiac concussion is a condition where there may be dysrhythmia in the absence of myocardial necrosis.

Recognizing the pattern

The patient may present with a dysrhythmia, heart failure or cardiac tamponade following a blow on the chest. There may be a pericardial friction rub on examination.

Proving the diagnosis

The electrocardiogram (ECG) may show changes typical of infarction if there is a large area of cardiac contusion. Any arrhythmia is possible. Cardiac enzymes are elevated. An echocardiogram shows the degree of cardiac dysfunction.

Management

It is most important to be aware of the possibility of a cardiac injury. The patients most at risk from complications are those with ECG changes, particularly if other major injuries are present.

The patient must be put on an ECG monitor. Care must be taken during intravenous infusion not to overload the circulation.

Measurement of the central venous pressure or intracardiac pressure may be useful. The patient should be examined frequently with particular care taken to auscultate the heart. A cardiothoracic surgeon should be warned about the case if it is severe and transfer considered.

Haemopericardium

The pericardial cavity fills with blood following a penetrating injury to the heart (e.g. stab wound) or following blunt trauma with rupture of the walls of the atria or right ventricle. The outer fibrous pericardium limits distension of the pericardial sac, and blood in the cavity therefore prevents ventricular filling, resulting in cardiac tamponade with decreased cardiac output, hypotension, cyanosis and elevated jugular venous pressure. The heart sounds are quiet on auscultation.

Proving the diagnosis

This is a life-threatening condition. Ultrasound will show the collection. Aspiration of the pericardial cavity with a needle inserted just under the seventh costal cartilage and to the left of the xiphoid process proves the diagnosis and provides temporary relief.

Management

The pericardial cavity is opened through either an anterolateral thoracotomy or a sternotomy, and the defect repaired.

Penetrating injuries to the chest

The rise in urban violence means that penetrating injuries from bullets, knives and other sharp weapons are no longer rare events. In addition, a variety of relatively sharp objects will penetrate the chest wall during a road traffic accident (e.g. railings). Any penetrating injury to the chest may cause serious complications but the most dangerous are those that occur within the midclavicular lines and between the jaw and xiphisternum. These need careful surgical exploration because of the risk to internal organs. The pleura, subcostal vessels, lung, heart, great vessels and main airways may all be involved. Remember that a low or angulated penetrating wound in the chest may have perforated the diaphragm and injured abdominal viscera, especially the liver, stomach and spleen.

Proving the diagnosis

Preoperatively a chest and abdominal X-ray may be taken to look for missiles. Thoracoabdominal CT will clarify the track, and underlying injury. Cross-match 6–10 units of blood but warn the laboratory that more may be needed urgently later.

Management

If a cardiothoracic surgeon is available, their help should be obtained. Set up at least two good intravenous infusion lines, a central venous pressure line to prevent overtransfusion and chest drainage if necessary.

OPERATION: EXPLORATORY THORACOTOMY FOR PENETRATING CHEST INJURY

The wound is excised and all dirt, rib fragments and debris are removed either through the same wound or through a separate thoracotomy. The pleural cavity is explored and any pulmonary lacerations repaired. Any other damage is treated as necessary.

Procedure profile

Blood requirement	6–10
Anaesthetic	GA
Operation time	2–3 hours
Hospital stay	7 days, depending on other injuries.
Return to normal activity	Variable

The postoperative care following thoracotomy is described in section 6.1.

Abdominal trauma

Abdominal trauma may be due to penetrating or blunt injuries. Different problems arise in these two categories.

Penetrating injuries to the abdomen

These include the following:

- stab wounds.
- gunshot wounds.
- penetration by other foreign bodies.

The patient complains of abdominal pain and may be shocked with signs of peritonism. Remember that penetrating injuries entering the chest or buttocks can easily extend to the peritoneal cavity.

Management

All penetrating injuries of the abdomen that go through the deep fascia should be formally explored after the patient has been resuscitated. A preoperative abdominal CT is useful if the patient is not shocked. A laparotomy is undertaken to exclude damage to any hollow viscus that may result in fluid leakage and peritonitis, and also to stop any haemorrhage.

Blunt injury to the abdomen

Injury occurs from compression, crushing, shearing or deceleration forces. The external visible damage may be minimal but the internal injuries serious. A high index of suspicion is therefore required. There may also be delay between a causative injury and the appearance of signs of damage. The internal injury may be at a different site from the site of the original trauma. A careful history will suggest which organ is injured.

Investigation is now either by ultrasound or CT (with contrast). Ultrasound (FAST scan – focused abdominal assessment by sonography in trauma) is a quick, portable bedside procedure. CT requires transport and time, and so is not safe with an unstable patient. It is however more specific. Diagnostic peritoneal lavage (DPL) to show free blood in the peritoneal cavity is rarely done now.

As a result of modern imaging most blunt abdominal trauma is managed conservatively with careful monitoring. Haemodynamic instability, clinical signs of peritonitis and specific radiological findings (e.g. intraperitoneal gas) are all indications for intervention.

The internal injuries to be considered are the following.

- Ruptured liver.
- Ruptured spleen.

- Traumatic bowel injury.
- Pancreatic injury.
- Renal injury.

Ruptured liver

In blunt abdominal trauma the liver is usually injured by rapid compression and decompression. This tends to produce a ragged tear in its substance. The condition must be suspected in any case of multiple trauma or abdominal injury. This is especially true if there are external marks over the liver such as a seatbelt bruise, or if the patient is shocked with no obvious sign of blood loss. Rapid deceleration tears the liver from its attachments; the most serious of which is tearing into or avulsion of the hepatic veins from the vena cava.

Recognizing the pattern

The conscious patient may complain of abdominal pain situated in the right upper quadrant. The pain is worse on breathing. On examination they will be shocked (pale, sweaty, anxious, with a tachycardia and sighing respiration). The abdomen may exhibit localized tenderness and rigidity in the right upper quadrant. There may also be more generalized tenderness due to a haemo-peritoneum. The abdomen is distended.

Proving the diagnosis

Ultrasound (FAST) or CT scanning will show the injury. CT is only indicated if the patient is stable. The urinary bladder is emptied by a catheter. Blood tests include full blood count, liver function, clotting and cross-match.

Management

The patient is resuscitated. Most isolated liver injuries can be managed conservatively. They stop bleeding as a result of a degree of internal tamponade. Major vertical splits close to the hilus or vena cava are more likely to involve large veins and it is these that tend to produce catastrophic haemorrhage. The CT scan is often informative. Early evidence of haemodynamic instability in the face of volume replacement is the main indication for surgery. Major bile leaks may be a late consequence of conservative management.

OPERATION: LAPAROTOMY FOR RUPTURED LIVER

The abdomen is opened and the abdominal viscera inspected. If a hepatic tear is confirmed, one of the following procedures is carried out.

- The liver is packed between its external surface and the body wall in order to appose the edges of the rupture. Such packs can be left in place for 24 h and then removed at a second laparotomy. An experienced hepatic surgeon should be available for this second operation.

- Some small tears can be sutured, but careful pack placement will approximate most of these anyway. Exploration of deep wounds near to major structures should not be attempted by an inexperienced surgeon. There are very real risks of exsanguination or causing massive air embolism if open major venous structures are exposed. Elevation of the legs and positive-pressure ventilation can help direct such air embolism into the lower body.

- Liver resection is appropriate when part of the liver has been avulsed to such a degree that it is clearly not viable (partial hepatectomy; see p. 339).

- A variety of anciliary measures can be used in the above procedures to gain more effective haemostasis. Maintaining a low central venous pressure is usually not difficult in the bleeding patient, but the anaesthetist must be instructed not to raise the CVP above 5 cm of water, as this increases venous bleeding dramatically. Argon plasma coagulation is an effective way of stopping bleeding from raw surfaces and topical haemostatic agents (Tisseel, Tachosyl) can also be placed on raw surfaces or to buttress sutures. If the patient's condition permits, it is always worthwhile ensuring that there is no major bile leak, as this is a major cause of late morbidity.

Procedure profile

Blood requirement	10
Anaesthetic	GA
Operation time	Variable, 2–3 hours
Hospital stay	14 days depending on other injuries
Return to normal activity	2–3 months

Urea and electrolytes, platelets and clotting must be measured frequently.

If there is a large haematoma within the liver substance, the progress of this haematoma can be monitored using repeat ultrasound.

Ruptured spleen

Splenic rupture may occur as part of an abdominal compression injury or due to a localized blow over the left lower ribs. Rupture may follow trivial injury if the spleen is already enlarged, e.g. due to malaria. Occasionally an injury is sufficient to bruise the spleen but not to rupture the capsule. The haematoma thus formed may rupture after 7–10 days (delayed rupture of the spleen).

Recognizing the pattern

There is pain in the left upper quadrant together with localized tenderness and guarding. The tenderness may be more marked on inspiration. Not infrequently there is an associated fracture of the left lower ribs. The patient also complains of pain in the left shoulder tip (Kehr's sign) and both flanks may be dull to percussion with the right flank exhibiting shifting dullness (Ballance's sign).

Proving the diagnosis

The diagnosis of intraperitoneal bleeding can be confirmed by ultrasound (FAST). A straight X-ray of the abdomen may show an elevation of the left hemidiaphragm and a diffuse splenic shadow with displacement of the gastric air bubble. An ultrasound or CT scan is also helpful in detecting a splenic haematoma.

Management

The patient is resuscitated. Conservative management can be undertaken if injury is essentially to the spleen alone, and any haematoma confined to the spleen and its immediate surroundings with little or no free blood elsewhere. Continued pain, haemodynamic instability, shock and abdominal distension all indicate the urgent need for laparotomy.

OPERATION: LAPAROTOMY FOR SPLENIC INJURY

The abdomen is opened and blood evacuated. If possible the damaged spleen should be repaired and this can usually be achieved with polar avulsion injuries. The spleen may be repaired by one of the following methods.

- Direct suture of a laceration over a haemostatic material such as Surgicel.
- Partial splenectomy. The feeding vessels of the damaged area are ligated, the damaged area excised and the cut organ repaired.

If these procedures are not possible, a splenectomy is performed. The thick peritoneum lateral to the spleen (the splenorenal ligament) is divided vertically. This allows the spleen and the tail of the pancreas to be delivered into the wound. It is then easy to control bleeding by grasping the splenic pedicle between the fingers of one hand. The splenic artery, splenic vein and short gastric arteries are ligated and the spleen is removed. Care is taken not to damage the tail of the pancreas, the fundus of the stomach or the splenic flexure of the colon.

Procedure profile

Blood requirement	6
Anaesthetic	GA
Operation time	60–90 minutes
Hospital stay	7–10 days
Return to normal activity	1 month

Postoperative care is described in section 8.2 (see p. 358).

Traumatic bowel injury

The bowel may be damaged either by direct injury or indirectly due to damage of its feeding vessels. In the latter case there is risk of rupture some days after the initial injury. Such injuries occur in road traffic accidents when the bowel is crushed against the spine by a seat belt.

Recognizing the pattern

The patient with a bowel injury may have minimal signs at first and the condition may not be suspected in view of other injuries.

If the patient deteriorates with increasing abdominal pain and distension after 2–3 days, think of this possibility.

Proving the diagnosis

The diagnosis is confirmed by an X-ray which shows free peritoneal gas. CT with contrast gives more detail. Aspiration of the abdomen produces bile-stained bowel contents.

Management

Ideally this is by early laparotomy and repair or resection of the damaged area together with careful exploration to exclude other abdominal trauma. With multiple injuries or when other intra-abdominal structures require attention, it is inadvisable to carry out multiple intestinal anastomoses. An appropriately sited loop stoma should be performed.

OPERATION: SMALL BOWEL RESECTION

The damaged bowel is resected and an end-to-end anastomosis performed.

Procedure profile

Blood requirement	2
Anaesthetic	GA
Operation time	90–120 minutes
Hospital stay	7 days
Return to normal activity	4–6 weeks

Postoperatively a nasogastric tube is aspirated regularly and the patient is kept on minimal oral fluids until flatus is passed. Anastomotic problems are rare.

Pancreatic injury

The pancreas may also be damaged by a crushing injury from a seat belt or steering wheel. The pancreas usually fractures vertically over the portal vein, producing a sizeable retroperitoneal haematoma. The diagnosis is usually made by CT scan. Pancreatic injury should be suspected when non-specific symptoms persist particularly in the presence of hyperamylasaemia or the detection of a high amylase content in peritoneal fluid. It may be necessary to prove integrity of the main pancreatic duct by MR pancreatography.

Management
A transected pancreatic duct is usually best managed by distal pancreatectomy (see p. 345).

Renal injury
The kidneys may be damaged by blunt injury to the loins or by compression from the front. The injury may then be extraperitoneal, although in children the peritoneum is more likely to be breached as there is little perinephric fat. The renal damage may be anything from a subcapsular haematoma to a complete tear. Occasionally the renal vessels are avulsed.

Recognizing the pattern
The patient is shocked and there is tenderness in the loin. Haematuria occurs but may be delayed. It may be microscopic and only detected by urinalysis. There may also be clot colic. On examination fullness in the loin may indicate a perinephric haematoma.

Proving the diagnosis
CT with contrast will show the degree of structural damage and renal dysfunction, and demonstrate a haematoma. It will also confirm a normally functioning kidney on the other side. Renal artery angiography is occasionally useful.

Management
Having excluded other abdominal trauma, the initial treatment is conservative, comprising bed rest and analgesia. If there is extravasation of urine, antibiotics such as ampicillin (500 mg 6-hourly) or co-trimoxazole (2 tablets 12-hourly) may be given. Laparotomy is indicated if there is continued uncontrolled bleeding.

OPERATION: LAPAROTOMY FOR RENAL INJURY
If possible, the damaged kidney is repaired, although a partial or complete nephrectomy is often required. A full laparotomy is undertaken to exclude other intra-abdominal injury.

Procedure profile

Blood requirement	6
Anaesthetic	GA
Operation time	1–2 hours
Hospital stay	Depends on the injuries
Return to normal activity	Depends on other injuries

Postoperatively a severe ileus may occur which may need treatment with a nasogastric tube and intravenous fluids. The long-term follow-up should include a repeat renal scanning after 3 months to check renal function.

15.4 Spinal and pelvic injuries

Fractured spine

The importance of spinal injury lies in the danger of associated trauma to the spinal cord or nerve roots. Injury is more common in the cervical or lumbar region because the vertebrae are relatively unsupported.

A stable spinal fracture will not displace further and there is no continuing danger to the spinal cord. With an unstable fracture abnormal movement can encroach on the vertebral canal with resulting spinal cord damage.

At the scene of the accident, before the patient is moved, a cervical collar should be applied and any movement of the spine kept to an absolute minimum with the patient placed on a spinal board. The head is secured with sand bags and tape.

Do not move the patient except 'as a log' until an unstable fracture has been excluded.

Recognizing the pattern

Always consider the possibility of spinal injury when a patient has suffered severe trauma.

The patient complains of severe localized pain at the site of the fracture, which may radiate along the distribution of the relevant nerve roots. The patient lies still and the pain is worse on any movement. Ask if there is any numbness, tingling or weakness in the limbs.

On examination there may be visible deformity of the spine. Palpation of the vertebrae may reveal discontinuity or displacement, and localized tenderness. Tenderness on one side of the midline suggests muscular or ligamentous injury or damaged transverse processes. If the cord has been damaged, you may find abnormalities in sensation, movement and reflexes in the limbs. In cervical injuries there may be abnormalities in the pulse, blood pressure and respiration.

Proving the diagnosis

Spinal X-rays must be done in any case of possible spinal injury. Anteroposterior and lateral views are usually taken. There are other specialist views for the odontoid peg or lumbar pedicles. A qualified doctor should be present to supervise the movement of the patient.

When inspecting X-rays check for the following.

- Ensure that all seven cervical vertebrae are seen including the C7–T1 junction. Sometimes special views are necessary to demonstrate this.
- Symmetry between the two sides.
- Any incongruities in the width of the vertebral bodies.
- Any incongruities of the joint spaces.
- On the lateral view look for a step in the posterior or anterior longitudinal ligament disclosing displacement of a vertebra. Loss of this alignment and widening of the gap between the spines are typical of an unstable fracture.
- Look carefully for evidence of injury to the bones themselves. CT scanning now provides an alternative to straight X-rays for

radiologically inaccessible parts of the vertebral column (e.g. C7–T1 junction, thoracic vertebrae, etc.).

Management

The patient can be rolled but the head, trunk and pelvis are supported so that there is no relative movement of one vertebra on another ('log rolled'). In a case of a suspected cervical fracture the head is immobilize in hard cervical collar, sandbags and tape. The whole spine is protected using a spinal board.

With muscular bruising or a fractured transverse process, the patient may be allowed home, given analgesics and advised to rest on a firm mattress for 7–10 days. Admission may be required if the pain is severe or movement severely restricted.

If there is a stable vertebral fracture, the patient is admitted, given analgesics and put on a bed with a rigid base. The patient is X-rayed again 2 or 3 weeks later and then mobilized slowly. In the case of an unstable fracture consider transferring the patient to a spinal centre. External support is needed, and active reduction may be required. Skeletal traction with skull calipers is used for unstable cervical fractures. Alternatively, vertebrae may be reduced and fused by open operation.

When there is damage to the spinal cord, attention must be paid to the paralysed limbs to prevent contractures or pressure sores. There may be an ileus for 3 or 4 days. A cervical cord injury may mask symptoms due to other abdominal trauma. Bladder and bowel function may need assistance.

Fractured pelvis

A fractured pelvis must always be considered and excluded after multiple trauma. When the pelvic ring is broken in two places the iliac crests may be mobile (an 'open book' fracture). Blood loss occurs from the iliac venous plexus, exposed bone, avulsed arteries and torn muscle. External evidence of pelvic fracture may be slight but this blood loss can be considerable (e.g. 4–5 L) and ongoing. There is a possibility of associated visceral injury to the urethra, vagina, bladder or rectum.

Recognizing the pattern

The patient complains of back pain, particularly if the sacroiliac joints are involved. Movements are painful. On examination there is pain on palpating the pelvis and deformity may be visible. In an open book pelvic fracture the iliac crests are mobile and compressible. Do not elicit this more than once because abnormal movement dislodges blood clot, causing more bleeding. A careful examination should be made of both legs, particularly of the arterial and nerve supply. A rectal examination should be performed. Ask about bleeding from the urethra or micturition problems, which may indicate associated visceral damage.

Proving the diagnosis

The fracture is seen on pelvic X-ray. This should be identified in the primary survey.

Management

The patient is given oxygen. He or she may be shocked and require initial transfusion. At least 8 units of blood should be cross-matched and two good intravenous lines set up. O-negative blood may be needed.

A stable pelvic fracture can be treated conservatively with bed rest, analgesia and lower limb exercises. The patient is mobilized as the improvement in pain permits.

Fractures in more than two places results in disruption of the pelvic ring and an unstable pelvis. An unstable pelvic fracture may result in severe blood loss and is a potentially life-threatening condition. Resuscitation is urgent. The fracture is held closed to try and stem blood loss by:

- compressing the iliac crests together
- suspending the patient in a rolled sheet placed under the buttocks
- fitting an external fixation device. This procedure is usually done in theatre, and is necessary before laparotomy.

Continuing haemorrhage may be controlled by radiological arterial embolization or surgical ligation. Management requires close collaboration between anaesthetist, orthopaedic and general surgeons, radiologist and the blood transfusion laboratory. Once the patient is stable, the fracture is scanned and internal fixation planned as needed. Fractures involving disruption of the acetabulum may later result in osteoarthritis. This risk is lessened if an accurate reduction and internal fixation of the fracture is achieved.

Associated injuries
Damage to the urethra
The urethra may be partially or completely torn. The two sites commonly affected are the membranous urethra at the apex of the prostate (following bilateral fracture of the pubic rami) or the bulbous urethra (following a blow in the perineum).

Recognizing the pattern
There is a history of inability to pass urine, meatal bleeding and a distended bladder. A high-riding, mobile prostate on rectal examination suggests a complete membranous urethral tear. When the bulbous urethra is ruptured, a tense perineal haematoma or a swollen, bruised penis and scrotum are seen. Urethral injury should always be suspected following pelvic fracture.

Proving the diagnosis
If the patient is conscious and can spontaneously pass urine, this is tested for the presence of blood. If the patient is unconscious or cannot pass urine an urethrogram is performed before a cautious attempt to pass a catheter is attempted.

Management
- Resuscitation of the patient is the first priority. The urethral repair can wait 12–24 h if necessary.
- Antibiotics.
- If catheterization was not attempted, or was unsuccessful, urine is drained through a suprapubic cystostomy.
- A ruptured membranous urethra is usually repaired around a catheter which is used as a splint. A ruptured bulbous urethra can be repaired or may be treated conservatively, in which case it should be reassessed at 10–14 days.

- If there is associated rectal damage, the definitive repair is delayed until any infection has been treated.
- Any collection in the retropubic space, such as extravasated blood or urine, is drained.
- Stricture is a common sequel to any urethral trauma, and a follow-up urethrogram or urethroscopy is required. The treatment of stricture is described on p. 465.

Trauma to the bladder

There are two mechanisms of bladder injury. A direct blow to the lower abdomen, when the bladder is distended, causes the viscus to burst with leakage of urine into the peritoneum. A fractured or dislocated symphysis pubis may also pierce the bladder causing extraperitoneal leakage.

When there is extraperitoneal leakage, the patient may have a strong desire to void urine but is unable to do so. Intraperitoneal leakage causes very few symptoms other than anuria, and the diagnosis may be missed, particularly in a trauma victim, where the anuria may be attributed to shock.

Proving the diagnosis

The diagnosis is proved by abdominal CT, an intravenous urogram or urethrogram. This should be done if there is any suspicion of bladder injury.

Management

Antibiotics should be commenced. Urgent laparotomy and repair are required. The urethra is catheterized at operation and the peritoneal and extraperitoneal spaces are drained. A follow-up urethroscopy must be done; 20% of patients have accompanying urethral damage and there is a risk of stricture formation.

Injuries to the rectum

These are rare. The damage is usually caused by a crushing or burst injury to the pelvis.

Recognizing the pattern

The patient may have bleeding from the anus and shows signs of a pelvic peritonitis. Rectal examination shows blood.

Management
The treatment is laparotomy, a defunctioning colostomy and washout of the bowel. The tear is repaired at a later date.

Injury to the vagina
These are rare, and usually caused by direct injury from bone fragments. There will be blood per vaginam. The patient will need an examination under anaesthetic (EUA) and repair.

Damage to blood vessels
Management
The internal or external iliac artery can be damaged but more commonly there is damage to the pelvic venous plexus. These injuries are associated with profuse blood loss and are a surgical emergency. They should be treated by blood transfusion (cross-match 6–10 units), and stabilization of the pelvis by external fixation to encourage tamponade. If these measures fail embolization of the affected vessels may be required.

Nervous injury
The sciatic nerve may be damaged by a traction force or posterior dislocation of the hip. This is usually a neuropraxia or axonotmesis (see p. 655) and eventual recovery is possible. Severe disruption of the sacroiliac joints can cause a nerve root injury, where the damage is permanent.

Recognizing the pattern
The presenting sign is of foot drop. There is a partial or complete loss of sensation down the leg, apart from the medial surface which is supplied by the long saphenous nerve (a branch of the femoral nerve).

Management
Neuropraxia or axonotmesis should eventually recover. Meanwhile, physiotherapy to the limb maintains the mobility and prevents any contracture deformity. The nerve must be explored if it is thought likely that it is severed, but this is unusual.

15.5 Trauma to the skin and limbs

Management of wounds

The management of skin wounds depends on whether they are clean or contaminated and whether the skin edges are intact (incisional wound) or damaged (crushed or torn wound). There may also be skin loss. The aim is to heal the wound as perfectly as possible and prevent secondary infection by pyogenic bacteria or organisms causing gas gangrene and tetanus. Always consider which structures lie underneath a wound. Are they damaged?

Wounds may be closed by:
- primary suture – immediate
- delayed primary suture – at 48 h
- secondary suture – at 5–7 days.

The gold standard closure is by suture. The is the best way to ensure haemostasis. Other ways to close wounds include clips, glue, and steristrips.

Recognizing the pattern
- Ask the patient the following.
  - How did it happen? Was it sharp (incisional) or blunt trauma? Could there be any foreign body or glass in the wound? (Glass indicates an X-ray.)
  - How long ago did it happen?
  - Is it known to be clean or dirty?
  - Are they immunized against tetanus, and if so when was the last injection of tetanus toxoid given (see p. 649)?
  - Is there any loss of function?
  - Is the patient diabetic, or suffering peripheral vascular disease?
  - Is the patient taking steroids or anticoagulants?
- Examine the wound edges and look for evidence of contamination or infection.
- Examine closely for any injury to underlying vessels, nerves, tendons, bones or joints – especially in the hand.

Management
All wounds are carefully cleaned and debrided, removing dead tissue and foreign matter. Haemostasis is secured. Further

management depends on the age of the wound and whether it is contaminated or not.

HISTORY OF LESS THAN 12 HOURS
A clean wound is closed by primary suture. If the skin defect cannot be closed, the area may be covered by a split-skin graft (see below).

A wound that was heavily contaminated is cleaned and irrigated, left open and dressed. It is then re-examined after 48 h and if no infection is present the wound closed by delayed primary suture.

HISTORY OF MORE THAN 12 HOURS
A clean wound cannot be closed as it must be assumed that any potential infection has become established. It should be treated with delayed primary suture as above.

A heavily contaminated or infected wound is thoroughly debrided and dressed. It is redressed daily after cleaning with further debridement and saline or chlorhexidine irrigation until the inflection has cleared. Then, when the wound is clean, the granulation tissue is removed, the skin edges freshened and the wound closed by secondary suture. Skin defects are closed by split-skin grafts.

OPERATION: SIMPLE SUTURE OF A SKIN WOUND
The skin is cleaned with a suitable agent. The area is draped off and local anaesthetic is injected around the edges of the wound, using a puncture site outside the wound. The skin edges are debrided of all dead and contaminated tissue. The wound edges are then opposed, using interrupted nylon sutures. In the head and neck multiple small sutures are used so as to minimize 'cross-hatching' in the scar later.

Procedure profile

Blood requirement	0
Anaesthetic	LA
Operation time	Minutes
Hospital stay	Outpatient
Return to normal activity	Variable – depends on job and site of wound

OPERATION: SPLIT-SKIN GRAFT

Donor sites are usually the upper arm or thigh and a graft may be taken using a special knife, under a local or general anaesthetic. It is important to learn how to do this by observing and assisting an experienced surgeon. The donor site is dressed with non-adherent dressing and left for 10 days. The split skin graft is placed raw face uppermost on paraffin gauze and then cut to size. Haemostasis in the recipient area is important to prevent blood from lifting the graft. If a mesh graft is used, a larger area can be covered and any haematoma can escape through the holes in the graft. The graft is applied and sutured at the edges with silk, one end of each stitch being left long enough to tie over a sponge or pad soaked in antiseptic lotion.

Procedure profile

Blood requirement	0
Anaesthetic	GA or LA
Operation time	30 minutes – 2 hours depending on size
Hospital stay	7–10 days
Return to normal activity	Variable

Postoperatively the top ties are divided and the sponge removed at between 5 and 7 days. The graft can then be inspected and if healing is satisfactory the rest of the sutures are removed.

TETANUS PROPHYLAXIS

Tetanus is a disease characterized by muscle spasm caused by the toxin of *Clostridium tetani*, a Gram-positive, anaerobic, sporing bacillus. The spores appear in animal faeces and therefore contaminate earth. Extensive wounds with heavy contamination are typically infected, although tetanus can follow small penetrating injuries. Active immunization with toxoid is now a routine part of the triple vaccine given to children. A booster dose should be given every 10 years. The organism is sensitive to penicillin, metronidazole or tetracycline.

A high-risk wound is one that is heavily contaminated, deep, more than 8 h old and containing dead/ischaemic tissue.

Management

Surgical debridement and toilet must be performed for all wounds.

The type of tetanus prophylaxis given depends on the nature and age of the wound and the immune category of the patient. The measures available include the following:

- a booster dose of tetanus toxoid
- a complete course of tetanus toxoid
- penicillin
- antitetanus globulin.

- Patients with active immunity who have received a dose of toxoid within the last 10 years need no further prophylaxis.
- Patients who last had toxoid more than 10 years ago require a tetanus toxoid booster and, if the wound is old or deep, or contamination is present, a course of penicillin.
- Non-immune patients should be given a tetanus toxoid course and a course of penicillin for all but the most minor wounds.
- Human antitetanus globulin has been produced for passive immunity in patients with high-risk wounds. It is expensive, not readily available and not without risks.

Hand injuries

These are commonly seen in the emergency department. The importance of careful assessment, particularly of associated injury to artery, tendon or nerve, has been mentioned. Remember to ask about the patient's occupation and handedness. Patients who work with their hands are often self-employed. When they injure them, they will be worried about their income. They will expect you to understand this. The hand should be cleaned and elevated to lessen swelling. Severe hand injuries should be referred for a specialist hand surgeon's opinion.

Amputated fingertips are commonly seen. If the bone is exposed it is best trimmed back and the wound allowed to granulate. If the wound is less than 1 cm in diameter, particularly in children, re-epithelialization will be satisfactory. If a whole finger has been amputated, reimplantation is possible. The finger should be cooled and the patient referred to a microsurgery unit.

Fractures

This section covers the general principles of fracture management as far as these may be required by the junior surgical trainee treating a patient with multiple trauma. For the management of specific fractures the reader should refer to a textbook of orthopaedics.

Individual fractures may be either closed, when the skin is intact (simple fracture), or open, when the skin surface over the fracture has been broken to however small an extent (compound fracture). Other terms, which may be applied to fractures, describe the type of break as either transverse, spiral, oblique or comminuted (Fig. 15.5.1).

Recognizing the pattern

The patient complains of localized pain at the fracture site and is unable to use the affected limb. Unlike a sprain when disability

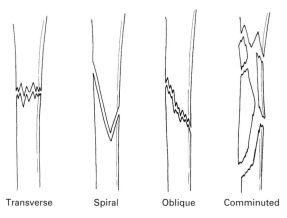

Transverse   Spiral   Oblique   Comminuted

Fig. 15.5.1 Types of fracture.

increases as the injured joint stiffens, a fracture causes immediate loss of function. The mechanism of injury should be ascertained, as this will give a clue to the type of fracture expected.

On examination there is swelling, bony deformity and loss of function of the affected limb. Abnormal mobility and crepitus at the fracture site may provide incontrovertible evidence of a fracture. Note whether there is a skin wound. If there is, the fracture must be regarded as compound whether or not the bone is visible.

Proving the diagnosis

Plain x-ray is the mainstay of fracture diagnosis having detected the site by clinical examination. Do not look at an x-ray until you have decided what you will see. At least two views should be obtained. Always ensure that the X-ray includes the joint above and below the fracture.

CT scan with reconstruction provides three-dimensional images of complex fractures, e.g. around the acetabulum.

Management

The precise management depends on the site of the fracture and other associated injuries. In general, however, the steps in management of any fracture are as follows.

RESUSCITATION AND TEMPORARY SPLINTING

Fractures of long bones are associated with a significant blood loss, which may require replacement. The pain resulting from a fracture is extreme and analgesic therapy is important. A temporary splint gives relief and protects against further damage whilst the patient is transferred to hospital and X-ray department.

REPAIR OF SKIN WOUNDS

If the fracture is compound any skin wound must be carefully explored under general anaesthesia and the bone ends exposed and cleaned. The soft tissue must be cleaned and all dirt and devitalized tissue must be removed. Associated arterial, nerve and tendon injuries will need to be repaired. The method of wound closure will depend on the time after the injury and the extent of contamination. Clean, recent wounds may be closed immediately, others may have to be closed by delayed primary suture. Antibiotics are given.

REDUCTION

If the deformity is putting the overlying skin or neighbouring artery or nerve under pressure, then reduction is urgent. Otherwise it can be delayed whilst more general resuscitative measures are carried out. Reduction may be achieved by closed manipulation under anaesthesia or by open operation.

FIXATION

The aim is to maintain the position of the reduced bone ends until they heal together.

External immobilization is often achieved with plaster of Paris. When immobilization is achieved with plaster of Paris, there is a danger of compression of the contents of the limb as the fracture continues to swell. This danger can be avoided by using an initial 'back slab', which can if necessary, be completed later. If a complete plaster has to be applied, it must not be too tight and should contain plenty of padding to allow the fracture to swell. A routine 'plaster check' must be carried out after 24 h and the circulation in the distal limb assessed. This can be performed by the patient after instruction. If there is any evidence of occlusion, then the plaster must be removed.

Another form of immobilization is the application of traction on each side of the fracture. This may be applied either to the skin or to a pin passed through the skeleton (e.g. a tibial pin for reduction of a fractured femur).

Internal fixation is used when the fracture is reduced by open operation. The bone ends are fixed either by a device placed within the cortex (intramedullary nail, screws or wires) or by a pin and plate placed on the outer cortex.

REHABILITATION

Any prolonged immobilization of the limb will lead to muscle wasting and joint stiffness. Regular physiotherapy is important therefore both during the period of immobilization and once the fracture has healed.

Fat embolism

Fat embolism can complicate major fracture. It occurs when droplets of fat get into the bloodstream. The fat may be derived from bone marrow or adipose tissue but may also be of metabolic origin, perhaps by aggregation of chylomicrons. The emboli may lodge in the pulmonary circulation or pass through the lungs and lodge in parts of the systemic circulation such as the brain, skin and kidney.

Recognizing the pattern
The patient is often a young adult with a lower limb fracture, but the condition can also occur in those with severe burns or extensive soft tissue trauma. There is sudden onset of respiratory distress, drowsiness, restlessness or disorientation 24–48 h following injury.

On examination mild pyrexia and tachycardia are early signs. Petechial haemorrhage due to skin emboli is a helpful sign but may not be present. Cyanosis and right heart failure may occur in severe cases.

Proving the diagnosis
Fat droplets may be found in the sputum and urine. The platelet count is invariably low. An arterial blood gas sample will show hypoxaemia, which is the major cause of death. A chest radiograph shows a 'snow-storm' appearance.

Management
Oxygen should be given. Other measures that have been advocated include heparinization and intravenous low molecular weight dextran. Severe respiratory distress may require sedation and assisted ventilation.

Arterial damage

Arteries may be damaged by direct trauma transecting the vessel, by external compression (e.g. from a nearby fracture) or by traction which disrupts the intima. Thrombosis and occlusion of the vessel often follow this latter injury, even though the outer wall of the artery is intact.

Recognizing the pattern
Penetrating arterial injury is unmistakable. Bright red pulsatile blood escapes from the wound.

With an acute arterial occlusion the patient complains of pain in the muscles distal to the damaged vessel. The affected tissues are pale and cold and there are paraesthesiae and paralysis. Distal pulses are absent.

Proving the diagnosis
An emergency arteriogram is always indicated when there is a suspicion of arterial injury. This is usually performed in the operating theatre by the surgical team.

Management
An occlusion of a main limb artery needs urgent exploration and repair.

OPERATION: EXPLORATION OF TRAUMATIC ARTERIAL OCCLUSION
The artery is exposed and the site of damage identified. If the artery has been transected, the damaged ends are resected and a vein graft used to bridge the gap created. Attention must also be paid to any venous damage. If the artery is intact, then an occlusion is due either to external compression or to an intimal tear. If any external compression has been relieved and the distal pulses do not return, an arteriotomy is performed and the damaged segment either excised or bypassed.

Procedure profile

Blood requirement	2–4
Anaesthetic	GA
Operation time	1–2 hours
Hospital stay	Depends on other injuries
Return to normal activity	Depends on other injuries

Nerve injuries

There are three types of nerve injury.
- Neuropraxia is caused by a blunt injury resulting in 'concussion' of the nerve.

- Axonotmesis is caused by a stretching injury which ruptures the axons but not the nerve sheath. The axons degenerate distal to the injury.
- Neurotmesis is complete severance of the nerve and its sheath.

Recognizing the pattern

The clinical signs of nerve injury are loss of sensation and flaccid paralysis with loss of reflexes. The precise clinical picture depends on the particular nerve which is damaged.

Management

NEUROPRAXIA AND AXONOTMESIS

If the injury is a neuropraxia, the treatment is conservative and the nerve usually recovers in 7–10 days. Axonotmesis takes longer because the axons have to grow back down the intact nerve sheath. Physiotherapy is required to prevent contractures and maintenance of normal posture until renervation occurs. The patient needs adequate reassurance and should be told that the nerves grow at the rate of about 1 mm/day (or 1 inch/month). Several weeks may therefore be needed for recovery of an axonotmesis in a limb.

NEUROTMESIS

When a nerve has been divided, the wound must be carefully explored to identify the nerve ends. These should be freshened and the nerve sheath resutured accurately to restore continuity. If this is done with care, there is a good chance that the axons will regrow down the distal nerve sheath. They regrow at the rate of 1 mm/day. A divided digital nerve can be repaired using a microsurgical technique. Digital nerve injuries particularly in the dominant hand involving the thumb, index or little finger (ulnar border) cause serious disabilities and should always be repaired.

Tendon injuries

Tendons may be partially or completely lacerated. Such tendon injuries are commonly seen after cuts over the dorsum of the fingers, back of the hand or the wrist. Careful repair is essential.

Recognizing the pattern

Complete division of a tendon is made obvious by the loss of function of the affected muscle. Partial division may present with pain and a sensation of weakness on contraction against resistance. Where there is a laceration over the anatomical site of a tendon, careful examination of the function of the extensors and flexors should be carried out. This is completed under the anaesthetic needed for wound closure.

Management

The treatment of partial or complete tendon rupture is surgical repair. The wound should be explored under a general anaesthetic. The wound may need to be extended. If necessary the patient can wait 6–8 h until the next morning's operating list, providing there is no associated arterial injury. A partial division of a tendon can be repaired by a continuous suture of fine Prolene or other similar material. A complete division needs end-to-end anastomosis.

Postoperatively the limb is splinted so as to relax the affected tendon and minimize any tension across the suture line. Physiotherapy is commenced early.

Burns

Major burns are a threat to life. Deterioration can be rapid and the management in the acute stage is critical. There are six types of burns:

- dry thermal – flame
- wet thermal – scald
- chemical
- electrical
- friction
- cold injury.

The damage is caused by coagulation of proteins with cell death. Burns can be of varying depth and any one burn is rarely uniform.

A mild burn causes vasodilatation and diffuse erythema (first degree). Kinins are released, which cause pain. Moderate burns cause some cell death with increased capillary permeability and blister and oedema formation (second degree). Sensation remains intact and as these burns are of partial thickness the skin will regrow. Severe burns cause death of cells involving the dermis and deeper tissues, and appear as white insensitive areas (third degree). The full thickness of the skin is damaged and the skin will not regrow as the germinal layers have been destroyed. Such a burn heals by fibrosis with resulting contractures.

The main early danger from major burns is the development of 'burn shock'. Burn shock is due to exudation of protein-rich fluid from the surface of the burn and oedema into the tissues beneath the burn. Both these follow increased capillary permeability. This is at its peak 6–12 h after a burn. The loss of fluid results in hypovolaemia which can develop rapidly, the extent depending on the size of the burn. A patient with 50% burns, for instance, can lose up to half their plasma volume within 3–4 h. This fluid loss must be replaced as rapidly.

Anaemia can develop due to blood loss, red cell destruction and bone marrow suppression.

Later, the damaged and necrotic tissue, lying in a protein-rich exudate, is an ideal site for infection, which can result in septicaemia.

ASSESSMENT

The precise history of the time and cause of the burn must be obtained including the length of time that the causative agent was active. A rapid initial examination is performed to assess the following.

- Whether or not the airway is affected by an inhalation burn – stridor, hoarseness, soot in nostrils, pharyngeal erythema.
- Signs of shock – apprehension, restlessness, thirst, pallor, sweating, tachycardia, hypotension and air hunger.
- The depth of the burn. Burns are classified as follows (see Table 15.5.1).
  - First degree – erythema.
  - Second degree – partial thickness.
  - Third degree – full thickness.
- The size of the burn (Fig. 15.5.2). The area of the burn is expressed as a percentage of the total body surface area. It is calculated using 'Wallace's rule of nines'. Areas of second and third

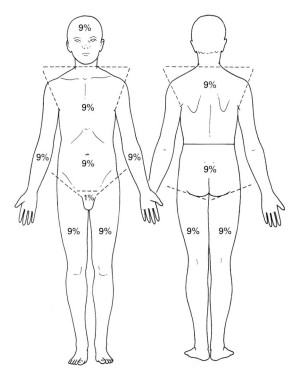

Fig. 15.5.2 A method for measuring the extent of burns on the body surface area. 'Wallace's rule of nines' (11 areas of the body, each equal to about 9% of the total surface area).

Table 15.5.1 The clinical features of different depths of burn.

	First degree – erythema	Second degree – partial thickness	Third degree – full thickness
Colour	Red	Red	White
Painful	Yes	Yes	No
Blisters	No	Yes	No
Wet or dry	Dry	Wet	Dry
Included in area calculation	No	Yes	Yes

degree burn are counted. It may be useful to remember that the patient's hand represents 1% of the adult body surface area.

This initial assessment allows burns to be divided into minor or major categories.

Minor burns

These are burns involving less than 10–15% of the adult body surface area (less than 10% in children), with little evidence of systemic upset or disturbance of the airway.

On examination, draw the size of the burn and map out the areas of definite full thickness, probable full thickness and partial thickness damage. These are judged by the appearance (erythema, blistering or white areas), and the presence or absence of sensation to pinprick (Table 15.5.1).

Management

Different centres have different regimes. Below is one possible scheme of management.

- Superficial burns of the face and superficial scalds are left exposed to the air. They heal in 10–14 days. Yellow soft paraffin can be applied to prevent cracking of the healing skin.
- Partial thickness burns cause erythema and superficial blistering with no break in the skin. They are cleaned with an antiseptic agent and dressed with tullegras. They are then re-examined in 3–5 days. Check that no areas have become full thickness. The wounds are then redressed and the burns usually heal with little scarring.
- Deeper burns will often require surgery. Initially, they must be cleaned with an antiseptic solution and all dirt, large blisters and dead tissue removed. Consideration must be made whether to refer the patient to a Burns Unit and their opinion asked about which dressing should be applied. Cling film is often used to cover the burn during transport to a burns unit.
- Full-thickness burns. These heal by fibrosis, causing contractures and scarring, and are best treated by skin grafting. This is done either at 3–5 days or after 3 weeks when the burnt skin is sloughing.
- Oral fluids containing sodium are sufficient to counteract any mild hypovolaemia.

Major burns

A burn is described as major when the area involved is more than 15% of the body surface area (10% in children). The regional burns centre should be contacted regarding all major burns.

Management

The main priority is maintenance of the airway and prevention of circulatory collapse. The patient must be assessed along ATLS guidelines. While this is undertaken, the burn is covered with cling film.

AIRWAY

Give all patients with major burns supplemental oxygen imme-diately. If the airway is obstructed or the patient has inhaled soot, an anaesthetist must assess the patient urgently as a definitive airway and the passage of an endotracheal tube may be necessary. If severe respiratory damage has occurred, an early tracheostomy may be indicated.

ANALGESIA

Burns are very painful and adequate analgesia must be given. Intravenous morphine (0.1 mg/kg) gives instant pain relief. Intravenous chlorpromazine (0.5 mg/kg) sedates the patient and acts as an antiemetic. Covering the burn with cling film reduces the pain significantly.

FLUID REPLACEMENT

Delay in replacing the fluid lost can lead to rapid deterioration, renal failure and death. Remember that the fluid loss is at its maximum 6–12 h *after the burn*, not after the time if admission. If a patient takes some time to reach the emergency department they may already be hypovolaemic with burn shock.

Set up at least one intravenous infusion with a wide-gauge cannula. Avoid using a central venous pressure line if possible, due to the risk of infection. Catheterize the patient to monitor the urine output. During cannulation take blood for haemoglobin, haematocrit, urea and electrolytes, and serum for grouping and cross-matching blood. The patient may need a nasogastric tube to decompress the stomach.

There are many formulae to help you calculate the fluid deficit. *Call your local burns unit to ask what regimen they use and follow their advice.* The patient will be referred to them. Formulae vary depending on the use of crystalloid or colloid. Two examples are given. The Parkland formula estimates the volume of crystalloid, and the Mount Vernon formula estimates the volume of plasma (colloid), required to replace the predicted fluid loss from burn shock. The Parkland formula is most often used.

The Parkland formula estimates that the volume of *crystalloid required* (in mL) in the first 24 h after a burn is:

$$4 \text{ mL} \times \text{body weight (kg)} \times \% \text{ burn}$$

A 70-kg man with a 50% burn would require 14 L in the first 24 h. Half is given in the first 8 h post burn, and the rest in the next 16 h. Hartmann's is better than normal saline because of its lower sodium concentration (see p. 85).

The Mount Vernon formula estimates the amount of *colloid required* (in mL) for each of 6 'time units' in the first 36 h after a burn (Fig. 15.5.3). This estimate is:

$$\frac{\% \text{ burn} \times \text{body weight (kg)}}{2}$$

A 50% burn in a 70-kg man needs 1750 mL of plasma in each time unit. That is, 10.5 L total of which half is given in the first 12 h, and 8.75 L in the first 24 h.

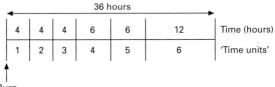

Fig. 15.5.3 Six 'time units' after a burn.

An extensive burn causes an ileus and the patient is not therefore able to take oral fluids. In this case the standard body requirements for water and electrolytes must be added to the burn formula regime.

If a patient arrives some hours after a burn then the initial fluid resuscitation must make up for lost time. Thereafter frequent clinical observations must be made to check on the patient's fluid status and urine output. Serial haematocrit estimations are invaluable. As a result of this reassessment, the amount of fluid required in each time unit can be modified accordingly.

BLOOD REQUIREMENTS

Blood replacement will be required if the burn is deep and more than 10% of the body area. Then, for each 1% burn, give 1% of the patient's total blood volume. The above patient would need 2.5 L of blood.

INFECTION

Systemic antibiotics should only be given on the advice of the local burns unit. The risk of multiresistant organisms is very significant if antibiotics are given prophylactically. They can be given to prevent bacteraemia during cleaning the wound; however, they should not be continued but be reserved for when the patient shows signs of clinical infection. The local management of the burn itself is described on p. 660.

MANAGEMENT OF BURNS IN SPECIAL SITES

Burns to these sites should be referred to the local burns unit for advice and possible transfer.

In deep circumferential burns of the limb or chest, the tight burnt skin may occlude the blood supply to the extremities or affect respiration. The burnt skin must be divided along the length of the limb or in a criss-cross pattern on the chest wall, to release this constricting pressure.

Burns around the eye rapidly result in extensive periorbital oedema. It is therefore essential to examine the eye early before the palpable fissure closes. If the eyelids have been destroyed, the eye must be bathed with artificial tears and the eyelids restored by plastic surgery at the earliest opportunity to prevent corneal scarring.

Burns of the head and neck with severe facial oedema or evidence of inhalation of soot or hot gases require urgent tracheostomy.

Severe burns to the hands must be cleaned, dressed with tulle-gras, and elevated to minimize oedema: Splintage and physiotherapy are likely to be needed.

Index

Page numbers in *italics* refer to figures; those in **bold** to tables.